Handbook of Secure Care

Edited by Geoffrey Dickens, Philip Sugarman and Marco Picchioni

RCPsych Publications

RCPsych Publications is an imprint of the Royal College of Psychiatrists,
21 Prescot Street, London E1 8BB
http://www.rcpsych.ac.uk

British Library Cataloguing-in-Publication Data.
A catalogue record for this book is available from the British Library.
ISBN 978-1-909726-36-9

Distributed in North America by Publishers Storage and Shipping Company.

The views presented in this book do not necessarily reflect those of the Royal College of
Psychiatrists, and the publishers are not responsible for any error of omission or fact.

The Royal College of Psychiatrists is a charity registered in England and Wales (228636) and in
Scotland (SC038369).

Printed by Bell & Bain Limited, Glasgow, UK.

Contents

Tables, boxes and figures

Tables

Boxes

Figures

Contributors

Nick Alderman   Director of Clinical Services, Partnerships in Care

Katina Anagnostakis   Associate Medical Director, Training and Education, and Consultant Psychiatrist, St Andrew's Healthcare

Ian Callaghan   National Service User Lead, My Shared Pathway

Eddie Chaplin   Research Lead, South London and Maudsley NHS Foundation Trust, and Visiting Researcher, Institute of Psychiatry, Psychology & Neuroscience, King's College London

Enys Delmage   Lead Psychiatrist, Adolescent Service, St Andrew's Healthcare

Geoffrey Dickens   Research Manager and Head of Nursing Research, St Andrew's Healthcare, and Professor in Psychiatric Nursing, University of Northampton

Tim Exworthy   Clinical Director and Consultant Forensic Psychiatrist, St Andrew's Healthcare

Nuwan Galappathie   Consultant Forensic Psychiatrist, St Andrew's Healthcare Birmingham

Theresa Gannon   Director of the Centre of Research and Education in Forensic Psychology and Professor of Forensic Psychology, University of Kent

Ernest Gralton   Clinical Director, St Andrew's Healthcare

Annette Greenwood   Trauma Service Manager, St Andrew's Healthcare

Camilla Haw   Consultant Psychiatrist, St Andrew's Healthcare and Professor in Mental Health, University of Northampton

Clive Long   Associate Director of Psychology and Psychological Therapies, St Andrew's Healthcare, and Professor in Clinical Psychology, University of Northampton

Fiona Mason   Chief Medical Officer, St Andrew's Healthcare

Jane McCarthy   Consultant Psychiatrist, East London NHS Foundation Trust, and Visiting Senior Lecturer, Institute of Psychiatry, Psychology & Neuroscience, King's College London

Shawn Mitchell   Associate Medical Director and Consultant Psychiatrist, St Andrew's Healthcare

Mark Morris Clinical Director and Consultant Psychiatrist, St Andrew's Healthcare

Muthusamy Natarajan Consultant Forensic Psychiatrist, St Andrew's Healthcare

Laura O'Shea Research Assistant, St Andrew's Healthcare

Catherine Penny Specialty Registrar in Forensic Psychiatry, South London and Maudsley Rotation, Visiting Teacher at the Institute of Psychiatry, Psychology & Neuroscience, King's College London

Marco Picchioni Honorary Consultant Forensic Psychiatrist, St Andrew's and Senior Lecturer, St Andrew's Academic Centre, Institute of Psychiatry, Psychology & Neuroscience, King's College London

Jane Radley Consultant Psychiatrist, St Andrew's Healthcare

Carol Rooney Director of Nursing, Partnerships in Care

Ashimesh Roychowdhury Associate Medical Director, Clinical Informatics and Consultant Forensic Psychiatrist, St Andrew's Healthcare

Piyal Sen Consultant Forensic Psychiatrist, St Andrew's Healthcare and Visiting Researcher, Institute of Psychiatry, Psychology & Neuroscience, King's College London

John Shine Consultant Psychologist, St Andrew's Healthcare

Philip Sugarman Chief Executive Officer, St Andrew's Healthcare

David Thomas Director of Quality and Governance

Huw Thomas previously Consultant Psychiatrist at St Andrew's Healthcare, Birmingham

Nichola Tyler Postgraduate Researcher, University of Kent

Lesley Wilson Head of Clinical Effectiveness, St Andrew's Healthcare

Graeme A. Yorston Consultant Forensic Psychiatrist, St Matthews Hospital

Preface

In any society a small proportion of people with mental disorder present with behaviour that transgresses norms and violates the rights of others. Concurrently, the same people are often vulnerable themselves – to violence, to abuse or exploitation by others – or at risk of neglect or self-harm. High rates of mortality are well documented. Long conceptualised as a 'forensic' population, they interface between mental health and criminal justice systems, and require containment for a time in secure services to manage risk. In recent years a growing realisation has been that both protection of the public and the personal recovery of these patients must be championed by progressive, specialist clinicians. The label 'forensic' is an insufficient descriptor of this group of services which provide care and treatment for mentally disordered offenders, but also for a range of individuals who have not been diverted from the criminal justice system. Many clinicians who work in secure services do not self-identify as 'forensic' practitioners. This book provides an overview of the clinical populations, professions, assessment and treatment approaches used in a wide range of specialist secure services. It does so with the intent of providing the broadest possible perspective and so we have opted to title our book the *Handbook of Secure Care*.

The aim of secure services has shifted over time from primarily containment to active programmes of therapy and rehabilitation within care pathways, which aim for less restrictive placements through levels of security, leading to open and community care and reintegration into wider society. Concurrently, services have grown, with an increase in the past decade in the number of secure mental health beds in many countries. In the 21st century this expanding sector has seen new super-specialisms (i.e. subspecialties) whose more bespoke skills reflect the needs of diverse niche groups. This diversity is expressed across diagnostic boundaries, from mental illness and intellectual disability to autism, brain injury and degenerative disorders. Distinct secure care pathways have evolved for men, women, adolescents and the elderly. Dedicated facilities also now exist for younger adults and the pre-lingually deaf.

Despite their diversity, these services share commonalities. Multi-professional assessment of risk, resilience and need is central, leading into outcome-focused recovery programmes. Secure services now include more psychiatrists, psychologists, nurses and occupational therapists than ever before, but also teachers, pharmacists, dieticians, language therapists and physical exercise technicians, a unique body of expertise bringing secure services into the mainstream, and providing these marginalised patient groups with equal access to the psychological, physical and social interventions they require.

The assurance of quality is a real challenge as secure services have a mixed and turbulent history of achievements and failures over many years. The new era of healthcare governance depends on transparency, and governments should and do demand reporting compliance and convincing evidence of higher standards and better outcomes, as well as controls on cost. The solution to providing more for less can only ever be the sharing of best practice from centres of excellence, together with clinical leadership in a spirit of challenge and ambition for what can be achieved.

Currently no single text within the wider forensic mental health field addresses secure specialist in-patient care. A team of clinicians from St Andrew's Healthcare, a multi-site hospital group and the largest charitable provider of public healthcare in the UK, has come together to produce this volume with a range of colleagues. As the only non-governmental teaching hospital in the UK, partnered with the Institute of Psychiatry, Psychology and Neuroscience at King's College London and several other leading universities, St Andrew's teaches a unique range of students across the professions, including postgraduate doctors and PhD students. Among many courses organised wholly or jointly by the charity's staff are masters modules in specialist care in Northampton and London, from which the idea for this work developed. We believe it represents the cutting edge of specialist secure care, and is intended as a much-needed resource for all students and professionals in the field of forensic care and challenging behaviour.

CHAPTER 1

The evolution of secure and forensic mental healthcare

Philip Sugarman and Geoffrey Dickens

Introduction and aims

It is in all likelihood a by-product of human evolution, and of the complexity of the human brain and of society, that there have always been dysfunctional individuals who present overtly with a mental or behavioural disorder. They may cause significant harm and disruption to others, as well as to themselves. The most seriously affected depend on the concerted efforts of those around them to provide a safe and supportive environment, or risk neglect, rejection, homelessness and even persecution. Perhaps there always will be such problems in our communities, and thus a continuing need for secure mental health services, at least until science and society have advanced greatly from their present position.

Mentally disordered offenders and others presenting serious challenging behaviour are more often successfully categorised and labelled by local juridical and medical practice, and subject to other processes of social stigmatisation, than they are helped towards recovery. In many instances temporary or indefinite containment is achieved, which may serve to protect the public, but alone this acts as a poor substitute for well-being and social recovery. Those with knowledge of social exclusion and those who work closely with this group will grasp both the immense long-term cost of this failure to society, in terms of morbidity and mortality, crime, social dependency and family breakdown, and the strategic value of early and late intervention. Governments, however, need to be persuaded that the investment involved will reap longer-term benefits (Sugarman, 2012).

It is important to appreciate how the very human need for secure containment of disturbed individuals transcends boundaries of time and place, of gender, age and developmental stage, and of diagnostic and criminal justice status. Very similar challenges of care, control and rehabilitation are seen in different cultures and in different groups. While the international psychiatric community is moving on with active information-sharing on areas such as service models (Maj, 2008), a fundamental debate is just beginning about how societies around the world can best catalyse effective

1

mental health service development (Sugarman & Kakabadse, 2011). We believe that local diversification in provision accelerates improvement in secure and forensic care, focused on service user need rather than organisational goals, with hospitals centred on the care and recovery of the most challenging and needy individuals, and on the promotion of excellence through teaching and research.

This chapter identifies the need, globally, for secure mental health provision and presents an overview of the history and development of secure care. It charts its social evolution, from origins in the earliest psychiatric hospitals, to growth into the complex pattern of forensic and secure mental health service specialisation that exists in the most advanced societies today. A narrative shape is given to historical patterns of innovation, differentiation and decline in secure services, within an appreciative critique of the achievements so far in this important area. We offer a sociological as much as a mental health professional view, although the chapter is intended as a balance to the abundance of critical sociology of psychiatric hospitals, for example as 'total institutions' (Goffman, 1961). A Whiggish view of inevitable progression is not offered, rather one of cycles of progression interspersed by periods of inertia or decline. We argue that we must be able to learn from the past, to identify and link coherent historical patterns with current trends and emerging developments.

Secure care is an expensive and intensive use of taxpayers' resources to deal with problems of a relatively small group. In the current financial climate it is more important than ever to develop the most efficient models of care possible. This requires an element of innovation as well as evaluation; we need to develop insight into how these services have changed so far, in order to be adept in engineering change for the future.

Background

The construction of a global overview of the development of secure care is challenging. Numerous reports on psychiatric services across the world are available, often identifying stretched, under-resourced or run-down (and traditionally locked) hospital facilities in low- and middle-income countries, as well as newer community services (e.g. Onokoko *et al*, 2010). New information is emerging about forensic and secure clinical practice in hitherto neglected areas, including the former Soviet Union (van Voren, 2006), China (Topiwala *et al*, 2011), Africa (Ogunlesi *et al*, 2012), Latin America (Taborda, 2006) and in Islamic countries (Pridmore & Pasha, 2004). Global reviews barely touch on the configuration of forensic psychiatry services, but they do identify how the growth of these services has been fuelled by deinstitutionalisation of the general mental health infrastructure and the related failure of services to keep those with a mental illness out of prison (e.g. Arboleda-Florez, 2006).

The need for forensic mental health provision around the world is underlined by numerous studies of the millions of mentally disordered people detained in prisons (Fazel & Danesh, 2002). In Europe there is a trend to increase forensic hospital provision (Priebe *et al*, 2008), with growing numbers of compulsory admissions visible in several countries, including larger jurisdictions such as Germany and France (Salize & Dressing, 2004) and the UK (Health and Social Care Information Centre, 2011). Different European nations have very varied patterns of forensic service provision, but there is an inverse relationship between the national rate of imprisonment and the number of forensic hospital beds (Priebe *et al*, 2005), the latter supplemented by specialist housing provision in several countries. A few European countries favour mental health treatment for prisoners in facilities outside prison – such as Cyprus, England and Wales, France, Iceland and Norway (Salize & Dressing, 2007). Forensic mental health provision in the Netherlands has been well described (e.g. Derks *et al*, 1993), and is notable for its early therapeutic focus, ahead of most other jurisdictions.

Secure and forensic mental health services in the USA are less advanced than other areas of healthcare (Bloom *et al*, 2000), although there are wide local variations. In some states there are equal numbers of mentally disordered offenders in hospital and prison, while in others there are as many as ten times more similar offenders in prison than in health services (Torrey *et al*, 2010). Elsewhere, a number of other English-speaking countries have been in the vanguard of forensic hospital and community service innovation, including Australia (Mullen *et al*, 2000), New Zealand (Brinded, 2000) and Canada (e.g. Livingston *et al*, 2012). The service in Victoria, Australia, is one of the leading examples of rapid development of a modern prestige service, drawing on the UK service model but with a strong emphasis on teaching, new clinical research and newly identified syndromes such as stalking, as well as multi-professional work, assessment and rehabilitation in both hospital and community (Ogloff, 2010). This 'teaching hospital' model is also well established in some of the larger providers of secure care in the UK, which run major specialist centres, such as the Bethlem (London), Rampton (Nottinghamshire), St Andrew's (Northampton) and St Bernard's (London, Ealing) hospital sites. The history of institutions such as these is worthy of study and can be instructive for the future.

Ideals and institutions

Psychiatric institutions typically begin as places of care and support, inspired by high spiritual and charitable ideals. The reception of the sick and the insane can be traced back to monastic healthcare facilities in the 5th c. BC in the Far East (Retief, 2005) and to temples in ancient Greece, where dream interpretation as a treatment foreshadowed its reappearance in European psychiatry 100 years ago. The separation of medical and psychiatric hospitals dates to the Golden Age of Islam, from the 9th to the 13th century AD (Retief, 2005), with the Persian language differentiating between psychiatric hospital (*maristan*) and medical hospital (*bimaristan*). *Maristans* are often said to have had tinkling fountains to calm the patients.

In Christian Europe of the Middle Ages, a few charitable hospitals were notably founded specifically for mental health use (e.g. López-Ibor, 2008), whereas in others such as the (Priory of St Mary of) Bethlem in London, this use evolved over time (Andrews *et al*, 1998). In the UK these origins have not been entirely lost. The largest secure care facility in the country, St Andrew's in Northampton, is a long-standing charity, as is the historic Retreat in York, also a secure care provider (Digby, 1984; Foss & Trick, 1989), and, interestingly they have Church of England and Quaker origins, respectively. Indeed, much of the secure care provision in the UK is still located on a surviving corner of large county asylum sites (such as St Bernard's and the Bethlem in London), most developed by local public authorities, and some founded as charities, but virtually all boasting a fine chapel, giving a sense of their original high-minded ethos.

The espoused values of mental health provision have, however, to be contrasted with the documented history of psychiatric hospitals and secure institutions, which catalogues numerous treatment interventions, of which some appear insightful and kindly to modern eyes, but many much less so. Initial high ideals at the laying of foundation stones later give way to more controlling and intrusive interventions in the face of practical necessity or custodial certitude. In spite of the values that inspired their creation, medieval infirmaries as well as later private madhouses became notorious bywords for stigmatisation and mistreatment (e.g. Scull, 2006).

Similarly, the Enlightenment values embodied in the 'moral treatment' movement and reflected in 'non-restraint' policies, were introduced at the Retreat and spread to the emerging county asylums (Yorston & Haw, 2004). However, Victorian doctors soon ran a national infrastructure, which by 1900 became a closed, sometimes abusive institutional world for 100 000 people (Porter, 2006) and the power base for medical superintendents whose association later became the Royal College of Psychiatrists (Bewley, 2008). The rise and decline of the British asylum system is well documented (e.g. Jones, 1991), and its direct influence can be seen in a wide international context of social, psychiatric and colonial control which is still playing out (Melling & Forsythe, 1999). In 1948 the nationalisation of hospitals in England inherited a system which peaked in the later 1950s at over 150 000 locked beds. Subsequent radical and progressive change introduced unlocked wards, voluntary, out-patient and community treatment. By 1990 the national combined capacity of government and independent hospitals had dipped below 35 000, a figure from which it is now again falling (Laing, 2012).

Provision for mentally disordered offenders

A parallel system to general mental health services has appeared in many jurisdictions. In England and Wales, after the Criminal Lunatics Act of 1800 empowered the courts to send those found insane to hospital, special wings at the Bethlem hospital were established. In 1863 a secure institution was opened at Broadmoor in Berkshire to house this burgeoning population, to become the first of the sites later known as 'special hospitals' in England. Twentieth-century expansion saw the addition of Rampton and Ashworth hospitals, together with Carstairs in Scotland forming the 'high secure' estate in modern parlance. These facilities suffered increasing isolation from broader progressive changes in psychiatric hospitals, their overly custodial culture exemplified by the power of the Prison Officers' Association as the main representative body for nursing staff. It was against this background that in the later 20th century these hospitals were troubled by repeated scandals about both public safety and abuse of patients, creating an impetus for new developments.

In 1971 Graham Young, a lethal poisoner, was released from Broadmoor into the community, deemed 'fully recovered'. Young was assisted in finding paid employment as quartermaster in a military equipment manufacturing company, with access to highly toxic chemicals. He poisoned many work colleagues, and was convicted on two counts each of murder and attempted murder just nine months after his release (Bowden, 1996). It was consequently recommended in the influential 'Butler report' that regional secure units (RSUs, later defined as 'medium secure' hospitals) were created as an innovative intermediate step-down between the special hospitals and the community (Home Office & Department of Health, 1975). At the same time, the 'Glancy report' (Department of Health and Social Security, 1974) recommended provision of secure services for those too disturbed to be cared for in a general mental health hospital. Concurrently, television programmes such as *The Secret Hospital* alleged institutionalised bullying and abuse of vulnerable patients in the special hospitals. The result was implementation of the Butler recommendations in the development of new, smaller, regional secure facilities from the 1980s, with patient transfers in from both sides, i.e. step-downs from higher security and admissions from courts and lower security. Thus the impetus for change was adverse publicity, an important pattern in secure services where service inertia and failure has developed.

The relatively open culture of the new regional medium secure services triggered the development of forensic psychiatry into a professionally and academically credible specialism, supporting multidisciplinary care, including forensic mental health in-patient nursing (Dale *et al*, 2001). Further innovation saw medium secure nursing, and medical and social work staff lead 'diversion' schemes for mentally disordered offenders, based in local courts, prisons and police stations. Later, the emerging ideas of closest-to-home care and the 'least restrictive alternative' as outlined in the 'Reed report' (Department of Health & Home Office, 1992), and escalating compulsory admissions both from prisons and the community (Rutherford & Duggan, 2007) fuelled demand for more local secure provision, which has since been codified as 'low security' (Department of Health, 2002). Allegations at the high secure hospital at Ashworth in the late 1980s of abusive regimes (Blom-Cooper, 1992), and later of security failures (Fallon *et al*, 1999), brought a renewed focus on security (Tilt *et al*, 2000) and acknowledgement that many patients, particularly women, were being held in inappropriately restrictive conditions. This initiated the development of regional 'enhanced medium secure' services for women.

The mix of individuals transferred from medium secure services, individuals diverted from custody and acutely disturbed non-offenders in local mental health services is a clinical challenge, now addressed by intensive care units, longer-term low secure units and newer 'enhanced' low secure units for acutely unwell prisoners. This is the current crux of the care pathway in England, between general and forensic services, with intense pressure to move patients through stepwise rehabilitation. Out-patient forensic psychiatry also grew with some RSUs, and after a slow start specialist community forensic teams now either work in parallel to, or are integrated with, general community mental health teams. These models represent the ongoing conflict between general and forensic mental health professional teams, which may resolve over time as professional identities regroup more functionally around secure and community care.

The growth of medium and low secure care has seen an increasing diversity of provision both from the state National Health Service (NHS) and from 'independent sector' companies and charities. In this century, Rampton Hospital in Nottinghamshire has emerged as the largest high secure hospital in the UK, with around 350 beds, including a unique collection of national specialist centres for women, people with intellectual disability, personality disorder and pre-lingually deaf patients. The high secure estate now sits at the tip of a pyramid of secure care encompassing around 20 000 beds (designated secure or locked). State-provided care is increasingly delivered by semi-autonomous, not-for-profit public bodies known as NHS foundation trusts, which are partially detached from state control and are increasingly taking on the characteristics of trading charities (Sugarman, 2010). These are not-for-profit, largely mental health-specific organisations, with the potential to be autonomous, effective and dedicated to service user need. Ideals and values, so often key in founding new care provision, must be embedded in their organisational mission and governance, to enable the innovation essential to service improvement in any jurisdiction (Sugarman, 2007; Sugarman & Kakabadse, 2011).

Effectiveness and outcomes

With the development of services and growth of admissions in this sector, at least in Europe (Priebe *et al*, 2005; Gordon & Lindqvist, 2007), and the current economic downturn, there is a debate to be had about resource allocation. For example, secure in-patient services in the UK have been castigated by some radical forensic psychiatrists as counter-therapeutic and self-perpetuating institutions which inhibit the development of wider systems of support for mentally disordered offenders (Wilson *et al*, 2011). In particular, the 'medium secure' level of care, which is the main powerbase of forensic mental health professionals, was caricatured as a financially unsustainable juggernaut, moving forward irrespective of the needs of patients or the realities of healthcare funding. This critique acknowledges that, at least in the UK, forensic in-patient services are well funded relative to local in-patient care, such that designated secure care takes a disproportionate part of the budget for psychiatric hospitals.

It can be argued, however, that the distinction between forensic secure and other hospitals is increasingly misleading in England, where the great majority of psychiatric wards are now physically locked even in the daytime, and the proportion of patients detained compulsorily has been climbing rapidly in recent years (Health and Social Care Information Centre, 2011). However, secure psychiatric care in England and Wales, broadly defined to encompass all psychiatric hospitals, still accounts for only around 15% of direct spending on mental health. Including community and social care, government spending on mental health has grown to well over £20 billion per annum (Centre for Mental Health, 2010).

Meanwhile there is limited evidence on the overall clinical, public safety and economic impact of secure care. In the absence of reliable service-wide data, a few focused studies have examined those with severe personality disorder, perhaps the most difficult to treat group (e.g. Dolan *et al*, 1996; Chiesa & Fonagy, 2002; Barrett & Byford, 2012), producing mixed conclusions on whether patients show significant improvement. Reconviction rates after discharge from secure care are much lower than for released prisoners (Coid *et al*, 2007), but are still significant for younger patients with substance misuse or personality disorder who have a criminal record. It is important there is a broad future social research effort in this area to inform national policy and service planning (Kane & Jordan, 2012).

In the absence of good evidence, a more emotional stance is likely, given that people have always had strong feelings about severe mental disturbance and locked psychiatric institutions. Taxpayers are entitled to know that these apparently advancing services are effectively protecting the community, and offering good value by helping patients to recovery ever more quickly through shorter, less costly stays. Mental health providers use their varied public, corporate and charitable governance systems to make sense of a complex legal, regulatory and commissioning (purchasing) environment, and must run coherent clinical governance infrastructures. The right cultural balance of audit processes, transparent information and innovative teamwork is crucial (Sugarman, 2007), supporting truly integrated governance that targets recovery outcomes (Sugarman & Kakabadse, 2008).

In England, health policy is now focused on patient choice, provider diversity, outcomes and payment by results, to identify variations in performance and improve effectiveness. In response to cost pressures the National Health Service (NHS) is encouraging earlier discharge, with falling lengths of stay in some secure providers (Partnerships in Care, 2011). This requires improving rates of recovery, to the level where care in the expanding range of less restrictive settings is practical. Adverse incidents are routinely reported to health purchasers, and payments linked to measures of quality are in place, including minimum volumes of weekly therapy, and standard risk, recovery and outcome tools. Advances in information technology may support future service comparison on a standardised 'dashboard' of clinical and service data, built up from protected clinical information. Current UK Department of Health work on 'payment by results' in mental health appears to be largely about price tariffs, built on a scheme of patient categorisation (Fairbairn, 2007). An appropriate model of 'forensic clusters' linked to this may be a basis for developing meaningful comparison between services on clinical performance for defined patient subgroups.

Important outcome domains for mentally disordered offenders (Cohen & Eastman, 2000) include symptom reduction, social rehabilitation, quality of life and public safety, as well as reconviction for offending. Health of the Nation Outcome Scales (HoNOS) data, measuring symptoms and functioning, are reported to the Department of Health and HoNOS-secure (Sugarman & Walker, 2007) has been adopted by forensic services in continental Europe, Australasia and North America, but ideally it should be superseded by similarly brief but more sensitive measures. Meanwhile it remains unproven whether measurement of clinical and risk outcomes improves 'real' outcomes such as patient-reported quality of life and recovery experience.

Reconviction and readmission have high face validity as real outcomes for policy makers and the public. High readmission rates indicate the need to support patients in the community, and high physical morbidity and mortality in this population must also be addressed. The ultimate outcome measures of the future might be shorter time in hospital by level of security and longer, healthy, crime-free survival time in the community. Using these as a basis for true 'payment by results' seems logical, but remains for the moment impractical.

Priorities and challenges

The identification of high psychiatric morbidity in prisons in the UK (Singleton *et al*, 1998), replicated in most countries studied (Fazel & Danesh, 2002), reinforces the need not only for transfer to hospital where appropriate, but also for prison in-reach services driven by the ideal of equivalence to community care. Importantly, there is a resurgent impetus for diversion into mental healthcare (Bradley, 2009), but regrettably a target to expedite prison transfers to hospital within 14 days has been dropped – apparently driven directly by the post-credit crunch NHS cost savings programme. There are many reports of reduced numbers of prison transfers as well as excessive delays (e.g. Wilson *et al*, 2010), falling foul of the equality principle between physical and mental health set out in recent government policy (HM Government 2011). It is reasonable to raise this with policy makers as both a human rights issue, on the grounds that people with cancer in prison would not be denied specialist hospital treatment in the same way, and an economic issue, highlighting the long-term cost of not meeting these needs (Sugarman, 2012).

In overview, rising demand for secure care, related to closure of old hospitals and worsening inner city deprivation, has stimulated the development of a hierarchy of new facilities, with risk management skills now central at every level of security. Some would see the forensic system as the 'new asylum', and certainly an intensive focus on length of stay and moving patients on is essential. Length of stay has fallen, as forensic care is increasingly a multi-directional pathway, from national specialist facilities to services with a presence in local communities and the criminal justice system. As specialist provision expands, it puts pressure on public expenditure but provides a diversity of care pathways, including some non-secure forensic care homes and hostels, with major potential to enable discharge from hospital.

We can see therefore that secure mental health service provision in England is in a state of transformation and innovation. Yet as we have shown, periods of innovation have historically been followed by periods of decline. The cycle of innovation and decline presents an opportunity to learn from history. Recent exposes of abuse, such as that perpetrated by care staff at the Winterbourne View unit in England for people with autism or intellectual disability (Care Quality Commission, 2011), indicates that progressive developments have not immunised the secure care sector from scandal when governance systems fail and when individual needs of patients are sidelined. The challenge for those involved in secure mental health facilities today is how to keep up a continual momentum of change driven by our ideals and ensure that descent into disreputable care and abusive practice is not the inevitable destiny for every generation of secure facilities. In the final part of this chapter we describe how diversification, technology and good governance can arm us for this challenge.

Emerging trends: specialisation, technology and recovery

Secure services are increasingly differentiating by gender, age, diagnosis and length of stay into new 'super-specialisms' – in the UK this is very visible at some larger specialist secure facilities. Bespoke programmes of care can meet the needs of forensic patients, who are often very different from the adult men with mental illness that standard secure services were designed for. These programmes increasingly build on the contribution of forensic and clinical psychologists in leading evidence-based intervention programmes, and on awareness of the importance of a high level of such patient-centred activity, integrated at the heart of services (Gudjonsson & Young, 2007).

Women in secure care have a distinct clinical profile and therapeutic needs, for which specialist services are effective (Long *et al*, 2010). The mental health needs of older prisoners have been poorly understood (Yorston, 1999) but specialist services are established, as are age-specific secure services for adolescents (Wheatley *et al*, 2004). Brain injury is associated with aggression and offending, for which effective neurobehavioural programmes are well evidenced (Alderman, 2001). Services are developing for groups such as young adults, the pre-lingually deaf and those with autism, in addition to established units for intellectual disability. The emerging picture is that highly specialist services are effective, offering improved outcomes and thereby shorter stays. The only exception to this may be signalled by England's Dangerous and Severe Personality Disorder Programme, which has struggled to demonstrate clinical and cost effectiveness (Tyrer *et al*, 2010), and is no longer a policy priority in an age of austerity.

There is a long established pattern in which adverse incidents have driven new thinking on safe and effective care, and this looks set to continue. Standardised security specifications now incorporate an expanding technology of safe design and materials solutions, which reduce many clinical risks. Information and communications technology is emerging in meeting new challenges and producing solutions in secure care, for issues such as media access, alarm systems and even GPS tagging of service users (Shaw, 2010). In Europe patients are protected under the Human Rights Act 1998 (Sugarman & Dickens, 2007), with restrictions imposed in proportion to risk, using evidenced approaches to professional judgement and control interventions. Active therapeutic regimes are based more and more on research and deployed across the range of needs. It seems as if practice in our specialty is finally beginning to have a tangible science and technology base.

In the meantime, the concept of health recovery, which can be traced to Greek sources such as Hippocrates (Coar, 1822), has seen something of a renaissance in mental health (Anthony, 1993). Recovery has been completely rehabilitated as a primary driver for the mission of mental health providers, defined in terms of hope, optimism and meaning, linked for some with spirituality (Leamy *et al*, 2011), and the role of chaplaincy in mental healthcare (Cook *et al*, 2009). Such changes seem therapeutic, against the rather austere tradition of science and therapeutic nihilism in psychiatry, but what matters is how such positive impulses are translated into the reality of service delivery. In all likelihood linking provider payments directly with outcomes will be key, enabling service users and commissioners to make the choice for 'front-loaded' packages, intended to have a transformational impact, boosting the prospects of swifter and fuller recovery.

Conclusions

High ideals such as recovery are driving continuing innovation in mental healthcare. The aim must be to successfully rehabilitate as many people as possible, with low reconviction and readmission rates. Health purchasers and public protection agencies need to be better engaged with services in enabling efficient movement through the system. Further integration of care pathways with mainstream psychiatry and the criminal justice system is essential. The future evolution of secure and forensic care is likely to be forged between specialist centres, which have the scale to support service diversification and innovation in rehabilitation, local secure services focused on shorter stays, and forensic community care and prison in-reach solutions which are still emerging. New technologies, clinical specialisation and closer-to-home services can improve the balance of control towards rights and liberty, whereas better governance and reporting can help support the choice of safer, more effective services.

References

Alderman, N. (2001) Management of challenging behaviour. In *Neurobehavioural Disability and Social Handicap following Traumatic Brain Injury* (eds R. Wood & T. McMillan). Psychology Press.

Andrews, J., Briggs, A., Porter, R., *et al* (1998) *The History of Bethlem*. Routledge.

Anthony, W. (1993) Recovery from mental illness: the guiding vision of the mental health service system in the 1990s. *Psychosocial Rehabilitation Journal*, **16**, 11–23.

Arboleda-Florez, J. (2006) Forensic psychiatry: contemporary scope, challenges and controversies. *World Psychiatry*, **5**, 87–91.

Barrett, B. & Byford, S. (2012) Costs and outcomes of an intervention programme for offenders with personality disorders. *British Journal of Psychiatry*, **200**, 336–341.

Bewley, T. (2008) *Madness to Mental Illness: A History of the Royal College of Psychiatrists*. RCPsych Publications.

Blom-Cooper, L. (1992) *Report of the Committee of Inquiry into Complaints about Ashworth Hospital (Cm 2028)*. HMSO.

Bloom, J., Williams, M. & Bigelow, D. (2000) The forensic psychiatric system in the United States. *International Journal of Law and Psychiatry*, **23**, 605–613.

Bowden, P. (1996) Graham Young (1947–90), the St. Albans poisoner: his life and times. *Criminal Behaviour and Mental Health*, **6**, 17–24.

Bradley, K. (2009) *The Bradley Report: Review of People with Mental Health Problems or Learning Disabilities In the Criminal Justice System*. Department of Health.

Brinded, P. (2000) Forensic psychiatry in New Zealand. *A review. International Journal of Law and Psychiatry*, **23**, 453–465.

Care Quality Commission (2011) *Review of Compliance, Castlebeck Care (Teesdale) Ltd*. Care Quality Commission.

Centre for Mental Health (2010) *The Economic and Social Costs of Mental Health Problems in 2009/10*. Centre for Mental Health.

Chiesa, M. & Fonagy, P. (2002) From the therapeutic community to the community: a preliminary evaluation of a psychosocial outpatient service for severe personality disorders. *Therapeutic Communities*, **23**, 247–258.

Coar, T. (1822) *The Aphorisms of Hippocrates*. Valpy.

Cohen, A. & Eastman, N. (2000) Needs assessment for mentally disordered offenders: measurement of 'ability to benefit' and outcome. *British Journal of Psychiatry*, **177**, 493–498.

Coid, J., Hickey, N., Kahtan, N., *et al* (2007) Patients discharged from medium secure forensic psychiatry services: reconvictions and risk factors. *British Journal of Psychiatry*, **190**, 223–229.

Cook, C., Powell, A. & Sims, A. (2009) *Spirituality and Psychiatry*. RCPsych Publications.

Dale, C., Woods, P. & Thompson, T. (2001) Nursing. In *Forensic Mental Health: Issues in Practice* (eds C. Dale, T. Thomson, P. Woods). Baillière Tindall.

Department of Health (2002) *National Minimum Standards for General Adult Services in Psychiatric Intensive Care Units (PICU) and Low Secure Environments*. Department of Health.

Department of Health & Home Office (1992) *Review of Health and Social Services for Mentally Disordered Offenders and Others Requiring Similar Services (Cm 2088)*. HMSO.

Department of Health and Social Security (1974) *Security in NHS Hospitals for the Mentally Ill and the Mentally Handicapped*. DHSS.

Derks, F.C., Blankstein, J.H. & Hendrickx, J.J. (1993) Treatment and security: the dual nature of forensic psychiatry. *International Journal of Law and Psychiatry*, **16**, 217–240.

Digby, A. (1984) The changing profile of a nineteenth-century asylum: the York Retreat. *Psychological Medicine*, **1**, 739–748.

Dolan, B.M., Warren, F.M., Menzies, D., *et al* (1996) Cost-offset following specialist treatment of severe personality disorders. *Psychiatric Bulletin*, **20**, 413–417.

Fairbairn, A. (2007) Payment by results in mental health: the current state of play in England. *Advances in Psychiatric Treatment*, **13**, 3–6.

Fallon, P., Bluglass, R., Edwards, B., *et al* (1999) *Report of the Committee of Inquiry into the Personality Disorder Unit, Ashworth Special Hospital (vol. 1) (Cm 4194, II)*. TSO (The Stationery Office).

Fazel, S. & Danesh, J. (2002) Serious mental disorder in 23 000 prisoners: a systematic review of 62 surveys. *Lancet*, **359**, 545–550.

Foss, A. & Trick, K. (1989) *St. Andrew's Hospital Northampton: the first 150 years, 1838–1988*. Granta Editions.

Goffman, E. (1961) *Asylums*. Penguin Books.

Gordon, H. & Lindqvist, P. (2007) Forensic psychiatry in Europe. *Psychiatric Bulletin*, **31**, 421–424.

Gudjonsson, G.H. & Young, S. (2007) The role and scope of forensic clinical psychology in secure unit provisions: a proposed service model for psychological therapies. *Journal of Forensic Psychiatry & Psychology*, **18**, 534–556.

Health and Social Care Information Centre (2011) *Mental Health Bulletin Fifth Report*. HSCIC.

HM Government (2011) *No Health without Mental Health*. Department of Health.

Home Office & Department of Health (1975) *Report of the Committee on Mentally Abnormal Offenders*. HMSO.

Jones, K. (1991) The culture of the mental hospital. In *150 years of British Psychiatry* (eds G. Berrios & H. Freeman), pp. 17–27. Gaskell.

Kane, E. & Jordan, M. (2012) *The Centre for Health and Justice – its raison d'être*. Newsletter no. 1. Institute of Mental Health (http://www.institutemh.org.uk/images/CHJ_Newsletter_no._1_FINAL.pdf).

Laing, W. (2012) *Mental Health and Specialist Care Services UK Market Report*. Laing & Buisson.

Leamy, M., Bird, V., Le Boutillier, C., *et al* (2011) Conceptual framework for personal recovery in mental health: systematic review and narrative synthesis. *British Journal of Psychiatry*, **199**, 445–452.

Livingston, J.D., Nijdam-Jones, A. & Brink, J. (2012) A tale of two cultures: examining patient-centred care in a forensic mental health hospital. *Journal of Forensic Psychiatry and Psychology*, **23**, 345–360.

Long, C., Dickens, G., Sugarman, P., *et al* (2010) Tracking risk profiles and outcome in a medium secure service for women: use of the HoNOS-secure. *International Journal of Forensic Mental Health*, **9**, 215–225.

López-Ibor, J. (2008) The founding of the first psychiatric hospital in the world in Valencia. *Actas Espanas Psiquiatrica*, **36**, 1–9.

Maj, M. (2008) The World Psychiatric Association Action Plan 2008–2011. *World Psychiatry*, **7**, 129–130.

Melling, J. & Forsythe, B. (eds.) (1999) *Insanity, Institutions and Society, 1800–1914: A Social History of Madness in Comparative Perspective*. Routledge.

Mullen, P.E., Briggs, S., Dalton, T., *et al* (2000) Forensic mental health services in Australia. *International Journal of Law and Psychiatry*, **23**, 433–452.

Ogloff, J. (2010) The evolution of forensic mental health services in Victoria, Australia: Contributions of Professor Paul Mullen. *Criminal Behaviour and Mental Health*, **20**, 232–241.

Ogunlesi, A.O., Ogunwale, A., De Wet, P., *et al* (2012) Forensic psychiatry in Africa: prospects and challenges. *African Journal of Psychiatry*, **15**, 3–7.

Onokoko, M., Jenkins, R., Miezi, S., *et al* (2010) Mental health in the Democratic Republic of Congo: a post-crisis country challenge. *International Psychiatry*, **7**, 41–43.

Partnerships in Care (2011) *Length of Stay Report Published*. Partnerships in Care (http://www.cinven.com/lib/docs/105715-pic-half-year-review-2011.pdf).

Porter, R. (2006) *Madmen: A Social History of Madhouses, Mad-Doctors & Lunatics*. Tempus.

Pridmore, S., & Pasha, M.I. (2004) Psychiatry and Islam. *Australasian Psychiatry*, **12**, 380–385.

Priebe, S., Badesconyi, A., Fioritti, A., *et al* (2005) Reinstitutionalisation in mental health care: comparison of data on service provision from six European countries. *BMJ*, **330**, 123–126.

Priebe, S., Frottier, P., Gaddini, A., *et al* (2008) Mental health care institutions in nine European countries, 2002 to 2006. *Psychiatric Services*, **59**, 570–573.

Retief, F. (2005) The evolution of hospitals from antiquity to the Renaissance. *Acta Theologica Supplementum*, **7**, 213–232.

Rutherford, M. & Duggan, S. (2007) *Forensic Mental Health Services: Facts and Figures on Current Provision*. Sainsbury Centre for Mental Health.

Salize, H.J. & Dressing, H. (2004) Epidemiology of involuntary placement of mentally ill people across the European Union. *British Journal of Psychiatry*, **184**, 163–168.

Salize, H.J. & Dressing, H. (2007) *Mentally Disordered Persons in European Prison Systems: Needs, Programmes and Outcome (EUPRIS)*. European Commission/Central Institute of Mental Health.

Scull, A. (2006) *The Insanity of Place/The Place of Insanity*. Essays on the History of Psychiatry. Routledge.

Shaw, D. (2010) Satellites used to track mentally-ill violent criminals. *BBC News*, 25 August. Available at http://www.bbc.co.uk/news/uk-11076823 (accessed January 2014).

Singleton, N., Meltzer, H., Gatward, R., *et al* (1998) *Psychiatric Morbidity among Prisoners: Summary Report*. Office for National Statistics.

Sugarman, P. (2007) Governance and innovation in mental health. *Psychiatric Bulletin*, **31**, 283–285.

Sugarman, P. (2010) On charity's big chance. *Health Service Journal*, **September**, 12.

Sugarman, P. (2012) Why we must not neglect mentally disordered offenders. *Parliamentary Brief*, **14**, 11.

Sugarman, P. & Dickens, G. (2007) Protecting patients in psychiatric care: the St Andrew's Human Rights Project. *Psychiatric Bulletin*, **31**, 52–55.

Sugarman, P. & Kakabadse, N. (2008) A model of mental health governance. *International Journal of Clinical Leadership*, **16**, 17–26.

Sugarman, P. & Kakabadse, A. (2011) Governance, choice and the global market for mental health. *International Psychiatry*, **8**, 53–54.

Sugarman, P. & Walker, L. (2007) *Health of the Nation Outcomes Scale for Users of Secure and Forensic Services: How to Use HoNOS-secure*. Royal College of Psychiatrists, St Andrew's Healthcare (http://www.rcpsych.ac.uk/pdf/HoNOS-secure%20v2b%20explanation.pdf).

Taborda, J.G.V. (2006) Forensic psychiatry today: a Latin American view. *World Psychiatry*, **5**, 96.

Tilt, R., Perry, B., Martin, C., *et al* (2000) *Report of the Review of Security at the High Security Hospitals*. Department of Health.

Topiwala, A., Wang, X. & Fazel, S. (2011) Chinese forensic psychiatry and its wider implications. *Journal of Forensic Psychiatry and Psychology*, **23**, 1–6.

Torrey, E.F., Kennard, A.D., Eslinger, D., *et al* (2010) *More Mentally Ill Persons are in Jails and Prisons Than Hospitals: A Survey of the States*. Treatment Advocacy Center, National Sheriffs' Association (http://www.treatmentadvocacycenter.org/storage/documents/final_jails_v_hospitals_study.pdf).

Tyrer, P., Duggan, C., Cooper, S., *et al* (2010) The successes and failures of the DSPD experiment: the assessment and management of severe personality disorder. *Medicine Science and the Law*, **50**, 95–99.

van Voren, R. (2006) Reforming forensic psychiatry and prison mental health in the former Soviet Union. *Psychiatrist*, **30**, 124–126.

Wheatley, M., Waine, J., Spence, K., *et al* (2004) Characteristics of 80 adolescents referred for secure inpatient care. *Clinical Psychology and Psychotherapy*, **11**, 83–89.

Wilson, S., Chiu, K., Parrott, J., *et al* (2010) Postcode lottery? Hospital transfers from one London prison and responsible catchment area. *Psychiatrist*, **34**, 140–142.

Wilson, S., James, D. & Forrester, A. (2011) The medium-secure project and criminal justice mental health. *Lancet*, **378**, 110–111.

Yorston, G. (1999) Aged and dangerous: old-age forensic psychiatry. *British Journal of Psychiatry*, **174**, 193–195.

Yorston, G. & Haw, C. (2004) Thomas Prichard and the non-restraint movement at the Northampton Asylum. *Psychiatric Bulletin*, **28**, 140–142.

CHAPTER 2

Mental disorder and offending

Nuwan Galappathie

Introduction

In the UK patients with mental illness who are convicted of criminal offences are termed mentally disordered offenders (MDOs). While the putative link between mental illness and violent offending attracts the attention of the media, politicians and clinicians (Mullen *et al*, 2000), its roots remain relatively poorly understood. The public perception of the link is undoubtedly influenced by media coverage of rare acts of serious violence committed by MDOs. In fact, while a robust body of research about MDOs, which is reviewed in this chapter, supports a link between mental illness and violent offending, the absolute risk is small and is accounted for by a very small number of patients (Walsh & Fahy, 2002). Despite the public's concerns, random acts of violence against strangers are vanishingly rare; indeed, those with mental health problems are more likely to be violent to relatives at home (Danielson *et al*, 1998), and are even more likely to be victims of violence, homelessness and financial disadvantage than perpetrators (Walsh *et al*, 2003).

Psychosis and violent offending

For many years, schizophrenia was considered not to be associated with an increased risk of violence. That notion has now been reliably rejected in the light of robust evidence of an association with violent offending (Eronen *et al*, 1996; Tiihonen *et al*, 1997). Notably, Wallace *et al* (1998) found that more than 7% in a UK sample of men convicted of homicide had previously received treatment for schizophrenia. Despite this statistical association between psychosis and violence, the nature and cause of the link remain contentious. Some authorities suggest a direct link, highlighting specific symptoms, including the feeling of being 'gravely threatened by someone who intends to cause harm' (Link & Stueve, 1994: p. 143) and of an override of self-control through external forces, termed collectively threat-control override (TCO) symptoms, as predictors and drivers of violence in psychosis. The TCO theory proposed that, acting on these symptoms, individuals take matters into their own hands in what is, in effect, a pre-emptive violent strike. The hypothesis has been supported by a modest amount of data; for example, Swanson *et al* (1996) found that psychotic patients with TCO symptoms were twice as likely to be violent as those without. However, the importance of TCO symptoms has been subsequently challenged. The MacArthur Violence Risk Assessment Study (Appelbaum *et al*, 2000) followed up 1136 patients discharged from psychiatric hospitals over 1 year and identified that future violence was best predicted by more general criminogenic factors, including past criminal and violent behaviour, childhood physical abuse, substance misuse and discharge into high-crime neighbourhoods. Delusions, including TCO symptoms, did not predict future violence. Instead, active substance misuse in the presence of schizophrenia doubled the risk of violence. Steadman *et al* (2000) in a similar study also failed to detect a significant relationship between TCO symptoms and violence in patients with psychosis. Despite uncertainty about the nature of the relationship between psychosis and violence the link remains strong. In a more recent study Swanson *et al* (2006) reported that of 1410 community and hospital patients diagnosed with schizophrenia, more than 19% had committed violent acts such as common assault, while 3.6% had committed more serious violence. Positive psychotic and depressive symptoms, childhood conduct difficulties and victimisation were linked to an increased risk of serious violence, while negative symptoms of schizophrenia were associated with a lower risk.

Psychosis and sexual offending

Any link between psychosis and increased risk of sexual offending is less well established than that for violence. High levels of psychiatric morbidity are commonly found among sex offenders but the disorders concerned are generally depression, substance misuse and personality disorder (Kafka, 2003; Långström *et al*, 2004). Fazel (2006), evaluating a Swedish sex offender cohort, found a prevalence of 4% for psychotic disorders. Smith & Taylor (1999) examined the records of 84 detained male patients with schizophrenia who had committed a sexual offence. They found that 80 were deemed to be actively psychotic at the time of the index offence. While they identified that almost half had delusions related to the index offence, only 18 had a specific delusional or hallucinatory drive for committing the offence, suggesting that other factors influenced the offending behaviour. They found that 67 of the men had a history of diverse offending but only 9 had previous convictions for sex offences. As a result, these data, as with those for general violence, suggest that a variety of criminogenic factors as well as some more illness-specific factors act as drivers for sexual offending in schizophrenia.

Substance misuse, mental disorder and offending

Substance misuse is associated with an increased risk of violence both in those with and without mental illness (Pernanen, 1991; Swartz et al, 1998). Alcohol is implicated in more than 50% of violent crime in the UK (Murdoch et al, 1990; English et al, 1995). Substance misuse and offending were linked in the US Epidemiological Catchment Area (ECA) study (Swanson et al, 1990), which found that violence was most closely associated with being young, male and of a low social status, whereas alcohol or substance misuse disorders were more strongly linked to violent conduct than schizophrenia alone. However, patients with schizophrenia appear more likely to misuse drugs: the ECA study reported a fourfold increased risk of substance misuse in schizophrenia (Regier et al, 1990) and up to 60% of those with psychosis may actively misuse drugs (Fowler et al, 1998). The presence, therefore, of both disorders together significantly increases the risk of violence (Scott et al, 1998). For example, Swartz et al (1998) reported on a series of over 300 involuntary US hospital admissions and found that of those with severe mental illness nearly 40% had drug and alcohol problems, often in the context of poor treatment adherence, with almost 20% being violent before admission. Fulwiler et al (1997) reported a similar relationship with early alcohol or drug misuse and violence in an urban assertive community treatment team.

The prevailing model at the present time therefore suggests an additive relationship such that comorbid substance misuse in the presence of schizophrenia is linked to a significantly greater risk of violence. In a study of almost 3000 patients with schizophrenia admitted to hospital in Australia, Wallace et al (2004) found that those diagnosed with schizophrenia were more likely to have been violent (8.2%) than healthy controls, with highest rates seen in those with comorbid substance misuse. The authors, however, emphasised that offending in schizophrenia cannot solely be explained by substance misuse; rather, it was more often linked to a range of factors that included symptomatic relapses. Hypothetically, substance misuse may also act as a marker of those patients who are most likely to disengage from monitoring and supervision, which may be independently related to an increased risk of violence.

In a Swedish cohort of over 8000 patients with schizophrenia admitted to hospital between 1973 and 2006 Fazel et al (2009) found that 13% had committed at least one violent offence, compared with just 5% of the general population. Substance misuse was again identified as a significant mediating factor for violence. That finding was further supported by Fazel et al's (2009) systematic review of 20 studies overall, including more than 18 000 patients, which endorsed the link between psychoses, including schizophrenia, and violent offending, particularly homicide (discussed below). Again, most of this excess risk was mediated by comorbid substance misuse.

Bipolar affective disorder is also associated with violent offending (Tiihonen *et al*, 1997; Arseneault *et al*, 2000; Brennan *et al*, 2000; Fazel & Grann, 2004). Fazel *et al* (2010) reported that in a Swedish longitudinal follow-up study between 1973 and 2004 of more than 3700 patients with the disorder nearly 8.5% had committed a violent offence, compared with 3.5% of general population controls. Again, the increased risk appeared primarily limited to those with comorbid substance misuse disorders.

Mental disorder and homicide

Coid (1983) estimated the number of homicides committed by people with mental disorder at 0.13 per 100000 population per year in the UK. More recently, others have found higher rates (Fazel & Grann, 2004; Simpson *et al*, 2004), while Large *et al* (2008) noted that homicide rates due to mental disorder peaked in the 1970s and have gradually declined to historic lows of 0.07 per 100000, while rates of homicides unrelated to mental disorder have continued to rise. It is generally considered that the reduction of mental illness-related homicides has been achieved through improvements in mental healthcare and in treatment. However, this may also be an artefact of the methods of data collection and could, for instance, be linked to changes in disposal thresholds at court. Shaw *et al* (2006) examined almost 1600 homicide convictions in England and Wales, between 1996 and 1999, and 15 cases in which the defendant was found to have committed the act but was not convicted on legal grounds. They found that 34% of homicide perpetrators had a mental disorder: 5% schizophrenia, 7% affective disorder, 9% personality disorder, 7% alcohol dependence and 6% drug dependence. However, only 5% were psychotic and 6% depressed at the time of the offence; 18% had a lifetime history of contact with mental health services but only half were actually in contact in the 12 months before the offence. The authors concluded that while there was an association between schizophrenia and homicide, many homicide perpetrators with a history of mental disorder were not being followed up by mental health services but also were not acutely ill at the time of the crime.

The most recent UK National Confidential Inquiry into Suicide and Homicide by People with Mental Illness (Appleby *et al*, 2012) reported on data for more than 6000 homicides committed between 1999 and 2009. At the time of the homicide 10% of perpetrators were found to have an abnormal mental state, with 6% being psychotic. Of the entire sample, 6% had schizophrenia, while 10% had been in contact with mental health services in the year before the offence. Only 16% of the sample committed a stranger homicide. Male patients were most likely to kill acquaintances, while female patients principally killed family members or partners, current or previous.

Personality disorder and offending

Antisocial personality disorder (ASPD) is associated with violent offending (Stone, 2007). Studies from the USA identify rates of between 4.5 and 6.8% in men in the community and around 0.8% in women (Robins *et al*, 1991; Swanson *et al*, 1994), whereas more recent UK data report rates of around 1.0 and 0.2% for men and women respectively (Coid *et al*, 2006*a*). These national differences may reflect international and cultural variations in diagnostic thresholds. In prison, the prevalence of ASPD may be as high as 50% (Fazel & Danesh, 2002). ASPD typically coincides with alcohol and substance use problems (Robins *et al*, 1991; Coid, 2003) as well as mood and anxiety disorders and brief psychotic episodes (Lenzenweger *et al*, 2007); further, ASPD increases the risk of offending, and in particular violent offending, across a variety of mental disorders (Moran *et al*, 2003).

Psychopathy describes, in part, offending of a more controlled or sadistic nature (Hare *et al*, 2000). It is not a mental disorder *per se* but typical of sadistic criminals who lack empathy and exhibit a range of other characteristics including manipulativeness, impulsivity, shallow affect and superficial charm. Initial descriptors were advanced by Cleckley (1976) and Hare (1980). The Psychopathy Checklist-Revised (PCL-R; Hare, 2003) has become the most commonly used rating scale to identify psychopathy. Hare *et al* (2000) found a prevalence of psychopathy in prisons at 4.5 and 13% based on PCL-R scores of greater than 30 and 25 respectively. Psychopathy is often associated with serious and persistent offending (Leistico *et al*, 2008; Campbell *et al*, 2009) that is likely to be attributable to impulsivity and cognitive distortions (Duggan, 2008).

A range of other personality disorders are also associated with violent offending: paranoid, narcissistic, schizoid and emotionally unstable subtypes. A smaller number of personality disorders (e.g. anankastic, avoidant and dependent personality disorder subtypes) have not been significantly associated with violent offending (Hart, 2001; Stone, 2007).

Community care and offending

In the UK, the move from institutional to community-based services began during the 1950s and has continued at increasing pace amidst changes in policy, legislation and practice (Leff, 2001). The development of community care was associated with concerns about the risks patients may pose to themselves and others outside of the institution. This conclusion was initially supported by the ECA data (Swanson *et al*, 1990), which showed that a mental disorder was associated with a fivefold increase in the risk of violence and substance misuse a tenfold increase. Other work has, however, challenged that conclusion. Wallace *et al* (1998) reported on a sample of more than 4000 people in Australia convicted in the equivalent of the English and Welsh Crown Courts. Among the men, approximately 25% had previous contact with mental health services. The majority did not attract a specific diagnosis, while of those who did, substance misuse and personality disorder diagnoses dominated, with only a modest number meeting criteria for mental disorders such as schizophrenia, affective psychosis and affective disorders. The findings in women were similar but with proportionally smaller numbers.

Recent community-based studies emphasise a modest link between mental disorder and offending in the community. Coid *et al* (2006*b*) reported data from the Psychiatric Morbidity Among Adults Living in Private Households in England, Wales and Scotland study. This community survey of 8397 people included self-reports of violence within the past 5 years. They found factors typically associated with violent offending such as male gender, lower socioeconomic status, younger age and single status. Of those with no mental disorder, less than 2% had been violent, causing injury to victims in the past 5 years. That rose to 7% for individuals with neurotic disorders, 7% for any personality disorder, 10% for hazardous drinking, 12% for psychosis, 18% for alcohol dependence, 25% for drug dependence and 26% for ASPD. However, when the population-attributable risk percentages were established for each condition it was found that hazardous drinking had a risk over 50%, drug dependence over 20%, ASPD 24%, but psychosis only 1.2%. This reflected both the high prevalence and greater impact of alcohol and substance misuse on offending in the community compared with psychosis.

The link between mental disorder and community offending was also explored by Grann *et al* (2008), who conducted a 5-year follow-up study of a cohort of almost 5000 offenders given community sentences. In total, almost a third of the sample reoffended: 22% of those with no psychiatric diagnosis, 23% of those with schizophrenia, 22% of those with depression, 36% of those with substance misuse disorder either as the principal or comorbid diagnosis, and 35% of those with personality disorder. After adjusting for sociodemographic and criminal history the researchers concluded that only substance misuse and personality disorders were associated with an independent increased risk of violent offending.

Females with psychotic disorders living in the community have a disproportionately increased risk of violent offending (Hiday *et al*, 1998; Wessely, 1998). Steadman *et al* (1993) found that women in the community reported committing violent offences more frequently than men. Dean *et al* (2006) prospectively followed over 300 female community patients with psychotic symptoms and reported that over 2 years, 17% of these women committed a violent assault. Risk factors included previous violence, other non-violent convictions, victimisation, African–Caribbean ethnicity, cluster B personality disorder and a high level of unmet need.

Hospital care, challenging behaviour and offending

Mentally disordered offenders can be admitted either voluntarily or under detention to the whole spectrum of in-patient mental health services in the UK, including to general adult in-patient services, secure mental health services and other specialist units. Within England and Wales a network of medium secure services developed following the 'Butler report' (Home Office & Department of Health, 1975) to act both as a step-down from high secure services and step-up from generic and low secure mental health services; in addition, they are the gateway for many prison transfers. The threshold for admission to in-patient services has risen at every security level over time, risk of harm to self or others being the most significant driver of admission (Commander *et al*, 1997). While psychiatric morbidity in the community principally comprises anxiety and affective disorders, those admitted to specialist in-patient services are more likely to experience psychotic disorders such as schizophrenia (Meltzer, 1995). In the UK, the National Service Framework for Mental Health introduced specialist community-based services, including assertive treatment teams, crisis resolution and home treatment services, in part to divert people away from in-patient admissions (Department of Health, 1999). Despite some initial positive findings (Issakidis *et al*, 1999; Johnson *et al*, 2005), more recent and robust data have not found evidence that these services prevent admissions (Killaspy *et al*, 2009; Jacobs & Barrenho, 2011), while the number of suicides in home treatment teams continues to rise (Appleby *et al*, 2012). Despite this evidence, the reduction in psychiatric in-patient beds continues, falling from 155 000 in 1954 to 27 000 in 2008, further increasing the threshold for admission (Tyrer, 2011) and consequently the pressure on bed occupancy rates. In this context, and together with ever-increasing significance attached to risk assessment and management, the debate around the structure and interface between forensic and general adult services continues (Turner & Salter, 2008).

Within the UK high secure estate, patients are more likely to be male, never married, of lower occupational level and without qualifications (McMiller *et al*, 2000). Walsh *et al* (2002) reported on 1740 in-patients in English high secure hospitals between January 1993 and June 1993: more than 900 had a psychotic illness, principally schizophrenia (81%) and schizoaffective disorder (6%), 25% had a comorbid personality disorder and 13% comorbid substance misuse. Of the patients with psychosis, 34% had committed a homicide, 53% another violent offence, 8% a sexual offence and 5% arson or property damage. The study contrasted that population with a community sample (Burns *et al*, 1999) and found a small excess of African–Caribbean patients but no other significant overrepresentation of ethnic minority groups.

Medium secure units provide an important recovery-focused graduated discharge pathway for MDOs (Coid & Kahtan, 2000). Coid *et al* (2001) reported on admissions to seven English medium secure units between 1988 and 1994. In a sample of more than 2600, nearly every patient was admitted under mental health legislation, 69% as a result of criminal offending, the remainder following non-criminal behaviour. The mean age at admission was below 32 years and most patients were single. The study identified regional differences in UK service provision. Follow-up data including community offending rates were later available on more than 1600 of the original cohort (Coid *et al*, 2007): more than a third of men but less than 15% of women were convicted of a criminal offence. The incidence of violence for discharged men was over 7%, with grave offences including homicide, serious wounding and rape in over 4%, sexual offences and less serious incidents of arson in less than 1%. Women had significantly lower offence rates, 2.5% for violence and 3% for grave offences and non-sexual offences, though there was a higher risk of non-serious arson at over 2%. The authors concluded that risk of post-discharge offending was predicted by gender, age, early offending, past convictions and the presence of personality disorder. Longer in-patient stay and placement on a restriction order were protective factors.

Prison population and mentally disordered offenders

In the UK, high levels of psychiatric morbidity are found among prisoners. Rates are highest in remand and female prisons. Maden *et al* (1994), in a cross-sectional survey of 258 female sentenced prisoners representing approximately a quarter of the sentenced female population, found that 16% had psychosis, 16% neurotic disorders, 18% personality disorder, 9% alcohol misuse and 26% drug dependence. In a comparison sample of 1751 men only about 2% had psychosis, 6% neurotic disorders, 10% personality disorder, 12% alcohol misuse and 12% drug dependence.

Many studies have since revealed very high rates of ASPD; Singleton *et al* (1998) found that 80% of male prisoners met criteria for diagnosis. Recently, Fazel & Seewald (2012) completed a comprehensive systematic review that examined 109 samples with more than 33 000 prisoners from 24 countries. The majority of studies were from the USA and over 80% of the sample were male. Prevalence of psychosis was 3.6% in men and 3.9% in women; prevalence of depression was 10.2% in men and 14.1% in women.

Hassan *et al* (2011) reported prospectively on rates of mental illness in newly convicted prisoners admitted to five local UK prisons. They sampled over 3000 prisoners within 3 days of reception; 1097 screened positive for mental illness and were re-interviewed within the first week and subsequently followed up at 1 month and then 2 months later. Clinical interviews were conducted with 980 inmates within the first week of admission, with 572 and 182 completing follow-up interviews; the majority were male. At first evaluation 10% suffered from psychosis, 32% from a major depressive disorder, 12% from other mental disorders, 67% from drug misuse and 52% from alcohol misuse. The rates of mental disorder remained stable over the first and second months; symptom severity was highest early on and gradually decreased in the men over time. Depressive symptoms reduced over time. Female prisoners and those on remand did not show the same reduction in symptom severity. The finding that mental illness symptoms did not worsen in prison is consistent with previous research in this area (Blaauw *et al*, 2007; Taylor *et al*, 2010).

Conclusions

Offending by individuals with a mental disorder has attracted a great deal of public and scientific interest during the past few decades. Research has highlighted high levels of mental disorder within the community, which has increasingly been shown to be associated both with offending and with challenging behaviours. The complexity of mental health problems has made conclusions about the mechanisms of causality, including the contribution of environmental, economic and societal factors, problematic. Whereas the great majority of people with mental health problems do not pose a specific risk to the public, the significant association that does exist between some mental disorders and violence requires careful understanding, increased research and the allocation of appropriate resources to ensure that MDOs are appropriately managed.

References

Appelbaum, P., Robbins, P. & Monahan, J. (2000) Violence and delusions: data from the MacArthur Violence Risk Assessment Study. *American Journal of Psychiatry*, **157**, 566–572.

Appleby, L., Kapur, N., Shaw, J., *et al* (2012) *The National Confidential Inquiry into Suicide and Homicide by People with Mental Illness, Annual Report*. University of Manchester.

Arseneault, L., Moffitt, T.E., Caspi, A., *et al* (2000) Mental disorders and violence in a total birth cohort: results from the Dunedin Study. *Archives of General Psychiatry*, **57**, 979–986.

Blaauw, E., Roozen, H. & Val Marle, H. (2007) Saved by structure? The course of psychosis within a prison population. *International Journal of Prison Health*, **3**, 248-256.

Brennan, P., Mednick, S. & Hodgins, S. (2000) Major mental disorders and criminal violence in a Danish birth cohort. *Archives of General Psychiatry*, **57**, 494–500.

Burns, T., Creed, F., Fahy, T., *et al* (1999) Intensive versus standard case management for severe psychotic illness: a randomised trial. *Lancet*, **353**, 2185–2189.

Campbell, M., French, S. & Grendreau, P. (2009) The prediction of violence in adult offenders: a meta-analytic comparison of instruments and methods of assessment. *Criminal Justice and Behaviour*, **36**, 657–590.

Cleckley, H. (1976) *The Mask of Sanity*, 5th edn. Mosby.

Coid, J. (1983) The epidemiology of abnormal homicide and murder followed by suicide. *Psychological Medicine*, **13**, 855–860.

Coid, J. (2003) Epidemiology, public health and the problem of personality disorder. *British Journal of Psychiatry*, **182**, 3–10.

Coid, J. & Kahtan, N. (2000) Are special hospitals needed? *Journal of Forensic Psychiatry*, **11**, 17–35.

Coid, J., Kahtan, N., Gault, S., *et al* (2001) Medium secure forensic psychiatry services: comparison of seven English health regions. *British Journal of Psychiatry*, **178**, 55–61.

Coid, J., Yang., M., Tyrer, P., *et al* (2006*a*) Prevalence and correlates of personality disorder in Great Britain. *The British Journal of Psychiatry*, **188**, 423–431.

Coid, J., Yang, M., Tyrer, P., *et al* (2006*b*) Violence and psychiatric morbidity in the national household population of Britain: public health implications. *British Journal of Psychiatry*, **189**, 12–19.

Coid, J., Hickey, N., Kahtan, N., *et al* (2007) Patients discharged from medium secure forensic psychiatry services: reconvictions and risk factors. *British Journal of Psychiatry*, **190**, 223–229.

Commander, M., Dharan, S., Odell, S., *et al* (1997) Access to mental health care in an inner-city health district. 1: Pathways into and within specialist psychiatric services. *British Journal of Psychiatry*, **170**, 312–316.

Danielson, K.K., Moffit, T.E., Caspi, A., *et al* (1998) Comorbidity between abuse of and adult and DSM-III-R mental disorders: evidence from an epidemiological study. *American Journal of Psychiatry*, **155**, 131–133.

Dean, K., Walsh, E., Moran, P., *et al* (2006) Violence in women with psychosis in the community: prospective study. *British Journal of Psychiatry*, **188**, 264–270.

Department of Health (1999) *The National Service Framework for Mental Health: Modern Standards and Service Models*. Department of Health.

Duggan, C. (2008) Why are programmes for offenders with personality disorder not informed by the relevant scientific findings? *Transcultural Sociology*, **363**, 2599–2612.

English, D.R., Holman, C.D'A.G., Milne. E., *et al* (1995) *The Quantification of Drug Caused Morbidity and Mortality in Australia*. Australian Government Publication Service.

Eronen, M., Hakola, P. & Tihonen, J. (1996) Mental disorders and homicidal behaviour in Finland. *Archives of General Psychiatry*, **53**, 497–501.

Fazel, S. (2006) *The Prevalence of Mental Illness and Personality Disorder among Convicted Sex Offenders*. NHS Forensic Mental Health Research Programme.

Fazel, S. & Danesh, J. (2002) Serious mental disorder in 23 000 prisoners: a systematic review of 62 surveys. *Lancet*, **359**, 545–550.

Fazel, S. & Grann, M. (2004) Psychiatric morbidity among homicide offenders: a Swedish population study. *American Journal of Psychiatry*, **161**, 2129–2131.

Fazel, S. & Seewald, K. (2012) Severe mental illness in 33 588 prisoners worldwide: systematic review and meta-regression analysis. *British Journal of Psychiatry*, **200**, 364–373.

Fazel, S., Långström, N., Hjern, A., *et al* (2009*a*) Schizophrenia, substance abuse, and violent crime. *JAMA*, **301**, 2016–2033.

Fazel, S., Gulati, G. & Linsell, L. (2009*b*) Schizophrenia and violence: systematic review and meta-analysis. *PLOS Medicine*, **6**, e1000120.

Fazel, S., Lichtenstein, P., Grann, M., *et al* (2010) Bipolar disorder and violent crime: new evidence from population-based longitudinal studies and systematic review. *Archives of General Psychiatry*, **67**, 931–938.

Fowler, I., Carr, V., Carter, N., *et al* (1998) Patterns of current and lifetime substance use in schizophrenia. *Schizophrenia Bulletin*, **24**, 443–455.

Fulwiler, C., Grossman, H., Frobes, C., *et al* (1997) Early onset substance abuse and community violence by outpatients with chronic mental illness. *Psychiatric Services*, **48**, 1181–1185.

Grann, M., Danesh, J. & Fazel, S. (2008) The association between psychiatric diagnosis and violent re-offending in adult offenders in the community. *BMC Psychiatry*, **8**, 92.

Hare, R. (1980) A research scale for the assessment of psychopathy in criminal populations. *Personality and Individual Differences*, **1**, 111–119.

Hare, R. (2003) *The Hare Psychopathy Checklist-Revised (PCL-R)* (2nd edn). Multi-Health Systems.

Hare, R.D., Clark, D., Grann, M., *et al* (2000) Psychopathy and the predictive validity of the PCL-R: an international perspective. *Behavioural Science and the Law*, **18**, 623–645.

Hart, S. (2001) Forensic issues. In *Handbook of Personality Disorders: Theory, Research and Treatment* (eds WJ Liversley), pp. 555–569. Guilford Press.

Hassan, L., Birmingham, L., Harty, M., *et al* (2011) Prospective cohort study of mental health during imprisonment. *British Journal of Psychiatry*, **198**, 37–42.

Hiday, V., Swartz, M., Swanson, J., *et al* (1998) Male-female differences in the setting and construction of violence among people with severe mental illness. *Social Psychiatry and Psychiatric Epidemiology*, **33**, 68–74.

Home Office & Department of Health (1975) *Report of the Committee on Mentally Abnormal Offenders*. HMSO.

Issakidis, C., Sanderson, K., Teeson, M., *et al* (1999) Intensive case management in Australia: a randomised controlled trial. *Acta Psychiatrica Scandinavica*, **99**, 360–370.

Jacobs, R. & Barrenho, E. (2011) Impact of crisis resolution and home treatment teams on psychiatric admissions in England. *British Journal of Psychiatry*, **199**, 71–76.

Johnson, S., Nolan, F., Pilling, S., *et al* (2005) Randomised controlled trial of acute mental health care by a crisis resolution team: the north Islington crisis study. *BMJ*, **331**, 599–602.

Kafka, M. (2003) The monoamine hypothesis for the pathophysiology of paraphilic disorders: an update. *Annals of the New York Academy of Sciences*, **989**, 86–94.

Killaspy, H., Kingett, S., Bebbington, P., *et al* (2009) Randomised evaluation of assertive community treatment: 3-year outcomes. *British Journal of Psychiatry*, **195**, 81–82.

Långström, N., Sjöstedt, G. & Grann, M. (2004) Psychiatric disorder and recidivism in sex offenders. *Sexual Abuse: A Journal of Research and Treatment*, **16**, 139–150.

Large, M., Smith, G., Swinson, N., *et al* (2008) Homicide due to mental disorder in England and Wales over 50 years. *British Journal of Psychiatry*, **193**, 130–133.

Leff, J. (2001) Why is care in the community perceived as a failure? *British Journal of Psychiatry*, **179**, 881–888.

Leistico, A., Salekin, R., DeCoster, J., *et al* (2008) A large-scale meta-analysis relating the Hare measures of psychopathy to antisocial conduct. *Law and Human Behaviour*, **24**, 335–346.

Lenzenweger, M., Lane, M., Loranger, A., *et al* (2007) DSM-IV personality disorders in the national comorbidity survey replication. *Biological Psychiatry*, **62**, 553–564.

Link, B. & Stueve, A. (1994) Psychotic symptoms and the violent/illegal behaviour of mental patients compared to community control. In *Violence and Mental Disorders: Developments in Risk Assessment* (eds J. Monahan & J. Steadman). University of Chicago Press.

Maden, T., Swinton, M. & Gunn, J. (1994) Psychiatric disorder in women serving a prison sentence. *British Journal of Psychiatry*, **164**, 44–54.

McMiller, P., Johnstone, E., Lang, F., *et al* (2000) Differences between patients with schizophrenia within and without a high security psychiatric hospital. *Acta Psychiatrica Scandinavica*, **102**, 12–18.

Meltzer, H., Gill, B., Petticrew, M., *et al* (1995) *The Prevalence of Psychiatric Morbidity among Adults Living in Private Households*. OPCS (Office of Population Censuses and Surveys) of Psychiatric Morbidity in Great Britain, Report 1. HMSO.

Moran, P., Walsh, E., Tyrer, P., *et al* (2003) Impact of comorbid personality disorder on violence in psychosis: report from the UK700 trial. *British Journal of Psychiatry*, **182**, 129–134.

Mullen, P.E., Burgess, P., Wallace, C., *et al* (2000) Community care and criminal offending in schizophrenia. *Lancet*, **355**, 614–617.

Murdoch, D., Pihl, R. & Ross, D. (1990) Alcohol and crimes of violence: present issues. *International Journal of the Addictions*, **25**, 1065–1081.

Pernanen, K. (1991) *Alcohol in Human Violence*. Guilford Press.

Regier, D.A., Farmer, M.E., Rae, D.S., *et al* (1990) Comorbidity of mental disorders with alcohol and other drug abuse: results from the epidemiologic catchment area (ECA) study. *Journal of the American Medical Association*, **264**, 2511–2518.

Robins, L.N., Tipp, J. & Przybeck, T. (1991) Antisocial personality. In *Psychiatric Disorders in America* (eds L.N. Robins & D.A. Regier), pp. 258–290. Free Press.

Scott, H., Johnson, S., Menezes, P., *et al* (1998) Substance misuse and risk of aggression and offending among the severely mentally ill. *British Journal of Psychiatry*, **172**, 345–350.

Shaw, J., Hunt, I., Flynn, S., *et al* (2006) Rates of mental disorder in people convicted of homicide: National clinical survey. *British Journal of Psychiatry*, **188**, 143–147.

Simpson, A., Mckenna, B., Moskowitz, A., *et al* (2004) Homicide and mental illness in New Zealand. *British Journal of Psychiatry*, **185**, 394–398.

Singleton, N., Meltzer, H., Gatward, R., *et al* (1998) *Psychiatric Morbidity among Prisoners in England and Wales*. TSO (The Stationery Office).

Smith, A.D. & Taylor, P.J. (1999) Serious sex offending against women by men with schizophrenia. Relationship of illness and psychotic symptoms to offending. *British Journal of Psychiatry*, **174**, 233–237.

Steadman, H., Monahan, J., Robbins, P., *et al* (1993) from dangerous to risk assessment: implications for appropriate research strategies. In *Mental Disorder and Crime* (ed. S. Hodgins), pp: 39–61. Sage.

Steadman, H., Silver, E., Monahan, J., *et al* (2000) A classification tree approach to the development of actuarial violence risk assessment tools. *Law and Human Behaviour*, **24**, 83–100.

Stone, M. (2007) Violent crimes and their relationship to personality disorders. *Personality and Mental Health*, **1**, 138–153.

Swanson, J., Holzer, C., Ganju, V., *et al* (1990) Violence and psychiatric disorder in the community: evidence from Epidemiologic Catchment Area surveys. *Hospital Community Psychiatry*, **7**, 761–770.

Swanson, J., Swartz, M., Van Dorn, R., *et al* (2006) A national study of violent behaviour in persons with schizophrenia. *Archives of General Psychiatry*, **63**, 490–499.

Swanson, J.W., Borum, R., Swartz, M., *et al* (1996) Psychotic symptoms and disorders and the risk of violent behaviour in the community.*Criminal Behaviour and Mental Health*, **6**, 309–329.

Swanson, M.C., Bland, R.C. & Newman, S.C. (1994) Epidemiology of psychiatric disorders in Edmonton, antisocial personality disorders. *Acta Psychiatrica Scandinavia*, **376**, 63–70.

Swartz, M. S., Swanson, J.W., Hiday, V.A., *et al* (1998) Violence and severe mental illness: the effects of substance abuse and non-adherence to medication. *American Journal of Psychiatry*, **155**, 226–231.

Taylor, P., Dunn, E., Kissell, A., *et al* (2010) Improving mental state in early imprisonment. *Criminal Behaviour and Mental Health*, **20**, 215–231.

Tiihonen, J., Isohanni, M., Räsänen, P., *et al* (1997) Specific major mental disorders and criminality: a 26-year prospective study of the 1966 northern Finland birth cohort. *American Journal of Psychiatry*, **154**, 840–845.

Turner, T. & Salter, M. (2008) Forensic psychiatry and general psychiatry: re-examining the relationship. *Psychiatrist*, **32**, 2–6.

Tyrer, P. (2011) Has the closure of psychiatric beds gone too far? Yes. *BMJ*, **343**, d7457.

Wallace, C., Mullen, P., Burgess, P., *et al* (1998) Serious criminal offending and mental disorder. *British Journal of Psychiatry*, **172**, 477–484.

Wallace, C., Mullen, P., Burgess, P. (2004) Criminal offending in schizophrenia over a 25-year period marked by deinstitutionalization and increasing prevalence of comorbid substance use disorders. *American Journal of Psychiatry*, **161**, 716–727.

Walsh, E. & Fahy, T. (2002) Violence in society: contribution of mental illness. *BMJ*, **325**, 507–508.

Walsh, E., Leese, M., Taykor, P., *et al* (2002) Psychosis in high-security and general psychiatric services: Report from the UK700 and Special Hospitals' Treatment Resistant Schizophrenia groups. *British Journal of Psychiatry*, **180**, 351–357.

Walsh, E., Moran, P., Scott, C., *et al* (2003) Prevalence of violent victimisation in severe mental illness. *British Journal of Psychiatry*, **183**, 233–238.

Wessely, S. (1998) The Camberwell Study of Crime and Schizophrenia. *Social Psychiatry and Psychiatric Epidemiology*, **33**, S24–28.

CHAPTER 3

Clinical risk assessment in secure care

Ashimesh Roychowdhury, Muthusamy Natarajan,
Laura O'Shea, Geoffrey Dickens

Introduction

Overview

This is the first of two linked chapters examining the closely related concepts of risk assessment and risk management in secure mental healthcare.

In this chapter, we consider the nature of risk in the context of secure mental healthcare, particularly the risk of physical violence but also that of suicide. We provide an overview of the epidemiology of violence and suicide risk in people with mental disorder. Next, we explain how risk assessment has developed over recent decades. We describe unstructured, actuarial and structured professional judgement methods of violence risk assessment, and discuss two of the main tools used in secure clinical practice. Finally, we review the evidence on risk assessment in relation to specialist or minority populations in secure care including women, those diagnosed with intellectual disability, autism spectrum disorder, Black and minority ethnic groups, adolescents and those in neuropsychiatry services. In Chapter 4 we discuss methods of risk management in the secure setting.

The importance of risk assessment

The assessment of risk should be a part of every clinical encounter. Public policy, such as the Department of Health's publication Improving Health, Supporting Justice (the 'Bradley report'; Department of Health, 2009), dictates that mental health services play a key role in public protection. Despite the fact that there is a duty of care to the patient to provide treatment in the least restrictive environment (Mental Health Act 1983), clinicians are also required to ensure the safety of the ward environment for staff and other patients, and the safety of the wider public. Certain adverse outcomes among mental health service users, including homicide or suicide, result in a mandatory inquiry. Significant third-party risk is one of the few situations in medical practice where doctor–patient confidentiality can be breached both in the UK and the USA (*Tarasoff v. Regents of the University of California*, 17 Cal. 3d 425, 551 P.2d 334, 131 Cal. Rptr. 14 (Cal. 1976); General Medical Council, 2009).

Defining risk in secure care

In the context of secure mental healthcare risk is commonly defined as the probability that physical or psychological harm will occur. It is important, however, that the concept of risk is also understood to encompass the likelihood of benefit: risk assessment requires scope to judge and balance the risk of benefit against the risk of harm. Risk comprises five dimensions: nature, probability, severity, imminence and frequency (Hart, 2001). Risk assessment must address all of these areas to enable a risk management plan to be formed. The risk of violence is the main focus of interest in forensic secure care, although other types of risk must also be assessed and managed, notably suicide and self-harm.

Violence is defined in the Historical, Clinical and Risk Management (HCR-20) manual as the 'actual, attempted, or threatened harm to a person or persons' (Webster *et al*, 1997). The authors state that violence is defined by the act rather than the damage inflicted, such that 'behaviour which would be fear-inducing to the average person may be counted as violence (e.g. stalking)' (Webster *et al*, 1997). Sexual violence is defined in the Risk of Sexual Violence Protocol (RSVP) manual as 'actual, attempted, or threatened sexual contact that is non-consensual' (Hart *et al*, 2003). Suicide is 'self-injurious behaviour with a fatal outcome for which there is evidence (either explicit or implicit) that the individual intended at some level to kill himself or herself' (Links *et al*, 2003). A suicide attempt similarly involves intention but has a non-fatal outcome and self-injurious behaviour involves deliberate harm to one's own body but with zero intention of fatality (Links *et al*, 2003). Assessed risk in secure mental healthcare is commonly ascribed a level such as 'high', 'medium' or 'low', which is clinically meaningful and easily communicable (Monahan & Steadman, 1996).

Mental disorder and risk

Mental disorder and violence

The MacArthur Violence Risk Assessment Study (Steadman *et al*, 1998) examined the prevalence of violence by patients recently discharged from psychiatric hospitals in the USA. It was found that at least one violent act was committed within 20 weeks of discharge in 18.7% of patients. Lower rates of violence were found in those who had a major mental disorder, such as schizophrenia, compared with those diagnosed with personality disorder, and a compounding increase was observed in those who misuse substances. Also, commands from voices specifically to commit violence were associated with increased violence, although there was no general association between command hallucinations and violence. Individuals who had violent thoughts or who were angry were more likely to commit a violent act. The study also provided empirical support for several major violence risk factors which may previously have only been assumed to be associated with risk of violence, including prior arrests (their seriousness and frequency), demographic factors (younger male, unemployed), history of child abuse (seriousness and frequency), diagnosis (antisocial personality disorder), family factors (e.g. a father who used drugs and who left home before the child reached 15 years of age) and other clinical factors (substance misuse, anger control, violent fantasies, loss of consciousness, involuntary hospital admission). Skeem & Mulvey (2001) found that elements of psychopathy, as measured using the Psychopathy Checklist: Screening Version (PCL:SV; Hart *et al*, 1995), significantly predicted violence in the MacArthur sample and that this was independent of antisocial behaviours and personality disorders other than psychopathy.

Elbogen & Johnson (2009) found, as part of the National Epidemiologic Survey on Alcohol and Related Conditions (NESARC), that the incidence of violence was higher in people with severe mental illness, but that was only significant for people with comorbid substance use/dependence. They found that historical factors such as past violence and dispositional (e.g. gender), clinical (e.g. perceived threats) and contextual (e.g. unemployment) factors were significantly associated with violence risk rather than severe mental illness alone. Similarly, Fazel *et al* (2009) found substance misuse to be a significant mediator of increased risk of violence among those with schizophrenia and other psychoses, although the risk is similar to risk in those with substance misuse alone without psychosis. They found that the odds ratio for a violent conviction in those with schizophrenia and substance misuse was 4.4, whereas without substance misuse it was 1.2.

In summary, mental disorder may be linked to some increased risk of violence but most increased risk appears to be related to other factors, notably substance misuse.

Mental disorder and suicide

At least 90% of people who die of suicide are suffering from a mental disorder at the time of death (Hawton & Herringen, 2009). Affective disorders are the most common, with more than half of individuals meeting criteria for current depressive disorder (Cavanagh *et al*, 2003). Of particular relevance to secure mental health services, schizophrenia and substance misuse (especially alcohol) increases risk, and comorbidity of disorders is also a major risk factor (Cavanagh *et al*, 2003). Other biopsychosocial risk factors include hopelessness, impulsive and aggressive tendencies, history of abuse, major physical illness, previous suicide attempt and family history of suicide. Environmental risk factors include job loss or financial loss, relationship loss, access to lethal suicide means and local suicide clustering. Sociocultural factors include lack of support, stigma associated with help-seeking, barriers to mental health treatment, cultural beliefs that emphasise suicide as noble, and exposure to media portrayals and real-world instances of suicide. Protective factors include social and family support, restricted access to lethal means of suicide, access to effective mental health/substance misuse treatment, and cultural beliefs that discourage suicide (US Department of Health and Human Services Public Health Service, 2001).

The annual report of the National Confidential Inquiry into Suicide and Homicide by People with Mental Illness (2012) revealed that there were 1556 in-patient suicides between 2000 and 2010 in England and Wales (average 141 per year, but on a decreasing trajectory). The risk of suicide for mental health service users is greatest in the first 7 days following discharge from hospital, when on authorised leave from hospital, after absconding, during the period following admission, or in the case of prison transfers, while waiting to be transferred. Risk assessment for suicide specifically is not discussed in depth in this chapter, though it is one of the risks covered by the Short Term Assessment of Risk and Treatability (START) risk assessment (Webster *et al*, 2004). Dedicated tools used in the assessment of risk of suicide/self-harm include the Risk Assessment Matrix (Hart *et al*, 2005), the SAD PERSONS scale (Patterson *et al*, 1983) and the Suicide Intent Scale (Beck *et al*, 1974). The ability of any of these tools to accurately predict risk is low (e.g. Harriss & Hawton, 2005; Bolton *et al*, 2012).

Risk assessment

Predictive validity

Table 3.1 shows the potential outcomes of a violence risk assessment. Patients assessed as being at high risk of violence may actually be violent ('true positive' outcome) or may desist from future violent behaviour ('false positive'). Similarly, patients assessed as being at low risk of future violence may actually be violent ('false negative') or they may desist ('true negative'). Clearly, the aim of accurate risk assessment is to maximise the frequency of true positive and true negative predictions. However, in the 1980s and 1990s the base rates of violence (i.e. the known prevalence of a specified type of violent behaviour within a given population over a period of time) in those with mental disorder were considered to be so low that even a highly accurate risk assessment instrument would result in significant errors, particularly false positives (Szmukler, 2003). To illustrate, example figures are shown in Table 3.2 for a sample of 1000 service users where the base rate of violence in that population is 10% and the sensitivity and specificity of the risk assessment is 90%. Using these numbers, the risk assessment appears to be highly accurate in that 90% of patients are allocated to true positive and true negative conditions. However, the positive predictive value (PPV), which is the proportion of those identified by the risk assessment

Table 3.1 2 × 2 contingency table showing potential outcomes of risk assessment for violence

		Outcome at follow-up	
		Violent	**Non-violent**
Risk assessment prediction	**High risk**	True positive (TP)	False positive (FP)
	Low risk	False negative (FN)	True negative (TN)
Sensitivity		TP/(TP+FN)	
Specificity		TN/(TN+FP)	
Positive predictive value (PPV)		TP/(TP+FP)	
Accuracy		TP+TN/(TP+FP+TN+FN)	

Table 3.2 2 × 2 contingency table showing potential outcomes of risk assessment for violence for 1000 service users where base rate of violence is 10%

		Outcome at follow-up	
		Violent (n=100)	**Non-violent (n=900)**
Risk assessment prediction	**High risk**	90	90
	Low risk	10	810
Sensitivity			
Specificity			
Positive predictive value (PPV)		50%	
Accuracy		90%	

FP:FN 9:1, TP:FP 1:0

instrument as high risk and who actually are violent, is only 50%, which is the level of chance prediction, in other words, only as accurate as tossing a coin.

This argument cast doubt on whether any form of violence risk assessment could be carried out with sufficient accuracy. This situation posed significant ethical challenges in the management of individual patients because it was difficult to confidently justify any restrictions as being proportionate to the risk.

More recently, this pessimism has been countered by studies showing that the base rates of violence in those with mental disorder are higher than first thought, as well as by advances in statistical methods. Risk assessment instrumentation accuracy is currently based on receiver operating characteristics (ROC) and the area under the curve (AUC), which provide an index of precision (Mossman, 1994). The ROC is a plot of the true positive rate on the y axis (the test sensitivity) against the false positive rate on the x axis (the test specificity) (Fig. 3.1). The AUC represents the likelihood of correct risk prediction with the chance level being 0.5 which is represented by a straight line, where for every true positive identified there is a false positive. For different cut-off points on the risk assessment instrument, the true positive and false positive rates can be plotted with the resulting curve representing the 'optimal fit' that gives the greatest AUC. An AUC of 1.0 gives perfect prediction and an AUC of 0.7 or above represents a large effect size. An AUC of 0.75 means that if someone was violent, there is a 75% chance that the risk assessment instrument would have identified him as being at higher risk for violence.

Unlike the PPV, the ROC method is unaffected by base rates (Mossman, 1994). However, the base rate of violence in risk assessment remains important because of the difficulty of translating the AUC value into clinically meaningful information by itself (Buchanan, 2008). To elaborate, if a risk assessment instrument was used as a screening test and those identified as likely to be violent remained in secure care, then, for any given period, the number of patients we require to be detained (numbers needed to detain (NND)) in order to prevent one violent act can be calculated.

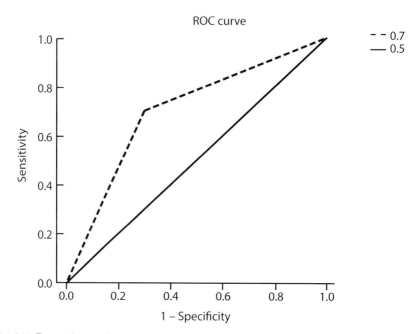

Fig. 3.1 Example receiver operating characteristic (ROC) curve.

NND is the inverse of PPV and, like the ROC, derives from sensitivity, specificity and the base rate. For example, with a violence base rate of 10% and an AUC of 0.75, a risk assessment tool would require the detention of five people to prevent one unwanted act, while chance prediction (AUC 0.5) would require detention of 10. The NND rises as the base rate of violence falls. Therefore, base rates, if known, provide a context in which to make proportionate decisions resulting from a risk assessment. In such circumstances the definition of the base rate is of some importance: for example, base rates that are contingent upon a definition that emphasises intentionality may be problematic when interpreting AUC curves for populations with intellectual disability.

Methods of risk assessment

There are three recognised approaches to risk assessment: unstructured clinical judgement, actuarial risk assessment tools and structured professional judgement (SPJ) (Hart, 2001).

Unstructured clinical judgement

Using this approach a clinical opinion on risk is formulated without necessarily following a predetermined and commonly agreed structure. The term unstructured may be misleading: a structure may be imposed on the evaluation but it will vary from clinician to clinician and/or between one patient and another even when assessed by the same clinician. This approach has the advantage of being flexible, quick and idiographic (person-centred) (Hart, 2001). However, it has been criticised for being subjective and impressionistic, lacking in transparency, reliability and validity, and for producing decisions based on the qualifications of the assessor (Grove & Meehl, 1996).

Actuarial approaches

Criticism of unstructured approaches led to interest in actuarial approaches to assessing risk. These are assessments that are based on validated statistical relationships between measurable predictor and outcome variables, and the outcome of the assessment is determined by fixed and explicit rules. Actuarial risk assessment is essentially atheoretical and there is no attempt to elucidate an explanatory causal relationship between predictor and outcome variables; the importance lies in the strength of the statistical correlation between the two. Actuarial tools are often based on static predictors that require little clinical judgement to rate, whereas some items still require clinical judgement. In the latter case then the process remains actuarial in that the total score is used to reflect the risk and gives rise to probabilistic statements.

One of the best known actuarial tools is the Violence Risk Appraisal Guide or VRAG (Quinsey *et al*, 1998). The VRAG was developed in a Canadian male high secure population and is based on follow-up data from more than 600 patients who were released or given a criminal justice disposal. Twelve items were weighted according to their ability to predict violence at 7- and then 10-year follow-up. Analysis of the VRAG using receiver operating characteristics yielded large AUC values of 0.73 to 0.77. The authors consequently argued for the replacement of clinical risk assessment with actuarial tools.

Mossman (1994) re-analysed 58 data-sets from 44 published studies and concluded that actuarial risk assessment had greater predictive accuracy than unstructured clinical assessment, particularly for violence over 1 year. The question of the relative predictive accuracy of actuarial *v.* clinical risk assessment was considered a 'dead horse' in favour of actuarial assessments (Monahan *et al*, 2001). Despite this, there ensued a resurgence of clinical risk assessment approaches, based on a number of factors. There was accumulating evidence that clinicians were fairly good at assessing risk of violence and suicide (Haim *et al*, 2002). Actuarial approaches were criticised for having a 'floor effect', assigning low to moderate risk to all groups, based on an inability to take into account dynamic situational factors pertinent to the individual (Hart, 1998). Further, scores on instruments such as the VRAG gave little guidance to services on treatment options or on which factors to focus on to achieve clinical change (Hanson & Harris, 2001). Actuarial tools ignored the importance of moderating factors (variables that affect the strength and direction of the relationship between the predictor and criterion variable), mediating factors (intervening factors between the independent and dependent variable) and protective factors (that reduce the likelihood of the outcome variable) (Rogers, 2000). Actuarial tools also lacked utility in helping make the range of decisions required in secure care. For example, in making a decision about continued detention or release, the assessing clinician is interested in only those types of violence that would have justified detention, as opposed to all types of violence. Further, actuarial tools only answer the question 'in a group with these characteristics, how likely is it that this member of the group will commit the act in question within the specified time period?' This is only applicable if the person is from a group similar to that in which the tool was validated. Issues that exercise clinicians, such as severity or imminence of risk in different situations, are not helped by actuarial scores.

These criticisms of the actuarial approach reveal that the methodology was based on the assumption that risk assessment is a predictive process with a single, dichotomous outcome variable. It is increasingly recognised that risk assessment is a much broader task that requires assessment of all five dimensions of risk, with the aim to stratify people into groups that will dictate the appropriate care and risk management strategy (Royal College of Psychiatrists, 2008).

Structured professional judgement

The emergence and evolution of the SPJ approach (Hart, 1998) reflected and addressed the problematic issues of actuarial approaches. The method provides clinical judgement with a structured application. There has been a proliferation of SPJ tools for different risks, such as the HCR-20 for violence (Webster *et al*, 1997), the Sexual Violence Risk-20 (SVR 20; Boer *et al*, 1997) and RSVP (Hart *et al*, 2003) for sexual offending, the Domestic Abuse, Stalking and Harassment and Honour Based Violence risk assessment (DASH; Richards *et al*, 2008), the Spousal Assault Risk Assessment (SARA; Kropp *et al*, 1999) and the Short-Term Assessment of Risk and Treatability (START; Webster *et al*, 2004) for multiple risk domains.

Each SPJ instrument follows a core six-step methodological process (Hart *et al*, 2003).

1   *Gather information.* First, there is collation of comprehensive background information, including multiple sources and clinical interview where possible.

2   *Identify risk factors.* A rating is made regarding the absence (0 or 'no'), partial presence (1 or 'maybe') or presence (2 or 'yes') in the individual of the risk factors identified on the SPJ tool. The items are derived from the empirical literature and selected for their association with the outcome variable, but, unlike actuarial tools, they are not optimised from one sample, which enhances generalisability. Each item is operationally defined to enhance inter-rater reliability. Most SPJ tools consider both historical/static and dynamic risk items. The relevance of each item to future risk can be rated and case-specific items can also be considered.

3   *Develop risk formulation.* Once items are rated, the next step is to construct an explanatory/causative model about how the risk items combine to produce the outcome.

4   *Consider risk scenarios.* Various risk scenarios are considered, including circumstances in which previous risk behaviour may be repeated, escalated or altered ('twist' scenarios). A risk specificity statement is made detailing the level, nature and imminence of the risk, factors that may increase or decrease the risk, situations in which the risk is likely to occur, and suggestions for management and treatment (Dernevik, 2004). Unlike actuarial tools, multiple scenarios can be considered, depending on the decision in question.

5   *Develop risk management strategies.* Options to reduce risk, including through treatment, monitoring and supervision, and to reduce impact of risk through victim safety planning are considered and strategies made. (Risk management in secure care is discussed in detail in Chapter 4.)

6   *Summary judgement of risk.* A summary judgement of risk as low, medium or high is made. Research suggests that the summary judgement, especially if agreed by a clinical team, adds incremental predictive

validity to SPJ approaches (Kropp *et al*, 1999). There is also evidence that communication of risk in this categorical manner leads to more action (in this case, risk management interventions) compared with probabilistic statements (Murphy, 1991).

Commonly used SPJ tools

HCR-20

The best known SPJ instrument is the HCR-20 (Webster *et al*, 1997). Twenty items were derived based on a review of the scientific and professional literature, along with consideration of a number of legal issues. The historical (H) scale comprises ten items that are thought to be relatively static and reflect the individual's psychosocial adjustment and history of violence. However, some of these variables are amenable to change; for example, items related to 'relationship instability' and 'employment problems' may both show some improvement over time, while the item 'previous violence' may change for an individual who commits a first serious violent offence. The clinical (C) scale includes five dynamic risk factors that reflect the individual's current or recent mental health-related functioning and the risk management (R) scale includes five dynamic risk factors that reflect professional opinions regarding

---

Box 3.1 HCR-20 items

- Historical items (the past)
  - Previous violence
  - Young age at first violent incident
  - Relationship instability
  - Employment problems
  - Substance use problems
  - Major mental illness
  - Psychopathy
  - Early maladjustment
  - Personality disorder
  - Prior supervision failure
- Clinical items (current)
  - Lack of insight
  - Negative attitudes
  - Active symptoms of major mental illness
  - Impulsivity
  - Unresponsive to treatment
- Risk management items (future/projected)
  - Plans lack feasibility
  - Exposure to destabilisers
  - Lack of personal support
  - Non-compliance with remediation attempts
  - Stress

Source: Webster *et al* (1997)

---

the individual's ability to adjust to the institution or community (Douglas *et al*, 2001). The three scales are shown in Box 3.1.

Research studies commonly use the actuarial data from the HCR-20 to test its predictive risk by summing the presence of risk factors to yield a total score (maximum score 40) (Douglas *et al*, 2001). Douglas and colleagues (1999) tested the use of the HCR-20 in the assessment of violence in a psychiatric out-patient sample. It produced AUCs greater than chance, ranging from 0.76 (for any violence and physical violence) to 0.77 (for threatening behaviour) to 0.80 (for violent crime). Research comparing the efficacy of risk assessment tools for predicting in-patient aggression has produced promising results for the HCR-20. A number of studies have found that the HCR-20 has incremental validity over the PCL-R (Morrissey *et al*, 2007; McDermott *et al*, 2008a) and the VRAG (McDermott *et al*, 2008a), such that it increases the ability to predict in-patient aggression above that achieved by the other measures (Haynes & Lench, 2003). Further, in a recent meta-analytic comparison of six risk assessment tools, the HCR-20 produced the largest mean effect size for prediction of institutional violence (Campbell *et al*, 2009). Even those who have not found the HCR-20 to have superior predictive validity have advocated its use on account of its capabilities of assessing risk at admission, throughout admission and upon consideration of release (Daffern, 2007).

It is generally accepted that the dynamic C and R scales are stronger predictors of in-patient aggression than the H scale. Research has provided mixed results regarding the relative efficacy of the C and R subscales, yet there is currently greater empirical support for the C subscale (O'Shea *et al*, 2012). There is some tentative evidence that efficacy may differ as a function of the type of aggression being predicted. For example, McDermott *et al* (2008b) found that the C scale was the strongest predictor of impulsive and psychotic aggression, while the R scale was the best predictor of predatory aggression.

Short-Term Assessment of Risk and Treatability (START)

The START (Webster *et al*, 2004, 2009) is a 20-item clinical guide designed to structure regular clinical assessments regarding the evaluation of mental disorder, monitoring of patient progress, planning of treatment and estimation of short-term (maximum of 3 months) risks to the self and others (Box 3.2). It is intended that START should be completed by a multidisciplinary team through a process of discussion and consensus (Webster *et al*, 2009). The START differs from previous risk assessment tools as it considers and individual's strengths in addition to their vulnerabilities. The tool is intended to guide decision-making related to seven specific risks: violence, self-harm, suicide, substance misuse, being victimised, self-neglect, and unauthorised absences.

An important feature of the START is that it allows clinicians to identify any critical vulnerabilities or key strengths, as well as any signature risk

---

Box 3.2 START items

Social skills	Material resources
Relationships	Attitudes
Occupational	Medication adherence
Recreational	Rule adherence
Self-care	Conduct
Mental state	Insight
Emotional state	Plans
Substance misuse	Coping
Impulse control	Social support
External triggers	Treatability
Case specific	Case specific

Source: Webster *et al* (2009)

---

signs an individual may have, which may serve as a reliable predictor of impending relapse and risk of violence towards the self or others. Finally, clinicians are required to make specific risk estimates with regard to the seven risk areas identified and to describe current management measures, in terms of the individual's current security level and privileges, and risk management plans (Webster *et al*, 2009).

START is a better predictor of verbal aggression and physical aggression towards others than the HCR-20 and PCL:SV (Desmarais *et al*, 2012). Interestingly, it was the vulnerability scale that was responsible for this incremental validity for verbal aggression, but for physical aggression towards others it was the strength scale.

Studies suggest a strong negative correlation between the strength and vulnerability scales, typically stronger than −0.80 (Braithwaite *et al*, 2010; Wilson *et al*, 2010; Chu *et al*, 2011), which raises a question about the value of rating items on both scales. The utility of the two scales can be further questioned by findings that neither have incremental validity over the other (Wilson *et al*, 2010; Chu *et al*, 2011) and that there appears to be very little difference in the predictive efficacy of the two scales (Braithwaite *et al*, 2010; Nonstad *et al*, 2010; Wilson *et al*, 2010). However, the vulnerability scale may be a stronger predictor of verbal aggression (Chu *et al*, 2011; Gray *et al*, 2011a; Desmarais *et al*, 2012) and the strength scale a stronger predictor of physical aggression (Gray *et al*, 2011a). Further, assessing strengths as well as vulnerabilities is clinically useful as it facilitates the integration of risk management and treatment plans (Nonstad *et al*, 2010).

Much of the research conducted into the predictive efficacy of START has focused on violence as the outcome, despite its intended purpose of guiding decision-making regarding a number of risky behaviours. This may be in part a result of the somewhat lower base rates of suicide and self-harm, compared with violence, in the populations studied (Nonstad *et al*, 2010; Nicholls *et al*, 2011) and of a lack of established measures for outcomes such as 'self-neglect' and 'being victimised' (Nonstad *et al*, 2010). The studies that have addressed the other risk areas identified by START have produced conflicting results. Braithwaite *et al* (2010) found that the vulnerability and strength scales both significantly predicted unauthorised leave and substance misuse, but not self-harm, suicide, victimisation or self-neglect. Other research has found that START does not significantly predict unauthorised leave (Nicholls *et al*, 2006; Desmarais *et al*, 2010) but does predict self-neglect (Gray *et al*, 2011*a*) and self-harm (Desmarais *et al*, 2010). This may be a result of using a measure designed to assess multiple outcomes; not all items are intuitively related to each category of challenging behaviour, for example, self-care is unlikely to affect the risk of aggression towards others. This was confirmed using logistic regression by Braithwaite *et al* (2010), and led to the development of optimised scales, allowing the prediction of each outcome using only a limited number of items that correlated with the outcome. The optimised vulnerability scales significantly predicted suicidality, self-neglect and victimisation, and increased the accuracy for predictions of unauthorised leave, substance misuse and aggression. Similarly, the optimised strength scales significantly predicted self-harm, suicidality and self-neglect and increased accuracy for the prediction of unauthorised leave and substance use. This finding may account for why summary judgements using START have been found to predict self-harm and victimisation where actuarial scores have failed to do so (Gray *et al*, 2011*a*), and have emerged as a stronger predictor of violence than scale totals alone (Wilson *et al* 2010; Desmarais *et al*, 2012), as it allows clinicians to consider the items most pertinent to the outcome in question.

SPJ *v.* actuarial assessment: summary

In summary, although some studies may show comparable rates of predictive validity between SPJ and actuarial tools (Yang *et al* 2010), the utility of SPJ tools to consider multiple scenarios of risk, incorporate mediating, moderating and protective factors and to help guide risk management plans, has led to their recommendation as the methodology of choice in secure care (Department of Health, 2007). However, returning to the issue of base rates, any method of risk assessment must be used in an appropriate way. Fazel *et al*'s (2012) meta-analysis of nine risk assessment instruments showed that, although negative predictive values were high (indicating that tools could successfully screen out low-risk cases), the positive predictive value was low (average PPV 0.41). Therefore, to use any risk assessment as the sole source of decision-making or as anything other than as part of a wider assessment of treatment and management was deemed 'not evidence based'.

Risk assessment in specialist populations in secure care

In this section we highlight how the predictive ability of risk assessment instruments may differ among specialist or minority groups with whom the majority of these tools were not developed. We also describe how the methodology of risk assessment could be modified to better reflect these differences.

Women

Research investigating the predictive validity of the HCR-20 with regard to in-patient aggression has been conducted predominantly among males. However, the risk factors for violence in women may differ from those in men. For example, the three most frequent other considerations listed by clinicians for men on the HCR-20 risk assessment were financial problems, lack of prospects for the future and violent fantasies, whereas for women they were forming a new intimate relationship, caring for children and prostitution (de Vogel & de Ruiter, 2005). This has led to research investigating whether the HCR-20 displays similar predictive efficacy for women as for men, producing inconsistent results (O'Shea *et al*, 2012). Nicholls *et al* (2004) found that the HCR-20 had a moderate – strong association with measures of both men's and women's in-patient aggression; de Vogel & and de Ruiter (2005) found that the HCR-20 was only a significant predictor of women's in-patient aggression when used in the SPJ process, but was significant for men when used both in this manner and actuarially. The Female Additional Manual (FAM) is a recently developed addition to the HCR-20 for assessing risk of violence in women. The FAM contains nine specific risk factors for women as well as additional guidelines to five HCR-20 items. The additional historical (H) items are 'prostitution', 'pregnancy at young age', 'victimisation after childhood', 'parenting difficulties' and 'suicidality/self-harm'; some additional C items are 'low self-esteem' and 'covert behaviour', and R items are 'problematic intimate relationship' and 'problematic child care responsibility'. In addition, FAM has extra risk estimates for self-destructive behaviour, non-violent criminal offences and victimisation. Preliminary research is positive in terms of predictive ability for violence and self-destructive behaviours in women.

Intellectual disability

Boer *et al* (2010) have suggested extensive adaptations of the HCR-20 for individuals with intellectual disability. However, these suggestions have not been empirically tested and recent research suggests that tools, including the HCR-20, have predictive efficacy for people with intellectual disability, possibly even more so than in those without. Gray *et al* (2007) investigated offenders with and without intellectual disability and found that the HCR-20 was a very good predictor of violent reconviction in the intellectual disability group over 5 years, achieving an AUC of 0.81, compared with 0.68 in the group without intellectual disability. Morrissey *et al* (2007), in a study of 212 offenders with intellectual disability, found that the HCR-20 total score was significantly correlated with in-patient aggression, whereas the PCL-R total score was not.

Autism spectrum disorder

The HCR-20 and other SPJ tools allow each of the triad of impairments in autism spectrum disorder (social and emotional reciprocity, language and communication, stereotyped and restricted behaviours and routines) to be considered as additional considerations and for a development of a narrative of the link between these features of the disorder and the risk of future violence. This is particularly important as, at a population level, the association between autism and violence is weak; however, in secure care, patients diagnosed with autism spectrum disorder may show significant violence that is believed to be functionally related to the disorder. The validation of HCR-20 in intellectual disability populations suggests likely validity in this population, but further research is needed for patients with autism spectrum disorder without intellectual disability.

Adolescents

There are a range of risk assessment tools for use with adolescents, such as the Structured Assessment of Violence Risk in Youth (SAVRY; Borum *et al* 2002), the Estimate of Risk of Adolescent Sexual Offence Recidivism (ERASOR; Worling & Curwen, 2001) and the Psychopathy Checklist Youth Version (PCL-YV; Forth *et al*, 2003). A key issue is which tool to use in the transition to adult services. Guidance from the Royal College of Psychiatrists suggests that, in those with intellectual disability, the SAVRY should continue to be used till the age of 21 as it contains more developmentally appropriate items (Royal College of Psychiatrists, 2001).

Personality disorder

Personality disorder is an item on the H scale of the HCR-20, as is psychopathy. The latter also forms part of the VRAG and is the single strongest predictor item for violence in both tools. However, surprisingly little research has been conducted into the predictive validity of tools for personality disorder as a diagnostic group. A recent study examining the prediction of future violence in patients discharged from secure psychiatric services found that while the HCR-20 was a significant predictor of future violent re-offences across all diagnoses, it was not equally accurate (Gray *et al*, 2011*b*). Only moderate to weak effects sizes were obtained for individuals diagnosed with substance use disorder, mood disorder and personality disorder. This result is of some concern given the established links both personality and substance use disorders have with violent behaviour (Steadman *et al*, 1998; Johnson *et al*, 2000; Elbogen & Johnson, 2009). However, research has found the HCR-20 to be an accurate predictor of in-patient aggression in patients with dangerous and severe personality disorder (DSPD), despite homogeneity of assessed risk scores within this population (Daffern *et al*, 2009; Langton *et al*, 2009).

Neuropsychiatry

There are no predictive validity studies of the HCR-20 or START in populations with acquired brain injury or progressive neurological conditions such as dementia. Some theoretical issues can be commented upon. In acquired brain injury, the injury event is often sudden and traumatic. It is not clear if the H scale of the HCR-20 remains predictive based on pre-injury information or whether it only becomes predictive once the post-brain injury picture has stabilised. Issues about the relevance of items and individualised scenario planning become vital in contextualising risk. For progressive neurological conditions, similar themes apply. In addition, the time frame over which any scenario is valid may need to be shortened, with regular reassessment, to reflect the changing clinical picture.

Older adults

Lewis *et al* (2006) found in a sample of forensic assessments of individuals aged 60 years plus that 68% had alcohol dependence, 44% had dementia and 32% had antisocial personality disorder. The majority were facing charges of violence (61%) and most were recidivists (81%). There are no violence risk assessment tools validated in older adult populations; however, Singh *et al* (2011) reported that studies with a mean sample age greater than 40 years produced significantly higher diagnostic odds ratios than those with a mean age of 25–40 years, which in turn were significantly greater than those with a mean of less than 25 years. This finding suggests that older age is associated with greater predictive validity. This is surprising given that many of the risk assessment instruments reviewed were developed in discharged prisoners in their late 20s and 30s (Singh *et al*, 2011) and one would expect them to perform most accurately with this age group.

Ethnicity

Another relatively under-researched area relates to the role of ethnicity and culture in relation to the predictive validity of risk assessment instruments. Although studies have been conducted in various countries, the vast majority of samples have been predominantly White (Daffern, 2007) and data from Black and minority ethnic groups have been reported in aggregate. One study that has directly investigated Black and minority ethnic differences in the predictive ability of the HCR-20 found no significant differences between Asian-Americans, European-Americans and Native Hawaiians (Fujii *et al*, 2005). However, a recent metaregression analysis found that the HCR-20 demonstrated higher predictive efficacy in samples with higher proportions of White in-patients (Singh *et al*, 2011). Although predictive efficacy as a function of ethnicity was not directly compared, this result seems to suggest that the HCR-20 may have greater validity for assessing White in-patients' risk for aggression, suggesting that potential ethnic differences warrant attention in future research.

Conclusions

Risk assessment instruments used in secure care are statistically proven to have greater predictive validity than chance. However, it is essential that clinicians understand what that actually means. It means that the instrument is 'predicting' if a person is in a high- or a low-risk group, not that the instrument is predicting the negative event itself. In a similar way, car insurance companies will stratify people into high- and low-risk groups and charge different premiums. The company makes profit by those in the high-risk group not claiming. The fact that a person from a high-risk group does not claim does not make the assessment incorrect. In this way, the tendency for a high false positive rate (if one erroneously assumes that the term high-risk meant that anyone with that label would have an incident that would lead to a claim) works in favour of the insurance company, but against the patient or healthcare professional. This has led to an emphasis on the word 'assessment' in risk assessment, as opposed to prediction. The assessment should answer several important questions such as:

- What are the key risk factors and how do they interact to lead to the behaviour in question?
- What are the key strengths that can prevent or mitigate any risk?
- What are the case-specific factors (such as different diagnostic groups) that are relevant to consider?
- What is the base rate of this risk in the population relevant to the patient?
- What is the actual quantum of loss (probability × harm) that could result from the risk occurring?

Taking into account all factors of the case, what is the most proportionate risk management plan? This includes assessing and weighing the risks of harm caused by intervention *v.* the original risk.

References

Beck, A.T., Schuyler, D. & Herman, I. (1974) Development of suicidal intent scales. In *The Prediction of Suicide* (eds A.T. Beck, H.L.P. Resnik & D. Lettieri), pp. 45–56. Charles Press.

Boer, D.P., Hart, S.D., Kropp, P.R., *et al* (1997) *Manual for the Sexual Violence Risk-20: Professional Guidelines for Assessing Risk of Sexual Violence*. British Columbia Institute against Family Violence.

Boer, D.P., Frize, M., Pappas, R., *et al* (2010) Suggested adaptations to the HCR 20 for offenders with intellectual disabilities. In *Assessment and Treatment of Sexual Offenders with Intellectual Disabilities: A Handbook* (eds L. Craig, W. Lindsay & K.D. Browne), pp. 177–192. Wiley-Blackwell.

Bolton, J.M., Spiwak, R. & Sareen, J. (2012) Predicting suicide attempts with the SAD PERSONS scale: a longitudinal analysis. *Journal of Clinical Psychiatry*, **73**, 735–741.

Borum, R., Bartel, P. & Forth, A. (2002) *Manual for the Structured Assessment of Violence Risk in Youth (SAVRY)*. University of South Florida.

Braithwaite, E., Charette, Y., Crocker, A.G., *et al* (2010) The predictive validity of clinical ratings of the Short-Term Assessment of Risk and Treatability (START). *International Journal of Forensic Mental Health*, **9**, 271–281.

Buchanan, A. (2008) Risk of violence by psychiatric patients: beyond the 'actuarial versus clinical' assessment debate. *Psychiatric Services*, **58**, 184–190.

Campbell, M.A., French, S. & Gendreau, P. (2009) The prediction of violence in adult offenders: A meta-analytic comparison of instruments and methods of assessment. *Criminal Justice and Behavior*, **36**, 567–590.

Cavanagh, J.T.O., Carson, A.J., Sharpe, M., *et al* (2003) Psychological autopsy studies of suicide: a systematic review. *Psychological Medicine*, **33**, 395–405.

Chu, C.M., Thomas, S.D.M., Ogloff, J.R.P., *et al* (2011) The predictive validity of the Short-Term Assessment of Risk and Treatability (START) in a secure forensic hospital: risk factors and strengths. *International Journal of Forensic Mental Health*, **10**, 337–345.

Daffern, M. (2007) The predictive validity and practical utility of structured schemes used to assess risk for aggression in psychiatric inpatient settings. *Aggression and Violent Behavior*, **12**, 116–130.

Daffern, M., Howells, K., Hamilton, L., *et al* (2009) The impact of structured risk assessments followed by management recommendations on aggression in patients with personality disorder. *Journal of Forensic Psychiatry and Psychology*, **20**, 661–679.

Department of Health (2007) *Best Practice in Managing Risk: Principles and Evidence for Best Practice in the Assessment and Management of Risk to Self and Others in Mental Health Services*. TSO (The Stationery Office).

Department of Health (2009) *Improving Health, Supporting Justice the National Delivery Plan of the Health and Criminal Justice Programme Board*. Department of Health.

Dernevik, M. (2004) *Structured Clinical Assessment and Management of Risk of Violent Recidivism in Mentally Disordered Offenders*. Karolinska University Press.

Desmarais, S.L., Nicholls, T.L., Read, J.D., *et al* (2010) Confidence and accuracy in assessment of short-term risks presented by forensic psychiatric patients. *Journal of Forensic Psychiatry and Psychology*, **21**, 1–22.

Desmarais, S.L., Nicholls, T.L., Wilson, C.M., *et al* (2012) Using dynamic risk and protective factors to predict inpatient aggression: reliability and validity of START assessments. *Psychological Assessment*, **24**, 685–700.

de Vogel, V. & de Ruiter, C. (2005) The HCR-20 in personality disordered female offenders: A comparison with a matched sample of males. *Clinical Psychology and Psychotherapy*, **12**, 226–240.

Douglas, K.S., Ogloff, J.R.P., Nicholls, T.L., *et al* (1999) Assessing risk for violence among psychiatric patients: the HCR-20 violence risk assessment scheme and the Psychopathy Checklist: Screening Version. *Journal of Consulting and Clinical Psychology*, **67**, 917–930.

Douglas, K.S., Webster, C.D., Hart, S.D., *et al* (eds) (2001) *HCR-20: Violence Risk Management Companion Guide*. Mental Health, Law, and Policy Institute, Simon Fraser University, and Department of Mental Health Law and Policy, University of South Florida.

Elbogen, E.B. & Johnson, S.C. (2009) The intricate link between violence and mental disorder results from the national epidemiologic survey on alcohol and related conditions. *Archives of General Psychiatry*, **66**, 151–161.

Fazel, S., Gulati, G., Linsell, L., *et al* (2009) Schizophrenia and violence: systematic review and meta-analysis. *PLoS Medicine*, **6**, e1000120.

Fazel, S., Singh, J.P., Grann, M., *et al* (2012) Use of risk assessment instruments to predict violence and antisocial behaviour in 73 samples involving 24 827 people: systematic review and meta-analysis. *BMJ*, **345**, e4692.

Forth, A.E., Kosson, D.S. & Hare, R.D. (2003) *Hare Psychopathy Checklist: Youth Version (PCL:YV)*. Multi-Health Systems.

Fujii, D.E.M., Tokioka, A.B., Lichton, A.I., *et al* (2005) Ethnic differences in prediction of violence risk with the HCR-20 among psychiatric inpatients. *Psychiatric Services*, **56**, 711–716.

General Medical Council (2009) *Confidentiality: Guidance for Doctors*. GMC.

Gray, N.S., Fitzgerald, S., Taylor, J., *et al* (2007) Predicting future reconviction in offenders with intellectual disabilities: the predictive efficacy of VRAG, PCL-SV, and the HCR-20. *Psychological Assessment*, **19**, 474–479.

Gray, N.S., Benson, R., Craig, R., *et al* (2011a) The Short-Term Assessment of Risk and Treatability (START): a prospective study of inpatient behavior. *International Journal of Forensic Mental Health*, **10**, 305–313.

Gray, N.S., Taylor, J. & Snowden, R.J. (2011b) Predicting violence using structured professional judgment in patients with different mental and behavioral disorders. *Psychiatry Research*, **187**, 248–253.

Grove, W.M. & Meehl, P.E. (1996) Comparative efficiency of informal (subjective, impressionistic) and formal (mechanical, algorithmic) prediction procedures: the clinical-statistical controversy. *Psychology, Public Policy, and Law*, **2**, 293–323.

Haim, R., Rabinowitz, J., Lereya, J., *et al* (2002) Predictions made by psychiatrists and psychiatric nurses of violence by patients. *Psychiatric Services*, **53**, 622–624.

Hanson, R.K. & Harris, A.J.R. (2001) A structured approach to evaluating change among sexual offenders. *Sexual Abuse*, **13**, 105–122.

Harriss, L. & Hawton, K. (2005) Suicidal intent in deliberate self-harm and the risk of suicide: the predictive power of the Suicide Intent Scale. *Journal of Affective Disorders*, **86**, 225–233.

Hart, S.D. (1998) Psychopathy and risk for violence. In *Psychopathy: Theory, Research and Implications for Society* (eds D.J. Cooke, A.E. Forth, & R.D. Hare), pp. 355–373. Kluwer Academic Publishers.

Hart, C., Colley, R. & Harrison, A. (2005) Using a risk assessment matrix. *Emergency Nurse*, **12**, 21–28.

Hart, S.D. (2001) Assessing and managing violence risk. In *HCR-20 Violence Risk Management Companion Guide* (eds K.S. Douglas, C.D. Webster, S.D. Hart, *et al*), pp. 13–25. Mental Health, Law, and Policy Institute, Simon Fraser University, and Department of Mental Health Law and Policy, Florida Mental Health Institute, University of South Florida.

Hart, S.D., Cox, D.N. & Hare, R.D. (1995) *The Hare Psychopathy Checklist: Screening Version (PCL:SV)*. Multi-Health Systems.

Hart, S.D., Kropp, R., Laws, D.R., *et al* (2003) *The Risk for Sexual Violence Protocol (RSVP) – Structured Professional Guideline for Assessing Risk of Sexual Violence*. Simon Fraser University, Mental Health, Law and Policy Institute.

Hawton, K. & van Heeringen, K. (2009) Suicide. *Lancet*, **373**, 1372–1381.

Haynes, S.N. & Lench, H.C. (2003) Incremental validity of new clinical assessment measures. *Psychological Assessment*, **15**, 456–466.

Johnson, J.G., Cohen, P., Smailes, E., *et al* (2000) Adolescent personality disorders associated with violence and criminal behavior during adolescence and early adulthood. *American Journal of Psychiatry*, **157**, 1406–1412.

Kropp, P.R., Hart, S.D., Webster, C.D., *et al* (1999) *Manual for the Spousal Assault Risk Assessment Guide, 3rd edn*. Multi-Health Systems.

Langton, C.M., Hogue, T.E., Daffern, M., *et al* (2009) Prediction of institutional aggression among personality disordered forensic patients using actuarial and structured clinical risk assessment tools: Prospective evaluation of the HCR-20, VRS, Static-99, and Risk Matrix 2000. *Psychology, Crime and Law*, **15**, 635–659.

Lewis, C.F., Fields, C. & Rainey, E. (2006) A study of geriatric forensic evaluees: who are the violent elderly? *Journal of the American Academy of Psychiatry and Law*, **34**, 324–332.

Links, P.S., Gould, B. & Ratnayake, R. (2003) Assessing suicidal youth with antisocial, borderline or narcissistic personality disorder. *Canadian Journal of Psychiatry*, **48**, 301–310.

McDermott, B.E., Edens, J.F., Quanbeck, C.D., *et al* (2008a) Examining the role of static and dynamic risk factors in the prediction of inpatient violence: variable- and person-focused analyses. *Law and Human Behaviour*, **32**, 325–338.

McDermott, B.E., Quanbeck, C.D., Busse, D., *et al* (2008b) The accuracy of risk assessment instruments in the prediction of impulsive versus predatory aggression. *Behavioral Sciences and the Law*, **26**, 759–777.

Monahan, J. & Steadman, H.J. (1996) Violent storms and violent people: how meteorology can inform risk communication in mental health. *American Psychologist*, **51**, 931–938.

Monahan, J., Steadman, H.J., Silver, F., *et al* (2001) *Rethinking Risk Assessment: The MacArthur Study of Mental Disorder and Violence*. Oxford University Press.

Morrissey, C., Hogue, T., Mooney, P., *et al* (2007) Predictive validity of the PCL-R in offenders with intellectual disability in a high secure hospital setting: Institutional aggression. *Journal of Forensic Psychiatry and Psychology*, **18**, 1–15.

Mossman, D. (1994) Assessing predictions of violence: being accurate about accuracy. *Journal of Consulting and Clinical Psychology*, **62**, 783–792.

Murphy, A. (1991) Probabilities, odds and forecasts of rare events. *Weather and Forecasting*, **6**, 302–307.

National Confidential Inquiry into Suicide and Homicide by People with Mental Illness (2012) *Annual Report: England and Wales*. University of Manchester (http://www.bbmh. manchester.ac.uk/cmhr/research/centreforsuicideprevention/nci/reports/annual_report_2012.pdf)

Nicholls, T.L., Ogloff, J.R.P. & Douglas, K.S. (2004) Assessing risk for violence among male and female civil psychiatric patients: the HCR-20. PCL:SV and VSC. *Behavioral Sciences and the Law*, **22**, 127–158.

Nicholls, T.L., Brink, J., Desmarais, S.L., *et al* (2006) The Short-Term Assessment of Risk and Treatability (START): a prospective validation study in a forensic psychiatric sample. *Assessment*, **13**, 313–327.

Nicholls, T.L., Petersen, K.L., Brink, J., *et al* (2011) A clinical and risk profile of forensic psychiatric patients: treatment team STARTs in a Canadian service. *International Journal of Forensic Mental Health*, **10**, 187–199.

Nonstad, K., Nesset, M.B., Kroppan, E., *et al* (2010) Predictive validity and other psychometric properties of the Short-Term Assessment of Risk and Treatability (START) in a Norwegian high secure hospital. *International Journal of Forensic Mental Health*, **9**, 294–299.

O'Shea, L.E., Mitchell, A.E., Picchioni, M.M., *et al* (2012) Moderators of the predictive efficacy of the Historical, Clinical and Risk Management-20 for aggression in psychiatric facilities: systematic review and meta-analysis. *Aggression and Violent Behavior*, **18**, 255–70.

Patterson, W.M., Dohn, H.H., Bird, J., *et al* (1983) Evaluation of suicidal patients: the SAD PERSONS scale. *Psychosomatics: Journal of Consultation Liaison Psychiatry*, **24**, 343–349.

Quinsey, V.L., Harris, G.T., Rice, M.E., *et al* (1998) *Violent Offenders: Appraising and Managing Risk*. American Psychological Association.

Richards, L., Letchford, S. & Stratton, S. (2008) *Policing Domestic Violence*. Oxford University Press.

Rogers, R. (2000) The uncritical acceptance of risk assessment in forensic practice. *Law and Human Behavior*, **24**, 595–605.

Royal College of Psychiatrists (2001) *Diagnostic Criteria for learning disability (DC-LD)*. Gaskell.

Royal College of Psychiatrists (2008) *Rethinking Risk to Others in Mental Health Services*. Final Report of a Scoping Group (CR150). Royal College of Psychiatrists.

Singh, J.P., Grann, M. & Fazel, S. (2011) A comparative study of violence risk assessment tools: a systematic review and metaregression analysis of 68 studies involving 25,980 participants. *Clinical Psychology Review*, **31**, 499–513.

Skeem, J.L. & Mulvey, E.P. (2001) Psychopathy and community violence among civil psychiatric patients: results from the MacArthur Violence Risk Assessment Study. *Journal of Consulting & Clinical Psychology*, **69**, 358–374.

Steadman, H., Mulvey, E., Monahan, J., *et al* (1998) Violence by people discharged from acute psychiatric inpatient facilities and by others in the same neighborhoods. *Archives of General Psychiatry*, **55**, 393–401.

Szmukler, G. (2003) Risk assessment: 'numbers' and 'values'. *Psychiatric Bulletin*, **27**, 205–207.

US Department of Health and Human Services Public Health Service (2001) *National Strategy for Suicide Prevention: Goals and Objectives for Action*. USDHHS (http://www.sprc.org/sites/sprc.org/files/library/nssp.pdf).

Webster, C.D., Douglas, K.S., Eaves, D., *et al* (1997) *HCR-20 Assessing Risk for Violence (Version 2)*. Mental Health, Law, and Policy Institute, Simon Fraser University.

Webster, C.D., Martin, M., Brink, J., *et al* (2004) *Short-Term Assessment of Risk and Treatability (START)*. St. Joseph's Healthcare Hamilton, Ontario, and Forensic Psychiatric Services Commission.

Webster, C.D., Martin, M., Brink, J., *et al* (2009) *Manual for the Short-Term Assessment of Risk and Treatability (START) (Version 1.1)*. British Columbia Mental Health & Addiction Services.

Wilson, C.M., Desmarais, S.L., Nicholls, T. L., *et al* (2010) The role of client strengths in assessments of violence risk using the Short-Term Assessment of Risk and Treatability (START). *International Journal of Forensic Mental Health*, **9**, 282–293.

Worling, J.R. & Curwen, T. (2001) *The 'ERASOR': Estimate of Risk of Adolescent Sexual Offence Recidivism (Version 2.0)*. Safe-T Program, Thistletown Regional Centre.

Yang, M., Wong, S.C.P. & Coid, J. (2010) The efficacy of violence prediction: a meta-analytic comparison of nine risk assessment tools. *Psychological Bulletin*, **136**, 740.

Tarasoff v. Regents of the University of California, 17 Cal. 3d 425, 551 P.2d 334, 131 Cal. Rptr. 14 (Cal. 1976).

CHAPTER 4

Risk management in secure care

Geoffrey Dickens, Ashimesh Roychowdhury, Muthusamy
Natarajan

Introduction

Risk management is central to clinical practice in secure settings and
should be determined by informed risk assessment. In the previous chapter
we identified that risk assessment should use the information gathered to
anticipate and plan for likely scenarios where the individual's risk might
be heightened. The subsequent development of risk management strategies
from that process is integral to, and is in many respects the most important
result of, that process. Risk management has both shorter- and longer-term
objectives. The immediate aim is to manage the patient on a day-to-day
basis, ensuring their safety and that of others. This should be supplemented
by the implementation of strategies to reduce risk over the longer term,
and to ameliorate and minimise the effects of risk behaviour when it
occurs. In the previous chapter we identified that structured professional
judgement (SPJ) involves a systematic approach to risk assessment (Box
4.1). Further, risk assessment is performed for a specific person, at a
particular time and for their own unique circumstances. In this chapter we
concentrate on risk management in the secure setting, where a considerable
proportion of the available risk management interventions are achieved by
the therapeutic application of security measures. We therefore provide an
overview of physical, procedural and relational security and discuss how
their proportionate use can ensure an appropriate level of security for the
individual. We describe approaches to the management of violence and
aggression in secure care, the management of suicidal and self-harming
behaviour and, briefly, a range of other risk behaviours relevant to the
secure setting.

Risk and security

In secure mental health settings the context for the safe delivery of care and
therapeutic interventions is, by definition, provided by the clinical security
arrangements. Importantly, security and therapy should be viewed as

> **Box 4.1** Six stages of structured professional judgement
>
> Step 1: Gather information
>
> Step 2: Consider presence and relevance of risk factors – historical, current, contextual, protective
>
> Step 3: Develop a risk formulation – motivators (drivers), (dis)inhibitors, destabilisers
>
> Step 4: Consider risk scenarios, e.g. repeat, escalation, twist
>
> Step 5: Develop risk management strategies
>
> Step 6: Summary of judgement
>
> Source: Hart *et al* (2003)

complementary rather than as mutually exclusive concepts (Kinsley, 1998). Security facilitates the delivery of therapy and simultaneously provides a mechanism to manage risk. It is, in itself, potentially therapeutic (Kennedy, 2002). Historically, the concept of security has encompassed different facets (Parker, 1985) but the contemporary view of security comprising physical, procedural and relational components dates to the Reed review of services for mentally disordered offenders (Department of Health & Home Office, 1992).

Physical security

This refers to the overt, visible security systems that are intended to prevent or deter unauthorised leave, including escape, and to prevent unauthorised ingress of people and/or contraband items. Most obviously, these are the perimeter fences or walls around a secure premise, but physical security also includes the designated entry and exit points through the secure perimeter. It includes internal structural elements such as the resilience of doors, windows and ceilings, and the types and amount of locks, alarms and CCTV cameras. Good design elements are incorporated into physical security measures to minimise risk, for example optimising lines of sight or toilets with integrated seats to reduce the risk of providing a hiding place for contraband items.

Procedural security

This describes the procedures within the physical environment that maintain security integrity. Procedural security includes the prohibition of items that could increase risk for violence, security breach, substance misuse or other unwanted behaviours. Commonly prohibited items include sharp implements, weapons, glass items, lighters/matches, alcohol, drugs and IT equipment including mobile phones, laptops and radio scanners. Additionally, procedural security encompasses the arrangements in place for searching patients, visitors and the environment for contraband items; the frequency and intensity of patient observations; and the supervision and restriction of visitors. The policies that are used to control access to potential weapons, for example counting cutlery in and out at mealtimes, or to control items that may be fashioned into weapons represent procedural security issues. Other issues include testing for illicit substances and procedures for supervising internal movement of patients. Sound physical and procedural security should provide the basis for a relatively relaxed social milieu within the unit (Kinsley, 1992).

Relational security

The concept of relational security has evolved considerably in recent years and refers to the detailed understanding of those who receive secure care, including their individual risk signals and behaviours, and to the possession of the skills required to prevent and manage violence and aggression (Collins & Davies, 2005). The UK Department of Health (2010*a*) guidance in *See Think Act: Your Guide to Relational Security* extends the concept further and describes relational security as comprising four components and eight sub-components, related to the team, the other patients, the inside world and the outside world (Table. 4.1). This provides a very comprehensive set of guidelines which define multiple, interconnected relational domains. Further, it suggests practical, proactive measures to promote therapeutic engagement and manage risk, for example by spending time with patients to discuss their personal risk triggers. Recent research (Tighe & Gudjonsson, 2012) suggests that the factors described in *See, Think, Act* comprise meaningful underlying constructs that are related to ward climate. Relational security is a wide-ranging concept and shares features with related concepts including therapeutic engagement, de-escalation and violence prevention strategies. Further, relational security encompasses concepts about appropriate staff–patient boundaries to promote a more therapeutic environment and reduce the risk of staff becoming, wittingly or unwittingly, involved in security breaches.

Security needs

In the UK, secure care is provided at levels of low, medium and high security. Patients are placed with regard to the severity and immediacy of the risk that they pose to the public, carers and themselves: high security is appropriate for those who pose a grave and immediate danger, medium security for those who display dangerous but less immediately risky behaviour, while low secure care is appropriate for those with disturbed behaviour (Department of Health, 2002, 2007; Rutherford & Duggan, 2007). The different security measures required at each level, largely

Table 4.1 Security domains and related risk considerations

Domain	Security considerations	Risk management plan considerations
Relational security: 'the knowledge and understanding staff have of a patient and of the environment, and the translation of that information into appropriate responses and care' (p. 5)	• Staff/patient ratio • Developing an understanding of risks using risk assessment tools • Regular meetings and discussions • Collecting intelligence (primarily in high security settings) (see also Table 4.2)	• Mental health information e.g. signs of relapse, level of monitoring • Risk information, e.g. SPJ tool completed, collection of risk data using an appropriate tool (e.g. Overt Aggression Scale) • Use of *See, Think, Act* principles (Table 4.2) • Safeguarding procedures • Support with establishing and maintaining relationships • Supporting diversity needs • Cognitive screening
Procedural security: 'the policies and procedures in place to maintain safety and security' (p. 5)	• Searches (person, e.g. rub-down searches, drug testing, and environmental, e.g. room or ward searches) • Contraband items • Procedures for visitor approval • Investigations • Policies and procedures to manage serious incidents • Routine monitoring of patient telephone calls and mail can only be done in high security	• Observations (nursing and physical health) • Procedural monitoring (e.g. regular checks dependent on risks including room searches, screening, pat-down search) and any special search or observation requirements • Behaviour management plan • Regular review of finances • Prevention and management of aggression and violence plan • Agreement of frequency of review in MDT setting, e.g. ward round
Physical security: 'the fences, locks, personal alarms and so on that keep people safe' (p. 5)	• Air lock (medium security) or dedicated entry point (low security) • Separate security facility which has an X-ray scanner and metal detector • High security has CCTV surveillance; other levels of security may have this • Staff have personal alarms in medium and high security; in low security a wall mounted or personal alarm system should be provided • Low secure standards specify a 3.2 m fence; medium secure standards specify a 5.2 m fence or building equivalent, and high security a 6 m high wall	• Needs for any special measures should be documented in the care plan, e.g. completion of perimeter checks, checking for tampering • Leave requirements should be fully documented, e.g. types of leave that can be taken, escorts and who can escort, vehicle used

MDT, multidisciplinary team; SPJ, structured professional judgement. Source of quotes: Department of Health (2010*a*).

Table 4.2 Elements of relational security

Key area	Subthemes	Good relational security practice
Team	Boundaries	• Full awareness of rules and policies related to security • Knowledge and application of interpersonal boundaries • Understanding of non-negotiable boundaries • Using appropriate flexibility • Consistency in decision-making • Knowledge and use of self-awareness • Clarity of communication
	Therapy	• Demonstration of caring and support • Setting a positive example • Show consideration and respect • Involve patients in planning own care • Encouraging and positive attitude • Managing transition and change
Other patients	Patient mix	• Understanding past histories of patients • Consideration how an individual patient can affect the whole ward risk profile • Being clear about the limits of the ward and team • Monitoring patient interactions • Being prepared to speak up about misgivings • Encouraging patients to speak up about misgivings • Being prepared to change the patient mix positively
	Patient dynamic	• Maintaining team efficacy • Detecting suspicious or unusual behaviour between patients • Monitoring for change in the patient dynamic • Provide patients with a safe space to report suspicious behaviour • Discussing patient dynamic at regular team meetings, including at handover
Inside world	Personal world	• Predicting and preparing for key 'trigger' events (anniversaries, events, people) • Offering regular time to talk to plan how to deal with trigger events • Knowing patients' histories and the associated risks • Staying alert and attentive to change • Don't over-pathologise patient's normal behaviour
	Physical environment	• Create opportunities for social engagement • Arrange environment to encourage observation and engagement • Encourage pride in the ward environment • Minimise noise and overcrowding • Be aware of ward areas that could be abused • Ensure access to fresh air

Table 4.2 *contd*

Key area	Subthemes	Good relational security practice
Outside world	Visitors	• Preparing for and supervising visits • Encouraging visits that are positive for the patient • Make visitors aware of rules and boundaries • Be aware of and prepared to act when visitors don't act in the interest of the patient • Ensure that physical and procedural security measures with visitors are applied consistently
	Outward connections	• Developing clear plans for leave • Being clear about non-negotiable rules and limits • Acting decisively if limits and rules are breached • Ensure consequences of unauthorised leave are understood • Awareness of changes in patient behaviour that may increase risk • Awareness of signs of increased risk

Source: Department of Health (2010*a*).

the physical and procedural security elements, are described in official documents, with some technical details restricted (Department of Health, 2002, 2007, 2010*b*). Some of the components of security are fixed and apply to all patients in a particular unit or ward. The most obvious examples include the height of the perimeter fence required or the intensity of the nurse/patient staffing ratio and the level of training required by staff in management of violence and aggression skills on a particular ward. Some elements are varied at individual patient level according to need and risk assessment, for example the level of monitoring of mail and telephone calls, access to the internet, the frequency and intensity of search procedures, and so on.

A decision on the overall level of security (low, medium or high) that a patient requires is made before admission and reviewed periodically as they progress through treatment. Certain types of risk, for example escape, could be minimised by subjecting every individual to the highest level of security. However, there is an ethical, practical and legal duty to ensure that risk management is proportionate and that patients are managed in the least restrictive environment possible (Department of Health, 1999). Inappropriately restrictive risk management may have the counterproductive effect of being disempowering, and precludes therapeutic risk-taking (Barker, 2012). The requirements of proportionate risk management translate into hierarchical levels of the physical and procedural elements of security, with more rigorous, risk-reducing measures found in higher secure settings. However, the relationship between security level and each security component is non-linear. For example, within a high secure setting there may be greater latitude for freedom of movement and independent living within the secure perimeter compared with lower secure placements precisely because the perimeter fence reduces risk of escape or absconsion. This means that, to an extent, security can be calibrated within each specific setting to meet the individual's own needs. For example, the amount of leave, and the conditions set on it, can be discussed and altered according to the assessed level of risk. Relational security, on the other hand, has a less obviously hierarchical structure and less easily translates into quantitative terms.

To restate, patients should be allocated to the appropriate level of security and, within that level of security, they should be managed according to their own level of assessed risk rather than to the level of the most risky individual patient. To help meet these demands, Collins & Davies (2005) developed the Secure Needs Assessment Profile (SNAP) to measure the security needs of individual patients. Comprising 22 items, each measuring one aspect of physical, procedural or relational security on a four-point, criterion-referenced Likert scale, the SNAP successfully distinguished patients believed to require high, medium and low security and those requiring open care. This suggested that particular groups of patients have security needs which map onto the security features of the three different security levels. An important consideration, of course, is that an actuarial score cannot reliably indicate the correct security placement for a patient; rather, it is their overall profile. For example, individual patients may have low security needs in many areas but presence of a specific 'trump' risk, such as high risk of absconding for a dangerous individual, in the absence of other security needs would contraindicate low secure care. Similarly, the Forensic Mental Health Services Managed Care Network (2005) drew on expert opinion to develop a matrix of security need with detailed advice about requirements at open, low/locked, medium and high security levels. This gives specific advice about design and construction, equipment, communications, restricted items, daily living items, access to money, valuables and belongings, people (visitors, child visitors and internal movement) and miscellaneous needs relating to need for detailed policies and required levels of contingency planning. Further, concrete recommendations about transfer between security levels are provided.

To summarise, security provides an important component of risk management that allows patients to be placed in an environment that best meets their overall level of security need and, within that security level, allows for appropriate variation proportionate to the risks posed.

Management of aggression and violence risk

Aggression and violence are problematic features of many mental health settings, though unsurprisingly more so in secure settings. Significantly higher rates of violence are reported in forensic in-patient settings (48% of patients and 4.1 events per patient) compared with acute in-patient settings (26% of patients and 0.7 events per patient) (Bowers *et al*, 2011). However, there is wide variation in incident rates across the range of security levels and specialist settings, for example higher rates in female wards and in those for people with an intellectual disability diagnosis (Uppal & McMurran, 2009; Dickens *et al*, 2013). The potential consequences of violence and aggression for victims are discussed in detail in Chapter 19, 'Psychological support following violent assault and trauma'.

The management of aggressive behaviour poses a significant challenge in secure services. Research in general adult acute psychiatry has found that the use of a structured risk assessment during the first days of treatment, and routinely throughout admission may in itself contribute to reducing incidents of aggression and reduce coercion, restraint and seclusion because risks are identified and management strategies implemented (Abderhalden *et al*, 2008; van de Sande *et al*, 2011). However, one study has shown that failing to provide healthcare workers with the resources necessary to prevent violence was associated with a failure to sustain the reductions in the longer term (Kling *et al*, 2011). Good management involves consistent application of relational security skills. Additionally, more formal observation of patients at risk of aggression may be instituted as a preventive measure. These may be calibrated according to the level of perceived risk from intermittent (e.g. every 15–30 minutes) to close observation within eyesight or within arm's length (National Institute for Health and Care Excellence (NICE), 2005).

Formal training in the prevention and management of aggression and violence is recommended for nursing staff who deal with potentially violent patients (National Institute for Mental Health in England (NIMHE), 2004). The interventions that can be employed fall into three broad categories: psychosocial, physical and pharmacological. Sometimes only one of these approaches is or can be adopted, but in reality good management will draw upon aspects of all three. Elements of each approach can be conceptualised as primary (actions taken before violence occurs), secondary (interventions to prevent imminent violence) and tertiary (minimising harm once violence has occurred) preventive interventions (Paterson *et al*, 2004). In the UK, NICE (2005) has issued guidance on the short-term management of disturbed and violent behaviour emphasising the value of prediction (e.g. risk assessment), prevention (e.g. using de-escalation techniques and observations, managing the environment to reduce stimulation) and interventions for continued management (e.g. rapid tranquillisation, seclusion, physical interventions).

Psychological and psychosocial interventions

De-escalation

Common law and professional guidance underscores the need for staff exposed to violent and aggressive behaviour to utilise verbal de-escalation as the first resort and whenever practicable (NICE, 2005). De-escalation is 'a gradual resolution of a potentially violent and/or aggressive situation through the use of verbal and physical expressions of empathy, alliance and non-confrontational limit setting that is based on respect' (Cowin *et al*, 2003: p. 66). More simply, de-escalation involves 'defusing' a situation or 'talking down' the agitated person with the intention of preventing aggression. De-escalation can be used as a primary or secondary intervention. There is, however, considerable variation in how de-escalation is operationally defined with a lack of consensus in the literature about the constituent components (Price & Baker, 2012). This may largely explain the absolute lack of evidence from randomised trials for any set of de-escalation techniques (Muralidharan & Fenton, 2006).

Despite the lack of trial evidence, de-escalation is intuitively an important intervention and one that nurses in particular have used for many years (Paterson *et al*, 1997). Thematic synthesis of qualitative studies (Price & Baker, 2012) suggests that the staff who are effective at de-escalation are open, honest, supportive, self-aware, coherent, non-judgemental and confident without being arrogant. They maintain personal control and convey calmness when faced with aggression. Effective de-escalators use a calm, gentle tone, tactful language and deploy humour sensitively. Engagement with the patient is the key, fostering mutual regard and removing the need for aggression. Rapport and dignity should be the targets. The timing of when to intervene can be important, as some studies indicate that unnecessary interventions can exacerbate problems (Lowe, 1992; Johnson & Hauser, 2001; Mackay *et al*, 2005; Delaney & Johnson, 2006; Johnson & Delaney, 2007). Note that effective de-escalation shares many features with effective relational security. Specific techniques include distraction, removing stimuli, including appropriate withdrawal from the situation, and adoption of a calm and controlled manner (Paterson *et al*, 1997; Muralidharan & Fenton, 2006). Interpersonal skills are especially important and include use of clear, calm, respectful language, the use of open-ended sentences, firmness and compassion, avoidance of challenges and provocation, and adoption of neutral expression and unthreatening posture (Cowin *et al*, 2003).

Psychological treatment programmes

Like other treatments, psychological interventions are intended to ameliorate harmful risk behaviours by acting on the deficits that are associated with them, while also aiming to increase the potency of protective factors. Psychological interventions include educational and cognitive–behavioural interventions to address criminogenic drivers. For example, antisocial attitudes, values and beliefs, lack of empathy, substance misuse and deficits in problem-solving skills are all highly correlated with criminal conduct, while recidivism is reduced when they are addressed in offender treatment programmes (Andrews *et al*, 2006). Promising results have been reported for similar programmes for mentally disordered offenders in secure hospitals (Tapp *et al*, 2009; Clarke *et al*, 2010; Cullen *et al*, 2012). It is well known that much of the increased risk for violence among people with mental disorder, and in particular psychosis, is related to substance misuse (Arsenault *et al*, 2000). For such patients psychological interventions can address substance misuse and psychiatric problems serially, in parallel or in an integrated manner. Unfortunately, the current evidence from a high-quality systematic review shows no advantage for any particular psychosocial dual-diagnosis intervention over treatment as usual across a range of outcomes (Cleary *et al*, 2008).

A more detailed account of psychological interventions in secure settings is provided in Chapter 14, 'Specialist psychological treatment programmes in secure mental healthcare'.

Physical interventions

Physical interventions are used to prevent imminent violence and to minimise the resulting harm when it does occur. They are also used in conjunction with pharmacological interventions (see below) to manage disturbed behaviour, including violence. Up to one third of patient assaults on care staff have no obvious, observable antecedent (Papadopoulos *et al*, 2012). This suggests that much, though not all, aggression can be detected and successfully de-escalated. Physical techniques, in the UK known as breakaway techniques, include skills to help a potential assault victim prevent an assault, by for example blocking a punch or kick, or escaping during a violent episode. While these techniques are widely taught to staff, they are poorly retained and of limited effectiveness (Wright *et al*, 2005; Rogers *et al*, 2006; Dickens *et al*, 2009, 2012). More coercive physical techniques involve restraint and seclusion, although again there is little high-quality trial evidence that demonstrates their effectiveness compared with alternatives (Sailas & Fenton, 2000). Despite this, they are commonly used in medium and high secure settings where 67% and 76% respectively of all aggressive incidents resulted in restraint (Larkin *et al*, 1988; Gudjonsson *et al*, 2000). While training is recommended for staff working with aggressive patients, including training in manual restraint (National Institute for Mental Health in England, 2004), most evaluation measures post-training increases in staff confidence but does not report on how this translates into practice (Stewart *et al*, 2009). A range of techniques are used involving restraining holds, for example wrist locks and restraining the patient on the floor in the prone position (Lancaster *et al*, 2008). The latter has been criticised as it has been implicated in 12 patient deaths between 1979 and 2000 (Paterson *et al*, 2003). NIMHE guidance (2004) now recommends it be used only in exceptional circumstances.

Seclusion involves the physical isolation of the patient within a designated fit-for-purpose room that is sufficiently robust to withstand damage. The purpose is to manage disturbed behaviour while avoiding prolonged manual restraint. NICE (2005) guidelines stipulate that the patient should be observed at all times and that the seclusion should be for the shortest time possible. Seclusion is used more frequently on psychiatric patients in the UK than in other European countries (Raboch *et al*, 2010), but other coercive measures are used more commonly outside the UK. Examples include mechanical restraint involving devices such as belts, harnesses, manacles, sheets and straps (Tanaghow, 2006), and a net bed, which is a lockable metal frame with side netting bolted to a bed (Tavcar *et al*, 2005).

Pharmacological interventions

The pharmacological management of aggression and violence, both as prophylaxis and in the acute setting, is reviewed in detail in Chapter 16, 'Prescribing for specialist populations'. In brief, there is some evidence for the use of medicines to manage aggression and violence; the strongest is for clozapine in schizophrenia (Frogley *et al*, 2012). The mechanism may be linked to its antipsychotic properties but also to reduced substance misuse and impulsivity, increased monitoring, and better surveillance compliance (Volavka & Citrome, 2008). There is also some evidence for the use of mood stabilisers such as valproate and carbamazepine, though the evidence is inconsistent (Jones *et al*, 2011).

Patient involvement and preference

NICE (2005) guidelines recommend that patients make advance directives about their personal preference for interventions when disturbed or violent. Whittington *et al* (2009) have found in acute psychiatric care that patients disapprove more of the net bed, mechanical and pharmacological restraint than of locked doors, seclusion and physical restraint. Haw *et al* (2011) found that just over half of patients thought they should be subjected to coercive treatment if necessary, and most preferred intramuscular injection to seclusion. The researchers concluded that patients' views on coercive treatments should be incorporated into their care plans with advance statements.

Management of suicide and self-harm risk

Admission to a secure hospital may be warranted for other risks, for example suicide or absconding, in addition to the risk of violence to others (Barraclough & Clare Harris, 2002). The National Confidential Inquiry into Suicide and Homicide by People with Mental Illness (2014) reported that the suicide rate in the UK was 9.4 per 100000: the highest rate was in males aged 35–44 years. There were 1360 in-patient suicides between 2002 and 2012 in England and Wales (average 136 per year, but on a decreasing trajectory). The risk of suicide was greatest in the first 7 days after discharge from hospital, while on authorised leave, when absconded, immediately after admission or, in the case of prison transfers, while waiting for transfer.

In 2011, of those who had died by suicide by hanging (14 individuals), 11 had used doors or a window as a ligature point and 6 had used sheets or towels. Self-harm (intentional, non-lethal self-harm) in secure units is common, accounting for about a third of all incidents in a high secure hospital (Uppal & McMurran, 2009).

Physical and procedural security can be used to manage risk of suicide and self-harm, chiefly to prevent access to the means (Mann *et al*, 2005; Gunnell & Miller, 2010) and to ensure an appropriate level of observation. Interventions to lower the risk include treatment of any underlying mental disorder and destabilising factors such as substance misuse and personality disorder. Staff need to be aware of a variety of psychosocial factors that can operate at the ward level, including bullying and targeting of vulnerable individuals. Management strategies will include the appropriate use of non-rip clothing, linen and bedding.

Other risks in secure care

Absconding and escape

'Escape' involves the breach of the physical security of the building and/or procedures, for example by scaling a perimeter fence. 'Absconding' occurs when a patient breaks away from custody/supervision while on escorted leave, while 'failure to return' involves a patient not returning from an authorised period of leave (Department of Health, 2009). Absconding and failure to return reflect deficits in relational and procedural security. The concern is that the individual could reoffend following an escape or absconding; although suicide, neglect and vulnerability are other risks (Hunt *et al*, 2010). There were 19 escapes from the three English high secure hospitals between 1976 and 1994 (Huws & Shubsachs, 1993; Moore, 2000) and a very low absconding rate from rehabilitation trips (Brook *et al*, 1999), but reliable figures for medium security are not available. Across patient groups in secure care, adolescents were most likely to abscond (Dickens & Campbell, 2001). The assessment of the risk of escape or absconding should begin before admission and be continually updated throughout the in-patient stay, and it should inform the decision about the level of security an individual requires. Points to consider include history of absconding or escape and the means used. Factors that may be relevant include acquaintances, evidence of money being saved or found on a person prior to leave, recent bad news, for example an adverse mental health tribunal hearing, mental state and behaviour deterioration, asylum and immigration status. The National Patient Safety Agency has indicated that escapes from within the secure perimeter of medium or high secure mental health services should be a 'never event' (Department of Health, 2011). Innovations such as GPS tracking tags (Shaw, 2010) have recently been introduced into some secure services to allow staff to track patients' whereabouts if leave conditions are violated. This may facilitate therapeutic risk-taking, but at present, while there is some promising evidence among offenders (Sapouna *et al*, 2011), the measure has not been subject to evaluation among mentally disordered offenders.

Hostage-taking

Hostage-taking is the unlawful detention of an individual against their will; in English statute this is the criminal offence of kidnapping (Alexander & Klein, 2010). There are very few reliable figures for incidents of hostage-taking within secure care but it appears to be a rare event – there were no reported incidents either in a high secure (Uppal & McMurran, 2009) or in low and medium secure setting (Dickens *et al*, 2013). Hostage-taking may represent an expression of a particular grievance or an instrumental means of effecting a change in circumstances, for example to facilitate an escape. Individuals with mental illness may take a hostage in response to changes in their mental state. Resolution of hostage-taking is a complex issue that depends on a number of environmental factors and knowledge of the hostage taker. Particular methods employed may include rescue by force and negotiation (utilising appropriate prevention and management of aggression and violence skills). In the UK, negotiating the release of a hostage is the responsibility of the police.

Substance misuse

As described in this chapter, substance misuse increases risk for violence, but over the longer term it may be amenable to psychological intervention. Other management strategies within the secure setting include physical and procedural measures to minimise the risk of illicit substances entering the premises. This may include searches, but also more targeted and effective interventions such as saliva or hair testing (Kintz *et al*, 2006), or the use of sniffer dogs (Khalifa *et al*, 2008). Secure care may represent an opportunity to detoxify and stabilise a patient who has been dependent on substances in the past.

Victimisation

Patient-on-patient victimisation undoubtedly occurs in secure settings, although reliable data are difficult to locate. This may reflect challenges of definitions which emphasise either covert/relational or overt/physical intimidation aspects of victimisation, and the inherent difficulties in obtaining accurate reports of covert patient-on-patient aggression. Ireland (2004, 2006) studied bullying in a high security setting and reported that a quarter of patient and staff respondents had seen patient-on-patient bullying within the past week, including instances of theft, verbal abuse, physical assault, intimidation or making another patient do chores.

Boundary violations

Like victimisation, boundary violation represents a potential hazard to both the patient and the therapeutic environment; however, in this instance the agent generating, or complicit in, the hazard are members of the clinical team rather than fellow patients. Serious boundary violations include inappropriate intimate sexual relationships between a member of staff and a patient. It may be that the sexual boundary violation is predicated on the differential power relationship between clinician and patient (Sarkar, 2004). However, there are instances where the staff member honestly believes that the relationship is predicated on a romantic footing and involves both partners as equals (Peternelj-Taylor, 2013). Relatively little is known about the prevalence of these serious violations specifically in secure settings. Self-report studies of psychiatrists in the USA indicate that 2–6% have a history of sexual involvement with patients (Gartrell *et al*, 1986; Quadrio, 1996) and an average 10 psychiatrists per year are expelled by the American Psychiatric Association for sexual misconduct with a patient (Sarkar, 2004). Interestingly, there is some suggestion that sexual boundary violations in secure settings are as likely to involve female staff as males (Garrett & Davis, 1998).

Forensic and secure psychiatric in-patients can be particularly vulnerable to sexual boundary violations because they have a frequent history of abuse; this can be compounded by disempowerment within the hospital system and by physical distance from their support systems. Further, given the nature of the population, there could be a tendency for management to dismiss allegations. Recent scandals involving abuse of patients by care staff at Winterbourne View (Department of Health, 2012) and potential historical abuse of patients at Broadmoor Hospital by the celebrity Jimmy Savile (West London Mental Health NHS Trust, 2014) have highlighted the potential for actual abuse by those placed in positions of trust. It is to be sincerely hoped that the emergence of these cases results in greater, and more intelligent, vigilance to ensure they do not reoccur. We note, however, the lesson from history is that the cycle of evolution in secure care is interspersed with episodes of decline sometimes associated with abuse of power (Chapter 1, 'The evolution of secure and forensic mental healthcare').

Less obviously serious, non-sexual, boundary violations include inappropriate self-disclosure, excessive advocacy for, or criticism of, individual patients, inappropriate physical touch, inappropriate emotional involvement, involvement in bartering or other financial transactions with patients, and lying to patients or lying to colleagues about a patient (Bartlett & McGauley, 2009). All may be considered clear transgressions of relational security, specifically of the boundaries subtheme of the 'team' domain (Table 4.2). Although vigilance is required, every attempt should be made to ensure that there is room for flexibility in individual relationships with patients. Prevention of boundary violations requires a clear education and training for all staff who are to have clinical contact with patients in secure settings; this may be particularly important for non-registered staff, including healthcare assistants who may not have worked in a mental health setting previously. Educational programmes should emphasise the need for self-awareness, for example being honest about one's own feelings and spotting warning signs such as discussing personal problems with patients, keeping secrets and bending rules, believing only yourself can help an individual patient, flirting or enaging in sexual banter (Peternelj-Taylor, 2013). Simultaneoulsy, senior managers with secure care organisations need to nurture a supportive working environment, provide clinical supervision, investigate alleged violations promptly, thoroughly and fairly, and faciliate continuing professional development.

Conclusions

In conclusion, common risks in secure settings include aggression and violence, self-harm, absconding and escape, substance misuse and vulnerability. The main mechanisms that are available for managing these risks in the secure environment involve physical, procedural and relational security. Effective implementation of security should aid day-to-day management and facilitate the delivery of psychological, psychosocial, pharmacological and other interventions aimed at reducing risk in the medium to longer term. Physical and procedural security should be carefully calibrated according to the assessed level of risk for an individual; there should be detailed consideration of the nature of presenting risk, and the scenarios in which risk is most likely to be heightened. Although physical and procedural security are important considerations, it is relational security that provides the opportunity for information-gathering to inform management and for interventions to reduce risk within the context of the ward milieu.

References

Abderhalden, C., Needham, I., Dassen, T., *et al* (2008) Structured risk assessment and violence in acute psychiatric wards: randomised controlled trial. *British Journal of Psychiatry*, **193**, 44–50.

Alexander, D.A. & Klein, S. (2010) Hostage-taking: motives, resolution, coping and effects. *Advances in Psychiatric Treatment*, **16**, 176–183.

Andrews, D.A., Bonta, J., & Stephen Wormith, J. (2006) The recent past and near future of risk and/or need assessment. *Crime and Delinquency*, **52**, 7–27.

Arsenault, L., Moffitt, T.E., Caspi, A., *et al* (2000) Mental disorders and violence in a total birth cohort: results from the Dunedin study. *Archives of General Psychiatry*, **57**, 979–986.

Barker, R. (2012) Recovery and risk: accepting the complexity. In *Secure Recovery: Approaches to Recovery in Forensic Mental Health Settings* (eds G. Drennan & D. Alred). Routledge.

Barraclough, B.M. & Clare Harris, E. (2002) Suicide preceded by murder: the epidemiology of homicide-suicide in England and Wales 1988–92. *Psychological Medicine*, **32**, 577–584.

Bartlett, A. & McGauley, G. (2009) *Forensic Mental Health: Concepts, Systems, and Practice.* Oxford University Press.

Bowers, L., Stewart, D., Papadopoulos, C., *et al* (2011) *Inpatient Violence and Aggression: A Literature Review. Report from the Conflict and Containment Reduction Research Programme.* King's College London (http://www.kcl.ac.uk/iop/depts/hspr/research/ciemh/mhn/projects/litreview/LitRevAgg.pdf).

Brook, R., Dolan, M. & Coorey, P. (1999) Absconding of patients detained in an English special hospital. *Journal of Forensic Psychiatry*, **10**, 46-58.

Clarke, A.Y., Cullen, A.E., Walwyn, R., *et al* (2010) A quasi-experimental pilot study of the Reasoning and Rehabilitation programme with mentally disordered offenders. *Journal of Forensic Psychiatry and Psychology*, **21**, 490–500.

Cleary, M., Hunt, G.E., Matheson, S.L., *et al* (2008) Psychosocial treatment programmes for people with both severe mental illness and substance misuse. *Cochrane Database of Systematic Reviews*, **1**, doi: 10.1002/14651858.CD001088.pub2

Collins, M. & Davies, S. (2005) The Security Needs Assessment Profile: a multidimensional approach to measuring security needs. *International Journal of Forensic Mental Health*, **4**, 39–52.

Cowin, L., Davies, R., Estall, G., *et al* (2003) De-escalating aggression and violence in the mental health setting. *International Journal of Mental Health Nursing*, **12**, 64–73.

Cullen, A.E., Clarke, A.Y., Kuipers, E., *et al* (2012) A multisite randomized trial of a cognitive skills program for male mentally disordered offenders: violence and antisocial behavior outcomes. *Journal of Consulting and Clinical Psychology*, 80, 1114–1120.

Delaney, K. R. & Johnson, M.E. (2006) Keeping the unit safe: mapping psychiatric nursing skills. *Journal of the American Psychiatric Nurses Association*, **12**, 1–10.

Department of Health (1999) *National Service Framework for Mental Health.* Department of Health.

Department of Health (2002) *Mental Health Policy Implementation Guide: National Minimum Standards for General Adult Services in Psychiatric Intensive Care Units (PICU) and Low Secure Environments.* Department of Health.

Department of Health (2007) *Best Practice Guidance: Specification for Adult Medium-secure Services.* Department of Health.

Department of Health (2009) *Absent without Leave: Definitions of Escape and Abscond.* Department of Health.

Department of Health (2010a) *See, Think, Act: Your Guide to Relational Security.* Department of Health.

Department of Health (2010b) *High Secure Building Design Guide: Overarching Principles for Ashworth, Broadmoor, Rampton Hospitals.* Department of Health.

Department of Health (2011) *The 'Never Events' List 2011/12: Policy Framework for Use in the NHS.* Department of Health.

Department of Health (2012) *Transforming Care: A National Response to Winterbourne View Hospital, Final Report.* Department of Health.

Department of Health & Home Office (1992) *Review of Health and Social Services for Mentally Disordered Offenders and Others Requiring Similar Services, Final Summary Report (Cm 2088).* HMSO.

Dickens, G. & Campbell, J. (2001) Absconding of patients from an independent UK psychiatric hospital: a 3-year retrospective analysis of events and characteristics of absconders. *Journal of Psychiatric and Mental Health Nursing*, **8**, 543–550.

Dickens, G., Rogers, G., Rooney, C., *et al* (2009) An audit of the use of breakaway techniques in a large psychiatric hospital: a replication study. *Journal of Psychiatric and Mental Health Nursing*, **16**, 777–783.

Dickens, G., Rooney, C. & Doyle, D. (2012) Breakaways in specialist secure psychiatry. *Journal of Psychiatric and Mental Health Nursing*, **19**, 281–284.

Dickens, G., Picchioni, M. & Long, C. (2013) Aggression in specialist secure and forensic inpatient mental health care: incidence across care pathways. *British Journal of Forensic Practice*, **15**, 206–217.

Forensic Mental Health Services Managed Care Network (2005) *Definition of Security Levels in Psychiatric Inpatient Facilities in Scotland*. FMHSMCN (http://www.forensicnetwork. scot.nhs.uk/documents/hdl/LevelsofSecurityReport.pdf).

Frogley, C., Taylor, D., Dickens, G., *et al* (2012) A systematic review of clozapine's anti-aggressive effects. *International Journal of Neuropsychopharmacology*, **15**, 1351–1371.

Garrett, T. & Davis, J. (1998) The prevalence of sexual contact between British clinical psychologists and their patients. *Clinical Psychology and Psychotherapy*, **5**, 253–256.

Gartrell, N., Herman, J., Olarte, S., *et al* (1986) Psychiatrist–patient sexual contact: results of a national survey. I: Prevalence. *American Journal of Psychiatry*, **143**, 1126–1131.

Gudjonsson, G., Rabe-Hesketh, S. & Wilson, C. (2000) Violent incidents on a medium secure unit: the target of assault and the management of incidents. *Journal of Forensic Psychiatry*, **11**, 105–118.

Gunnell, D. & Miller, M. (2010) Strategies to prevent suicide. *BMJ*, **340**, c3054.

Hart, S.D., Kropp, R., Laws, D.R., *et al* (2003) *The Risk for Sexual Violence Protocol (RSVP) – Structured Professional Guideline for Assessing Risk of Sexual Violence*. Simon Fraser University, Mental Health, Law and Policy Institute.

Haw, C., Stubbs, J., Bickle, A., *et al* (2011) Coercive treatments in forensic psychiatry: a study of patients' experiences and preferences. *Journal of Forensic Psychiatry and Psychology*, **22**, 564–585.

Hunt, I.M., Windfuhr, K., Swinson, N., *et al* (2010) Suicide among psychiatric in-patients who abscond from the ward: a national clinical survey. *BMC Psychiatry*, **10**, 14.

Huws, R. & Shubsachs, A. (1993) A study of absconding by special hospital patients 1976–1988. *Journal of Forensic Psychiatry*, **4**, 45–48.

Ireland, J.L. (2004) Nature, extent, and causes of bullying among personality-disordered patients in a high-secure hospital. *Aggressive Behavior*, **30**, 229–242.

Ireland, J.L. (2006) Bullying among mentally-ill patients detained in a high-secure hospital: an exploratory study of the perceptions of staff and patients into how bullying is defined. *Aggressive Behavior*, **32**, 451–463.

Johnson, M. E. & Delaney, K.R. (2007) Keeping the unit safe: the anatomy of escalation. *Journal of the American Psychiatric Nurses Association*, **13**, 42–52.

Johnson, M.E. & Hauser, P.M. (2001) The practice of expert nurses: accompanying the patient to a calmer space. *Issues in Mental Health Nursing*, **22**, 651–668.

Jones, R.M., Arlidge, J., Gillham, R., *et al* (2011) Efficacy of mood stabilisers in the treatment of impulsive or repetitive aggression: systematic review and meta-analysis. *British Journal of Psychiatry*, **198**, 93–98.

Kennedy, H.G. (2002) Therapeutic uses of security: mapping forensic mental health services by stratifying risk. *Advances in Psychiatric Treatment*, **8**, 433–443.

Khalifa, N., Gibbon, S. & Duggan, C. (2008) Police and sniffer dogs in psychiatric settings. *Psychiatrist*, **32**, 253–256.

Kinsley, J. (1992) *Security in The Special Hospitals a Special Task*. Service and Hospitality Safety Association.

Kinsley, J. (1998) Security and therapy. In *Managing High Security Psychiatric Care* (eds C. Kaye & A. Franey), pp. 75–84. Jessica Kingsley.

Kintz, P., Villain, M. & Cirimele, V. (2006) Hair analysis for drug detection. *Therapeutic Drug Monitoring*, **28**, 442–446.

Kling, R.N., Yassi, A., Smailes, E., *et al* (2011) Evaluation of a violence risk assessment system (the ALERT system) for reducing violence in an acute hospital: a before and after study. *International Journal of Nursing Studies*, **48**, 534–539.

Lancaster, G.A., Whittington, R., Lane S., *et al* (2008) Does the position of restraint of disturbed psychiatric patients have any association with staff and patient injuries? *Journal of Psychiatric and Mental Health Nursing*, **15**, 306–312.

Larkin, E., Silvester, M. & Jones, S. (1988) A preliminary study of violent incidents in a special hospital (Rampton). *British Journal of Psychiatry*, **153**, 226–231.

Lowe, T. (1992) Characteristics of effective nursing interventions in the management of challenging behavior. *Journal of Advanced Nursing*, **17**, 1226–1232.

Mackay, I., Paterson, B. & Cassells, C. (2005) Constant or special observations of inpatients presenting a risk of aggression or violence: nurses' perceptions of the rules of engagement. *Journal of Psychiatric and Mental Health Nursing*, **12**, 464–471.

Mann J.J., Apter, A., Bertolete, J., *et al* (2005) Suicide prevention strategies: a systematic review. *Journal of the American Medical Association*, **294**, 2064–2074,

Moore, E. (2000) A descriptive analysis of incidents of absconding and escape from English high security hospitals 1989–1994. *Journal of Forensic Psychiatry*, **11**, 344–358.

Muralidharan, S. & Fenton, M. (2006) Containment strategies for people with serious mental illness. *Cochrane Database of Systematic Reviews*, **3**, doi: 10.1002/14651858.CD002084.pub2.

National Confidential Inquiry into Suicide and Homicide by People with Mental Illness (2014) *Annual Report: England, Northern Ireland, Scotland and Wales*. University of Manchester (http://www.bbmh.manchester.ac.uk/cmhr/centreforsuicideprevention/nci/reports/Annualreport2014.pdf).

National Institute for Health and Care Excellence (2005) *Violence: The Short-Term Management of Disturbed/Violent Behaviour in Inpatient Psychiatric Settings and Emergency Departments*. NICE.

National Institute for Mental Health in England (2004) *Mental Health Policy Implementation Guide: Developing Positive Practice to Support the Safe and Therapeutic Management of Aggression and Violence in Mental Health In-Patient Settings*. Department of Health.

Papadopoulos, C., Ross, J., Stewart, D., *et al* (2012) The antecedents of violence and aggression within psychiatric in-patient settings. *Acta Psychiatrica Scandinavica*, **125**, 425–439.

Parker, E. (1985) The development of secure provision. In *Secure Provision* (ed. L. Gostin), pp. 15–65. Tavistock.

Paterson, B., Leadbetter, D. & McComish, A. (1997) De-escalation in the management of aggression and violence. *Nursing Times*, **93**, 58–61.

Paterson, B., Bradley, P., Stark C., *et al* (2003) Deaths associated with restraint use in health and social care in the UK: the results of a preliminary survey. *Journal of Psychiatric and Mental Health Nursing*, **10**, 3–15.

Paterson, B., Leadbetter, D. & Miller, G. (2004) *Workplace Violence in Health and Social Care as an International Problem: A Public Health Perspective on the 'Total Organisational Response'*. Stirling University (http://www.nm.stir.ac.uk/documents/ld-integrated-response.pdf).

Peternelj-Taylor, C. (2013) Forbidden Love: Sexual Boundary Violations in Forensic Psychiatric Nursing. 1st Federal Conference on Forensic Psychiatric Nursing, 1–2 July, 2013 (http://www.fh-diakonie.de/obj/Bilder_und_Dokumente/Aktuelles/Forbidden-Love_Peternelj-Taylor_JournalofForensicNursing.pdf).

Price, O. & Baker, J. (2012) Key components of de-escalation techniques: a thematic synthesis. *International Journal of Mental Health Nursing*, **21**, 310–319.

Quadrio, C. (1996) Sexual abuse in therapy: gender issues. *Australian and New Zealand Journal of Psychiatry*, **30**, 125–133.

Raboch, J., Kalisova, L., Nawka, A., *et al* (2010) Use of coercive measures during involuntary hospitalization: findings from ten European countries. *Psychiatric Services*, **61**, 1012–1017.

Rogers P., Ghroum P., Benson R., *et al* (2006) Is breakaway training effective? An audit of one medium secure unit. *Journal of Forensic Psychiatry and Psychology*, **17**, 593–602.

Rutherford, M. & Duggan, S. (2007) *Forensic Mental Health Services: Facts and Figures on Current Provision*. Sainsbury Centre for Mental Health (http://www.centreformentalhealth.org.uk/pdfs/scmh_forensic_factfile_2007.pdf).

Sailas, E. & Fenton, M. (2000) Seclusion and restraint for people with serious mental illnesses. *Cochrane Database of Systematic Reviews*, **1**, doi: 10.1002/14651858.CD001163.

Sapouna, M., Bisset, C. & Conlong, A.M. (2011) *What Works to Reduce Reoffending: A Summary of the Evidence*. Justice Analytical Services, Scottish Government (http://www.huckfield.com/wp-content/uploads/2012/11/11-SG-What-Works-to-Reduce-Reoffending-Oct1.pdf).

Sarkar, S.P. (2004) Boundary violation and sexual exploitation in psychiatry and psychotherapy: a review. *Advances in Psychiatric Treatment*, **10**, 312–320.

Shaw, D. (2010) Satellites used to track mentally-ill violent criminals. *BBC News*, 25 August.

Stewart, D., Bowers, L., Simpson, A., *et al* (2009) Manual restraint of adult psychiatric inpatients: a literature review. *Journal of Psychiatric and Mental Health Nursing*, **16**, 749–757.

Tanaghow, A. (2006) *Mechanical Restraint: Chief Psychiatrist's Guideline*. Mental Health Branch, Metropolitan Health and Aged Care Services Division, Victorian Department of Human Services (http://www.health.vic.gov.au/mentalhealth/cpg/restraint.pdf).

Tapp, J., Fellowes, E., Wallis, N., *et al* (2009) An evaluation of the Enhanced Thinking Skills (ETS) programme with mentally disordered offenders in a high security hospital. *Legal and Criminological Psychology*, **14**, 201–212.

Tavcar, R., Dernovsek, M.Z. & Grubic, V.N. (2005) Use of coercive measures in a psychiatric intensive care unit in Slovenia. *Psychiatric Services*, **56**, 491–492.

Tighe, J. & Gudjonsson, G.T. (2012) See, Think, Act scale: preliminary development and validation of a measure of relational security in medium- and low-secure units. *Journal of Forensic Psychiatry and Psychology*, **23**, 184–199.

Uppal. G. & McMurran, M. (2009) Recorded incidents in a high-secure hospital: a descriptive analysis. *Criminal Behaviour and Mental Health*, **19**, 265–276.

van de Sande, R., Nijman, H.L.I, Noorthoorn, E.O., *et al* (2011) Aggression and seclusion on acute psychiatric wards: effect of short-term risk assessment. *British Journal of Psychiatry*, **199**, 473–478.

Volavka, J. & Citrome, L. (2008) Heterogeneity of violence in schizophrenia and implications for long-term treatment. *International Journal of Clinical Practice*, **62**, 1237–1245.

West London Mental Health NHS Trust (2014) *Jimmy Savile Investigation: Broadmoor Hospital*. Report to the West London Mental Health NHS Trust and the Department of Health. West London Mental Health NHS Trust.

Whittington, R., Bowers, L., Nolan, P., *et al* (2009) Approval ratings of inpatient coercive interventions in a national sample of mental health service users and staff in England. *Psychiatric Services*, **60**, 792–798.

Wright, S., Sayer, J., Parr, A.M., *et al* (2005) Breakaway and physical restraint techniques in acute psychiatric nursing. *Journal of Forensic Psychiatry and Psychology*, **16**, 380–398.

CHAPTER 5

Recovery in secure environments

Shawn Mitchell and Ian Callaghan

Introduction

The concept of recovery in mental health can be encapsulated by three words: hope, opportunity and control. Hope is essential in sustaining all people through times of difficulty. The opportunity to make friends, sustain relationships, to work and to partake in educational and recreational activities is key in helping people to develop a sense of personal identity. Being in control of matters that are significant in one's everyday life is psychologically important, as is maintaining one's self-control.

In the past decade, recovery has become the clinical model for the delivery of mental health services in the UK. Following from previous guidance such as *A Common Purpose: Recovery in Future Mental Health Services* (Care Services Improvement Partnership *et al*, 2007) and *Refocusing the Care Programme Approach* (Department of Health, 2008), which promoted recovery-oriented mental health services, the cross-government mental health outcomes strategy for England (*No Health without Mental Health*; HM Government, 2011) placed recovery-based practice at the centre of mental health service delivery. Recovery-oriented services have been further supported through *Implementing Recovery: A Methodology for Organisational Change*, a joint project between the NHS Confederation and the Centre for Mental Health, using the ten organisational challenges identified by the Centre for Mental Health (Shepherd *et al*, 2009).

In this chapter we examine what the concept of recovery means for users of secure mental health services. We discuss the barriers to recovery and identify how hope, opportunity and choice can be supported. We then examine how changes can be embedded at an organisational level to support patient recovery in secure settings on a personal level.

Recovery and mental health

There are a number of definitions of recovery; a comprehensive and commonly used one is:

'a deeply personal, unique process of changing one's attitudes, values, feelings, goals, skills and/or roles. It is a way of living a satisfying, hopeful and contributing life, even with limitations caused by illness. Recovery involves the development of new meaning and purpose in one's life' (Anthony, 1993).

The key differences between a conventional medical approach and a recovery-focused approach to mental health are summarised in Table 5.1. Although it can be argued that the concept of recovery in mental health is nothing new and that most mental health services could make a claim to recovery-based practice, the key to truly recovery-oriented services involves a fundamental shift from 'being done to' to 'doing with', summarised in the well-known statement 'no decision about me without me'.

In many areas of healthcare provision – notably, of services for long-term conditions – the model of service users as 'experts by experience' has become an accepted approach. In this respect, mental health conditions do not differ from other long-term conditions and therefore the goals of a recovery-oriented mental health service will be similar to those for services for other long-term conditions. The shared goals of the Department of Health (2012) *Draft Strategy for Long Term Conditions* are:

- people will be supported to stay healthy and avoid developing a long-term condition, where possible
- people will have their conditions diagnosed early and quickly
- services will be joined up, and based around individuals' biological, psychological and social needs
- people with long-term conditions will be socially included, including succeeding in work and education
- people with long-term conditions will be as independent as possible and in control of their lives (up to and including the end of life)
- people with long-term conditions will be supported to stay as well as possible.

Criticisms of recovery approaches are often focused on the lack of a theoretical or empirical evidence base (Stickley & Wright, 2011). A riposte to this is that there is little evidence for any specific model of delivery of mental health services. In the absence of such an evidence base the driving factors for recovery-focused practice become ethical and moral.

Mental health recovery in secure services

Secure services provide mental healthcare in conditions of low, medium and high security. Though they are sometimes referred to as forensic services, not all their patients have committed offences. Most are likely to be detained primarily due to the risks posed to others, but a small percentage of service users in low secure accommodation may be detained due to concerns about risks to themselves. In England and Wales, these services work with approximately 7000 patients at any one time, around 4000 in

Table 5.1 Differences between conventional approach to mental health and recovery-oriented services

	Conventional approach	Recovery approach
Basic concepts	Diagnosis	Personal meaning
	Pathology	Biography
	Psychopathology	Distressing experience
	Treatment	Growth and discovery
	Staff and patients	Experts by training and experts by experience
Working practices	Focus on disorder	Focus on person
	Illness based	Strengths based
	Based on reducing adverse events	Based on hopes and dreams
	Individual adapts to the programme	Provider adapts to the individual
	Rewards passivity and compliance	Fosters empowerment
	Expert care coordinators	Self-management
Goals of service	Anti-disease	Pro-health
	Bringing under control	Self-control
	Compliance	Choice
	Return to normal	Transformation

Adapted from Slade (2009*a*).

high and medium security and the remainder in low secure services (Pereira *et al*, 2006; Sainsbury Centre for Mental Health, 2007). Secure services have generally been reluctant to adopt the recovery model, the main reasons being, first, that recovery is often regarded as being incompatible with risk management, and second, that it does not address offending behaviour. To address this, Drennan & Alred (2012) use the term 'secure recovery' and define it as follows:

> 'Secure recovery acknowledges the challenges of recovery from mental illness and emotional difficulties that can lead to offending behaviour. It recognises that the careful management of risk is a necessary part of recovery in our service but this can happen alongside working towards the restoration of a meaningful, safe and satisfying life' (p. x).

In *Pathways to Unlocking Secure Mental Health*, the Centre for Mental Health (2011) argues that the recovery approach should be promoted across secure care settings and that training should be available to all staff.

Challenges to recovery in secure services

Effects of detention

Being detained can be a significant barrier to recovery. When detained, choice is limited over a range of aspects of daily life, including matters such as food, access to fresh air or autonomy to choose one's own bedtime. Likewise, opportunities to social activities, including employment, are restricted, and patients are largely excluded from society. All these factors, added to the longer length of stay in hospital that users of secure services experience compared with those without an offending history, can result in institutionalisation, which is arguably the antithesis of personal recovery. It is also possible that the restrictive nature of secure environments can inhibit the recovery process and individual patient's recovery journey, thereby potentially increasing risk. However, some would argue that detention under mental health legislation can create the potential for recovery that would not otherwise exist in community settings. Rather than being considered to have 'maximal choice', patients who are detained can be considered to have 'optimal choice' (Roberts et al, 2008).

One of the potential difficulties for patients in secure environments is that their behaviours, emotions and thoughts are constantly observed and recorded in detail by professionals and any variation may be viewed as pathological. Patients themselves may also be susceptible to such an interpretation and, therefore, an understanding or an appreciation of normal variation can be lost. This may restrict the patient's ability to be able to 'live with' their mental health difficulties and, instead, maintains the focus on symptom reduction, which for a number of patients is not always possible.

Employment following discharge for secure patients can be difficult. A follow-up study of patients who were admitted to medium secure services found that 51% of their sample had been in employment, mostly unskilled work, prior to admission, but after discharge the employment rate fell to 14.5% and work was usually found through family members (Davies et al, 2007).

Stigma

Stigma can be a significant disadvantage to mental health patients. Individuals who also have a history of offending behaviour are faced with an additional stigma which can result in negative effects on the person's sense of self. Some authors hold the view that meaning of hope and life following an offence is crucial to counter despair and chronic alienation (Hillbrand & Young, 2008). The journey to recovery for patients who require secure mental healthcare often commences from a more disadvantaged starting point. This can result in longer periods of institutionalisation and a consequent lack of opportunities.

It is known that violent behaviour occurs less in mentally disordered offenders than in other offender groups, and is much lower than in individuals with substance misuse problems (Slade, 2009b). However, where patients have been violent in the past they may fulfil the stereotype of the 'typical' violent mentally disordered person. This dual stigma could pose a challenge to professionals working with this group because they might find it easier to be accepting and supporting of patients' mental health problems than of their offending behaviour.

Recovery and risk

Risk and recovery have often been regarded as opposing concepts. In secure services 'risk' usually refers to behaviours that cause harm to others and that may be illegal; but the term may also refer to harm to self. Risk may refer to behaviours that potentially lead to relapse, such as not taking medication, which may in turn lead to other risky behaviours. At the time of their admission individuals often experience high levels of distress. This can result in risky behaviour which in turn leads to significant restrictions that are intended to manage the risk. This can lead to patients experiencing increased feelings of hopelessness and frustration, which in turn can cause an increase in risky behaviour. From this perspective the overemphasis on risk within secure services may exacerbate a vicious circle of risk behaviour and restriction. Some patients have expressed concern at the lack of attention to their wider social care needs, particularly when the focus has been on problems and risk, rather than building on their strengths towards recovery (Department of Health, 2006).

Supporting recovery in secure environments

Hope

Maintaining hope

Maintaining a sense of hope can be a challenge at times in secure settings, particularly at the time of admission, when the individual has typically been transferred from prison or another secure setting. The restrictions imposed by a secure setting can further engender these feelings of hopelessness. In such circumstances maintaining hope may initially be the responsibility of mental health professionals in the secure service. This can be difficult for staff, particularly when patients manifest their hopelessness in challenging behaviour. In such circumstances, to avoid staff reacting negatively to patients and thereby amplifying their feeling of hopelessness, staff support is key to ensuring that therapeutic relationships are maintained. Peer support workers, or peer 'buddies', can also play a vital role at the time of admission, holding hope for the recently admitted individual (Ashcraft & Anthony, 2008).

Instilling hope

A number of factors can contribute to the instillation of hope. Honesty is important and discussions engendering hope need to be realistic and balanced. Hope-supporting factors include:

- Processes that support identifying care pathways through secure services, thereby helping the patient to look to a future in conditions of lower security with a positive attitude.
- Maintaining therapeutic relationships is key to promoting recovery and maintaining hope. The care coordinator or key worker is the person with whom the patient has the most significant therapeutic relationship, therefore it is important that consideration is given as to who this person will be, and once identified, consistency needs to be ensured.
- Peer workers can play a valuable role, providing personal examples of what can be achieved and giving guidance as to how to achieve personal goals. Some patients may find being challenged by a peer worker more acceptable than by a staff member who does not have lived experience.
- Ironically, restriction orders, as used in England and Wales, can act as an external locus of control, leading to mental health workers and patients working collaboratively to achieve goals that would reassure the Ministry of Justice, resulting in the patient being able to move to a less restrictive environment.

Learning from negative experiences

To maintain hope it is important that responses to untoward events are proportionate and supportive, and avoid catastrophisation. At the same time responses should ensure that the patient's responsibility in the situation is clear, and that it can be viewed as a learning experience for both the patient and the supporting mental health workers. For mental health workers to feel confident in responding in such a manner there should be a supportive organisational culture that promotes learning rather than apportioning blame. This approach is supported by the document *Independence, Choice and Risk: A Guide to Best Practice in Supported Decision Making* (Department of Health, 2007), which states that the approach to risk that an organisation takes overwhelmingly influences the practice of the workforce, and that the most effective organisations are those with good systems in place to support positive approaches to risk rather than defensive ones.

Opportunity

The very nature of secure environments means that patients are excluded from local communities and community activities, thereby reducing their opportunities for social inclusion. The communal aspect of a secure service can be used to provide opportunities. All opportunities should be community based as far as is possible, taking into consideration any safety issues. When such activities cannot be accessed consideration needs to be given as to how social inclusion can be best achieved within the secure environment.

Social activities

Secure environments are often geographically centralised, thereby isolating patients from family and friends. Consideration needs to be given as to how best to support them in maintaining social contacts, providing environments within the secure environments for socialising, and encouraging local communities and services to organise activities for patients.

Recreation

Recreational activities can be provided in various areas within secure environments and can be further augmented by volunteers and recreational organisations delivering such activities. Recreational activities can enhance patients' experience of secure environments by providing opportunities in the evenings and weekends, which are often times when there is little structured activity.

Vocation and education

Finding employment can be even more difficult for mental health patients if they have been to prison or have an offending history. Secure services need to identify vocational opportunities that start within the secure environment, either volunteering opportunities or more formal work experience. Examples of this include patient-run canteens or shops and peer training. Peer mentoring or 'buddying' and involvement in patient representation or advocacy can provide valuable opportunities for individuals to draw on their lived experience. A number of secure services have education arranged by local colleges within the secure environment, which helps continuity when individuals are able to access community-based education.

Information technology

Information technology is increasingly used as a form of social communication, both through email and social networking websites. Mobile phone text messaging has also become an important means of communicating with friends and family. In addition, a number of educational activities are available through the internet, including Open University courses. Therefore, information technology can be used to increase patients' educational opportunities and social inclusion even while resident in secure environments with limited community access. Patient access to information technology needs to be risk assessed and environmental and procedural security needs to be reviewed to enable patients' safe use of mobile phones and computers.

Recovery education centre (REC)

Recovery education centres, as described in *Transforming from a Day Treatment to a Recovery Education Centre* (META Services, 2005), have been developed in the UK in places such as Nottingham and south-west London. RECs view therapy as education and therefore anxiety management or social confidence groups, traditionally viewed as psychological therapy, become part of a college curriculum. Education is viewed as transformative, facilitating users' identity shift from patient to student to citizen. The colleges are registered as educational facilities. In the USA, the Recovery Innovations Arizona REC offers a degree course in mental health recovery. Courses offered by recovery education centres are co-developed, co-delivered and co-attended by mental health services staff and patients. Patients can choose which courses to attend, thus changing the dynamic from being told which therapies they need to attend to one in which they identify their own goals in collaboration with the clinical team. In secure environments RECs can provide an opportunity for patients to have roles as contributors and co-facilitators. Co-attendance creates the opportunity for more socially inclusive activities within the secure environment, with both staff and patients being students within the college session. In secure services, restrictions on patients leaving the secure environment can present some barriers to full participation in all aspects of the REC. Where this is the case, consideration needs to be given to how to deliver courses within the secure setting.

All training, where possible and appropriate, should be co-developed, co-delivered and co-attended by patients and staff. While RECs are still a relatively new concept and have not been universally adopted, a recovery approach can be taken to all training. Staff training events which would benefit patients, or which would benefit from patient input in development and delivery, should be identified. This can have a number of benefits, including cost efficiency and providing an opportunity for staff and patients to be in a situation in which they have different roles.

Control

Responsibility

A lack of insight into and/or a lack of acceptance of past risk behaviours can often be a hindrance, preventing patients owning responsibility for their own safety. This can impede their recovery. For some patients who have experienced mental health difficulties from a young age, the process of learning to take responsibility can be considered a 'growing up' or maturational process. Growing up involves accepting the past, rather than just participating in therapeutic activities, and thereby developing a sense of responsibility. Secure services need to be aware of this and provide patients with increasing opportunities to be responsible, while also learning from their own mistakes.

Choice

Having a choice as to which therapeutic groups or activities to undertake can enhance motivation compared with a more traditional manner of secure service delivery in which patients are directed to undertake specific interventions. Recovery education colleges can provide the means of achieving this.

Approaches to safety and risk: a recovery perspective

In the Department of Health (2006) consultation document *Reviewing the Care Programme Approach*, mental health patients expressed their concern at the lack of attention to their wider social care needs, with the focus being on problems and risks rather than building on their strengths towards recovery. From our experience, many patients hold the opinion that the term 'risk' has negative connotations, emphasising negatives and reinforcing stigma. The term 'safety' can be viewed as a less value-laden term. The goal of risk assessment and management from a recovery perspective is working towards patients being responsible for their own safety and well-being, as well as ensuring that they do not compromise the safety of others. Guiding principles underpinning risk management are as follows (Department of Health, 2007):

- people have the right to live their lives to the full as long as that does not stop others from doing the same
- fear of supporting people to take reasonable risks in their daily lives can prevent them from doing the things that most people take for granted
- what needs to be considered is the consequence of an action and the likelihood of any harm from it
- by taking account of the benefits in terms of independence, well-being and choice, it should be possible for a person to have a support plan which enables them to manage identified risks and to live their lives in a way that best suits them.

The aim of good risk management should be to allow and encourage the patient to take full responsibility for and control of their own safety and their safety with others. To achieve this, the patient should be integral to the process of risk assessment and management.

Recovery-focused risk assessment and management requires that discussions about risk be characterised by enhanced trust, honesty and transparency between staff and patients. For many, this will be a significant departure from a more traditional approach where risk assessments have been done behind closed doors, often without input from the patient themselves and often in language and tone that can seem critical of the patient.

In the past, risk assessments have tended to emphasise risk deficits rather than considering potentially positive and protective attributes. While structured professional judgement (SPJ) tools such as the HCR-20 (Webster *et al*, 1997) focus on historical factors, taking into consideration current clinical and other risk factors, newer SPJ tools, such as the Short

Term Assessment of Risk and Treatability (START; Webster *et al*, 2004) and the Structured Assessment of PROtective Factors for violence risk (SAPROF; Vogel *et al*, 2009), also consider strengths and protective factors respectively. With both of these the focus has moved from attempting to predict risk to active risk management in a more constructive framework in an attempt to reduce rather than minimise risk. This has also been considered in newer versions of the HCR-20 Revision (Version 3) (Douglas, no date), which focuses on formulating plans to manage and reduce risks to others. Strengths-based risk assessment tools have the potential to be much less stigmatising and to prompt discussion of how strengths may be increased, thereby reducing risk further and providing greater hope for change (Ullrich & Coid, 2011).

Principles guiding the development of standardised frameworks for risk assessment can be summarised as follows (Royal College of Psychiatrists, 2008):

- risk assessment should include the clinical experience and knowledge of the patient's own view of his or her experience
- patients' views of their level of risk, and their personal risk 'triggers', should be fully considered
- risk assessments should be linked with needs assessments
- good relationships make assessment easier and more accurate and may reduce risk
- risk management should be conducted in a spirit of collaboration between the mental health team, the patient and carers.

The timing of patient involvement in managing their risk is often key to successful risk assessment and management. There needs to be a gradual transfer of responsibility for maintaining safety and reducing risk in an open, supportive and collaborative relationship between staff and patient. On admission, the patient may be too unwell, distressed or disengaged to take a role in assessing and managing their risk, and therefore their safety and security may have to be maintained by others. However, if left too late in someone's stay in secure services the transfer of responsibility for maintaining safety may be rejected by a patient who by such time could hold the view that they have no role at all in managing their risks.

Some secure services in England have introduced safety planning groups in which patients are introduced to the meaning of safety and risk and risk assessment tools. Using role-play and case studies, patients become accustomed to performing risk assessments, deciding on ways to manage risk and how to risk assess their own and others' behaviour. In this way, patients' knowledge and understanding of risk, its assessment and management has increased and they are much more able to engage in their own risk assessment and management with their clinical team.

Another example of patients' collaborative role in risk and safety is through their involvement in self-assessment of mental state and safety prior to taking leave. This places greater responsibility on the patient to self-monitor and self-assess their safety. In England and Wales, patients who are detained under restriction orders of the Mental Health Act 1983 require the permission of the Ministry of Justice for leave. Application for this has to be made by the responsible clinician (usually, but not always, a consultant psychiatrist). Some services attach a patient statement to support the application.

It needs to be emphasised that risk assessment is merely part of safety management, with the assessment being continually reviewed in light of the outcomes of safety management plans. It can be argued that not considering this, and clinicians focusing their attention on the risk assessment, is a risk in itself.

Recovery and security

Security is one of the processes by which risk is managed and can be considered as having three different elements – physical, procedural and relational. Physical security refers to the fences, locks, alarms and other physical barriers; procedural security refers to all the policies and procedures that are in place to maintain safety and security, while relational security refers to the knowledge and understanding staff have of a patient and of their environment. The Department of Health (2010) guidance *See, Think, Act: Your Guide to Relational Security* puts recovery and the management of risk in the context of relational security. This suggests that risk is not only managed by physical and procedural boundary-setting, but also by the quality of the daily interactions between staff and patients. Although written at a time before a recovery approach was common in secure services, its focus on the quality of the therapeutic relationship encourages staff and services to see the management of risk in a more recovery-focused way.

Reducing seclusion and restraint

Ensuring safety should be driven by relational and procedural security. Physical interventions such as seclusion and restraint should only be used as a last resort. Ashcraft & Anthony (2008) describe how this was achieved in a recovery-oriented crisis service in Arizona. While this was not a secure service, there are principles that can be applied to secure services. The researchers identified that barriers to changing culture included previous staff training, staff and patient fear, hopelessness and prejudice. These are all factors that recovery-oriented practice addresses. Strategies employed to remove the barriers included strong leadership direction, policy and procedural change, and new staff training. The last emphasised building relationships, validating everyday experiences as frustrating being a normal part of life and not a psychiatric problem, and focusing training on shifts that had higher levels of restraint. Debriefing was also important, with discussion of any incidents occurring with the patient as soon as possible after the event, even while in seclusion. The final strategy was promoting a learning culture as to how to avoid restraint and seclusion.

Recovery and offending behaviour

Recovery approaches have been used in working with offenders, maintaining a focus on achieving social goals such as good housing, employment and social contacts as key to success and continued desistance from offending. The Good Lives model of offender rehabilitation takes the view that a necessary condition for the reduction of offending is the instillation of ways of living that are more fulfilling and coherent (Ward, 2002). This model places the responsibility on the offender to motivate themselves to work towards maintaining safety. There is a focus on the offender's goals and on helping them achieve these in a safe and adaptive way.

National guidelines for mental healthcare and delivery can support recovery. In England and Wales, My Shared Pathway – developed as part of the National Health Service's (NHS's) Quality Innovation, Productivity and Prevention (QIPP) programme – is an example of this (NHS Networks, 2012). My Shared Pathway provides guidance on how to make the clinical process and planning in secure services focused on the patient. This is done through having clearly identified goals that are shared by the patient and professional staff, clearly identified actions that are needed to help the patient achieve these goals, and by identifying a likely timescale to achieve this in order for the patient to be able to move to a lower level of security. My Shared Pathway aims to embed the recovery approach into everyday practice while focusing on specific outcomes. By having both patient and staff rating these outcomes the process can act as an outcome measure.

Organisational facilitation of recovery

Role of mental healthcare professionals

Recovery-oriented practice requires a significant shift in the attitudes of secure service mental health workers, from a position that is frequently directive and based on power and control to one where they provide a source of professional information and guidance, while respecting and supporting the patient's own experience and expertise. Safety is a key issue in the reason for the patient's admission to secure services and therefore risk and safety must be an explicit part of mental health workers' interaction with them. There should be a clear understanding that this will always underpin interactions and decisions, with the clear goal of the patient being ultimately responsible for their own safety and the safety of others.

The *Ten Essential Shared Capabilities* (NIHME, 2004) lists ten shared capabilities for all staff working in mental health services, which if followed will ensure that practitioners work in a recovery-oriented way:

1   Working in partnership
2   Respecting diversity
3   Practising ethically
4   Challenging inequality
5   Promoting recovery
6   Identifying people's needs and strengths
7   Providing patient-centred care
8   Making a difference
9   Promoting safety and positive risk-taking
10 Personal development and learning.

Peer support workers

Peer workers can be paid salaried or voluntary multidisciplinary team members who are required to explicitly draw on and share their own experiences of mental distress and mental health service use. Peer workers are a key component of recovery-oriented services. Recovery Innovations Arizona (reported by Working Together for Recovery, 2011) describe the key elements of the peer worker role as:

- *mutuality* – giving and receiving help and support with respect based on a shared experience
- *empathy* – understanding through the personal experience of 'having been there'
- *engagement* – sharing personal recovery experiences ('If he can do it, so can I')
- *wellness* – focusing on each person's strengths and wellness
- *friendship* – promoting recovery through relationship and friendship.

A study undertaken by Ashcraft & Anthony (2008) into eliminating seclusion and restraint in a recovery-oriented crisis service identified that employing peer workers appeared to have a significant role in reducing patient arousal, leading to a reduction and even cessation of seclusion and restraint.

Currently, there are no clear guidelines about the required lived experience for peer support workers in secure services; however, those who have not had personal experience of a secure environment may be less accepted by patients. Jacobsen *et al* (2012), in a study of the roles and functions of peer workers, identified that they do direct and indirect work with clients and also conduct work with staff. Direct work involves advocacy, connecting to resources, experiential sharing, building community, relationship building, group facilitation, skills building/mentoring/goal-setting, and socialisation/self-esteem building. Indirect work involved group planning and development, administration, team communication, supervision/training, receiving support, education/awareness building, and information-gathering and verification. Work with staff aimed to build relationships and legitimise the peer role.

Peer support – buddying

Buddying has been advocated to improve quality in in-patient mental health services. A buddy is a nominated patient allocated to support a new/transferring patient from an 'expert patient' perspective. The buddy would ideally meet the new patient prior to admission, but there may be practical problems about security that prevent this. The buddy would be present on the day of admission to show the new patient around the ward, offer continuing support and answer any questions they may have.

Patient involvement and partnership working: the future

For more than a decade, the value of patient involvement has been reflected in guidance for mental health services. In 1999, the National Service Framework for Mental Health identified the importance of involving patients in all aspects of improving services (Department of Health, 1999). The NHS Plan (Department of Health, 2000) placed patients at the centre of the NHS and the Health and Social Care Act (2001) stated that patients need to be consulted about all service provision. The Commission for Patient and Public Involvement in Health was established in 2003 to ensure involvement in decision-making about health services. Making true patient involvement a reality is a real challenge and requires more than simply inviting patients to meetings or asking for a signature on a form. For patient involvement to be meaningful a culture shift is required at all levels (Perkins & Goddard 2004), from individual treatment decisions, through to the development, planning and organisation of services.

Patient involvement is a key component for ensuring the success of recovery-oriented services. Users are already involved in services and the focus should be on working with them as equals, in partnership to help build their lives in the way they wish (Sainsbury Centre for Mental Health, 2009). Indeed, rather than calling it involvement, a more recovery-based approach would be to see patients as partners in their own care. Getting this partnership right can bring many benefits: patients bring experiences of both their mental health problems and of the mental health service itself. This experience can be empowering not only for patients, individually and collectively, but also for the mental health system on the whole (Williamson, 2004).

There are, of course, barriers to partnership-working with patients. Some think that true patient involvement is too time-consuming or costly. Others are wary of allowing patients to participate as equals in mental health services; and some do not see the value of patient involvement at all. Indeed, some patients are wary of mental health services and service providers and do not want to be engaged either individually or collectively. Nevertheless, 'participative approaches will enhance staff understanding and awareness of patient-centred working and ensures that recovery services are relevant to the people using them' (Care Services Improvement Partnership *et al*, 2007: p. 14).

Conclusions

Users of secure services frequently feel that their care is done *to* them rather than *with* them. There is often disengagement from staff and services, and patients may not understand their place as co-facilitators of their care. Involvement begins with engagement with the clinical team and the co-production of care plans and treatment schedules. It is important that patients feel they have a place among the other members of the multidisciplinary team and that their views and experiences are taken into account at all levels of the decision-making process. Ward rounds and other ward-based meetings can be anxiety-provoking for patients and it can be difficult for them to feel part of the proceedings. Some patients are unsure of the purpose of ward rounds and say they do not feel listened to. This may be helped by the use of simple but effective forms for the patient to record their concerns and requests and the feedback they received in the ward round. To work in a recovery-focused way, the patient should ideally be present for the whole of the ward round meeting, but in a secure setting this may be difficult if there is sensitive information to be discussed by the rest of the team.

The care programme approach (CPA) was introduced in 1991 and emphasises the importance of placing the patient at the centre of the planning, delivery and review of their care and treatment. This approach aims to promote recovery and 'will involve the user and the carer, where appropriate, as central participants in the process' (Department of Health, 2009: p. 24). Unfortunately, the reality can be quite different from this and many patients report that they do not feel part of the process. These meetings can seem even more daunting than ward rounds and the patient is again often not present for the whole meeting. To put the patient truly at the centre of the process, modifications could include the patient sending out invitations, choosing the time and location, chairing the meeting, taking part in drawing up pre- and post-CPA reports, and being present for the whole meeting, including for drawing up future plans and revising risk assessments.

References

Anthony, W.A. (1993) Recovery from mental illness: the guiding vision of the mental health system in the 1990s. *Psychosocial Rehabilitation Journal*, **16**, 11–23.
Ashcraft, L. & Anthony, W. (2008) Eliminating seclusion and restraint in recovery-orientated crisis service. *Psychiatric Services*, **59**, 1198–1202.

Care Services Improvement Partnership, Royal College of Psychiatrists, Social Care Institute for Excellence (2007) *A Common Purpose: Recovery in Future Mental Health Services.* RCPsych & SCIE.

Centre for Mental Health (2011) *Pathways to Unlocking Secure Mental Health.* Centre for Mental Health.

Davies, S., Clarke, M., Hollin, C., *et al* (2007) Long-term outcomes after discharge from medium secure care: a cause for concern. *British Journal of Psychiatry,* **191**, 70–74.

Department of Health (1999) *National Service Framework for Mental Health: Modern Standards and Service Models.* Department of Health.

Department of Health (2000) *The NHS Plan.* Department of Health.

Department of Health (2006) *Reviewing the Care Programme Approach 2006: A Consultation Document.* Department of Health.

Department of Health (2007) *Independence, Choice and Risk: A Guide to Best Practice in Supported Decision Making.* Department of Health.

Department of Health (2008) *Refocusing the Care Programme Approach: Policy and Positive Practice Guidance.* Department of Health.

Department of Health (2009) *Effective Care Co-Ordination in Mental Health Services: Modernising the Care Programme Approach.* Department of Health.

Department of Health (2010) *See, Think, Act: Your Guide to Relational Security.* Department of Health.

Department of Health (2012) *Draft Strategy for Long-Term Conditions.* Department of Health.

Douglas, K. HCR-20 Revision (Version 3) [blog]. Available at: http://kdouglas.wordpress.com/hcr-20/hcr-20/ (accessed 9 March 2015).

Drennan, G. & Alred, D. (2012) Preface. In *Secure Recovery: Approaches to Recovery in Forensic Mental Health Settings* (eds G. Drennan & D. Alred). Routeledge.

Hillbrand, M. & Young, J.L. (2008) Instilling hope into forensic treatment: the antidote to despair and desperation. *Journal of the American Academy of Psychiatry and the Law,* **36**, 90–94.

HM Government (2011) *No Health Without Mental Health: A Cross-Government Mental Health Outcomes Strategy for People of All Ages.* Department of Health.

Jacobsen, N., Trojanowski, L. & Dewa, C.S. (2012) What do peer support workers do? A job description. *BMC Health Services Research,* **12**, 205.

META Services (2005) *Transforming from a Day Treatment to a Recovery Education Centre.* Recovery Innovations.

National Institute for Mental Health in England (2004) *The Ten Essential Shared Capabilities: A Framework for the Whole of the Mental Health Workforce.* Department of Health.

NHS Networks (2012) *My Shared Pathway.* NHS Networks (http://www.networks.nhs.uk/nhs-networks/my-shared-pathway).

Pereira, S., Dawson, P. & Sarsam, M. (2006) The national survey of PICU and low secure services. *Journal of Psychiatric Intensive Care,* **2**, 7–12.

Perkins, R. & Goddard, K. (2004) Reality out of rhetoric: increasing user involvement in a mental health trust. *Mental Health Review,* **9**, 21–4.

Roberts, G., Dorkins, E., Wooldridge, J., *et al* (2008) Detained – what is my choice? *Advances in Psychiatric Treatment,* **14**, 172–180.

Royal College of Psychiatrists (2008) *Rethinking Risk to Others in Mental Health Services.* Final Report of a Scoping Group (CR150). RCPsych.

Sainsbury Centre for Mental Health (2007) *Forensic Mental Health Services, Facts and Figures on Current Provision.* Sainsbury Centre for Mental Health.

Sainsbury Centre for Mental Health (2009) *Implementing Recovery: A New Framework for Organisational Change* (Position Paper). Sainsbury Centre for Mental Health.

Shepherd, G., Boardman, J. & Burns, M. (2009) *Implementing Recovery: A Methodology for Organisational Change.* Centre for Mental Health.

Slade, M. (2009a) *100 Ways to Support Recovery: A Guide for Mental Health Professionals.* Rethink.

Slade, M. (2009*b*) *Personal Recovery and Mental Illness: A Guide for Mental Health Professionals.* Cambridge University Press.

Stickley, T. & Wright, N. (2011) The British research evidence for recovery, papers published between 2006 and 2009 (inclusive). Part One: a review of the peer-reviewed literature using a systematic approach. *Journal of Psychiatric and Mental Health Nursing,* **18**, 247–256.

Ullrich, S. & Coid, J. (2011) Protective factors for violence among released prisoners – effects over time and interactions with static risk. *Journal of Consulting and Clinical Psychology,* **79**, 381–390.

Vogel, V., de Ruiter, C., de Bouman, Y., *et al* (2009) *SAPROF: Guidelines for the Assessment of Protective Factors for Violence Risk (English Version).* Forum Educatief.

Ward, T. (2002) Good lives and the rehabilitation of sexual offenders: promises and problems. *Aggression and Violent Behaviour,* **7**, 513–528.

Webster, C.D., Douglas, K.S., Eaves, D., *et al* (1997) *HCR-20: Assessing the Risk of Violence (Version 2).* Simon Fraser University & Forensic Psychiatric Services Commission of British Columbia.

Webster, C.D., Martin, M.L., Brink, J., *et al* (2004) *Short-Term Assessment of Risk and Treatability (START).* St Joseph's Healthcare.

Williamson, T. (2004) User involvement – a contemporary overview. *Mental Health Review Journal,* **9**, 6–12.

Working Together for Recovery (2011) *Peer Support Worker* (http://www.workingtogetherforrecovery.co.uk/peersupportworker.htm).

CHAPTER 6

Personality disorder

Piyal Sen and Mark Morris

Introduction

In this chapter we introduce and explore the concept, nature and classification of personality disorder. We then briefly explore theories of aetiology and the controversial issues raised by this, and then turn our attention to the practice of clinical and risk assessment with people with personality disorder. Finally, we provide an account of the theory and practice of treatment.

Personality disorder is a common and often disabling collection of conditions. Studies have estimated community prevalence to be between 4 and 11% of the UK population (Moran, 2002; Coid et al, 2006), but in forensic settings like prisons those figures are much higher. The prevalence was estimated to be 78% for male remand, 64% for male sentenced and 50% for female prisoners (Singleton et al, 1998). Personality disorder is often found in association with other psychiatric conditions (Tyrer et al, 1997), where it is generally accepted to complicate recovery (Stevenson et al, 2011).

Modern psychiatry exists in a neurophysiological model of health and an expanding pathological model of illness; effective treatments exist for conditions such as psychosis and affective disorders, such that there is also a pragmatic paradigm underpinning the medical model. With personality disorder, one cannot yet make these pragmatic arguments owing to the absence of a coherent pathological model or empirically validated treatment regimes.

The conceptual difficulties with personality disorder begin with the definition. There is broad agreement about what personality is, in terms of characteristic and long-standing behaviours and attitudes that remain pretty fixed, starting from adolescence or even before. Adding the concept of disorder to this invokes notions of the behaviours being maladaptive and causing the self or others to suffer – but this is more a matter of degree rather than type, and of subjective judgement. We will explore definitions, assessment, aetiology and treatment issues – notwithstanding that this approach assumes a medical model approach which belies the controversies that surround the issue.

Nature and classification

The current *Diagnostic and Statistical Manual, Fifth Edition* (DSM-5) (American Psychiatric Association, 2013) defines personality disorders as 'enduring patterns of cognition, affectivity, interpersonal behaviour and impulse control, which are culturally deviant, pervasive and inflexible, and lead to distress or social impairment'. The important issues for diagnosis are its enduring pattern, starting at least from adolescence, its pervasive nature, affecting different areas of the person's life, and causing distress or social impairment. There are some differences between the DSM-5 and the *International Classification of Diseases, 10th Revision* (ICD-10; World Health Organization, 2010) classificatory systems' categories, as illustrated in Table 6.1. Each category is operationally defined by between seven and nine specific criteria, a set number required for diagnosis of the disorder. Individuals may meet criteria for more than one disorder. The DSM-5 clusters the categories into three groups, based on similarity of symptoms. ICD-10 does not use clusters, though an attempt has been made in Table 6.1 to match the equivalent diagnoses in both classification systems.

Typically, people accessing mental health services for the first time meet criteria for at least two, and often four or more, categories of personality disorder (Stuart *et al*, 1998). This categorical classification of personality disorder has been criticised repeatedly, as it implies clear boundaries between categories and qualitative distinctions between normality and abnormality as being present or absent. The reality is that symptoms specific to personality disorder are continuously distributed across clinical and healthy samples and the threshold for disorders is relatively arbitrary (Livesley *et al*, 1994; Blackburn, 2000). Inter-rater reliability ratings are poor, raising concerns about the validity of the diagnosis (Blais *et al*, 1998; Clark & Harrison, 2001; Livesley, 2007). They are also of limited utility when devising a management plan.

The alternative would be a dimensional approach that proposes a classification system based on the normal dimensions of human personality, though there is some debate on whether these collapse into three (Eysenck, 1990), four (Leese *et al*, 1997; Livesley, 2007) or five (McCrae & Costa, 1987) basic dimensions. Within such a classification structure, a disorder would be classified as an extreme position on a personality continuum, though it is the manifestation of the disorder in different areas of the person's life and the level of distress or social impairment that would determine the diagnosis. This leads to better inter-rater reliability and is more grounded in empirical research (Torgersen, 2000) and helps to identify behavioural markers for treatment. However, a detailed assessment of all the traits which make up the dimensions would simply be too complex for everyday use, and thus of unlikely clinical utility (First, 2005).

A possible solution which is currently being debated for future classification is an integrated system with the following components:

- an agreed measure of severity
- categories derived from empirical evidence
- an assessment of current personality status based on an evaluation of traits (Sarkar & Duggan, 2012).

The current principles by which personality disorder is distinguished from mental illness is that the latter has an identifiable onset and is not persistent generally from before adulthood. However, distinguishing between personality disorder and other persistent developmental conditions such as intellectual disability is more difficult. In the case of intellectual disability, it is the inherent cognitive ability that is affected, whereas for personality disorder this is more linked to the impairment of emotional, cognitive and interpersonal states (Alexander & Cooray, 2003).

Table 6.1 Comparison of DSM-5 and ICD-10 classification of personality disorder

	DSM-5	**ICD-10**
Cluster A	*Paranoid* Distrust and suspiciouness	*Paranoid* Sensitivity and suspiciousness
	Schizoid Socially and emotionally detached	*Schizoid* Emotionally cold and detached
	Schizotypal Social and interpersonal deficits; cognitive or perceptual distortions	No equivalent
Cluster B	*Antisocial* Violation of the rights of others	*Dissocial* Callous disregard of others, irresponsibility and irritability
	Borderline Instability of relationships, self-image and mood	*Emotionally unstable* (a) Borderline (unclear self-image and intense, unstable relationships) (b) Impulsive (inability to control anger, quarrelsome and unpredictable)
	Histrionic Excessive emotionality and atttention-seeking	*Histrionic* Dramatic, egocentric and manipulative
	Narcissistic Grandiose, lack of empathy, need for admiration	No equivalent
Cluster C	*Avoidant* Socially inhibited, feelings of inadequacy, hypersensitivity	*Anxious* Tense, self-conscious and hypersensitive
	Dependent Clinging and submissive	*Dependent* Subordinates personal needs and needs constant reassurance
	Obsessive–compulsive Perfectionist and inflexible	*Anankastic* Indecisive, pedantic and rigid

Other controversies

In the UK, mental health legislation has specifically been amended to ensure that psychiatrists cannot avoid treating personality disorder where public safety is an important concern (Mental Health Act 1983, revised 2007). The former legal distinction between 'mental illness' and 'psychopathic disorder', where the latter had to be 'treatable', has been removed so that both conditions are defined as 'mental disorder'. The 'treatability test' has been amended such that the requirement now is that appropriate treatment is available whether or not it is effective or whether the patient is engaging with it. It has been argued that the revised legislation offers similar opportunities for psychiatrists, only presented differently (Sen & Irons, 2010).

The controversy was further fuelled by the government-driven establishment of a separate classification, dangerous and severe personality disorder (DSPD), for the treatment of which specialist units in prisons and hospitals were established (e.g. Probation Circular, 2005), the primary focus being risk (Maden, 2007). Cost concerns and lack of evidence of treatment efficacy have now phased these units out, but this illustrates the political sensitivity in this area (Barrett et al, 2009; Duggan, 2011).

Race is another controversial area, with significant under-diagnosis of personality disorder among Black people within prisons and secure services in the UK (Coid et al, 2000, 2002; McGilloway et al, 2010). However, this difference is not noted in community samples (Crawford et al, 2012). For Asians, community studies in the USA and the UK show lower rates of personality disorder, but this is not a consistent finding (de Bernier et al, 2014). There is also some suggestion that Black patients receive a significantly narrower range of treatments for personality disorder (Bender et al, 2007). This suggests a possible issue with the operation of treatment filters for such patients, but further research is required in this area. The racial backgrounds of staff also cannot be ignored in personality disorder treatment (Sen & Ramaswamy, 2011).

Aetiology

Personality disorder probably has a multifactorial aetiology and develops as a result of interactions between:

- biologically based vulnerabilities
- early experiences with significant others
- the role of social factors in buffering or intensifying problematic personality traits.

Recent work indicates aetiological (genetic and environmental) overlap (Jang et al, 1996; Markon et al, 2002) and a common structural model between normal and abnormal personality (O'Connor, 2002; Markon et al,

2005). A significant contributor to personality characteristics is genetic and a product of the gene–environment interaction (Kendler & Eaves, 1986; Rutter, 2007). Evidence from twin and adoption studies suggests that normal personality dimesions have an inherited component of 40 to 50% (Paris, 1996). Core psychopathic features such as callousness and unemotionality have up to 60% heritability (Viding, 2005; Waldman & Rhee, 2007; Viding *et al*, 2008; Ferguson, 2010; Skeem *et al*, 2011). There is a huge body of research supportive of an association between psychopathic traits and genetic factors (Rhee & Waldman, 2002; Taylor *et al*, 2003; Viding, 2005; Waldman & Rhee, 2007) and research is now moving on to explore the link between genes and certain types of behaviour such as impulsivity and affective instability (Siever, 2005; Reichborn-Kjennerud, 2010).

Neuroimaging is identifying links between poor facial expression recognition and amygdala and other limbic functioning (Wilson *et al*, 2011). Other findings include differences in responding to and learning about emotive stimuli and deficits in the prefrontal cortex, which contributes to the risk of impulsive behaviour (Sarkar *et al*, 2012). This contributes further to the aetiological understanding of personality disorder.

A history of adverse attachments in childhood, particularly with the primary caregiver, followed by experiences during adolescence, leads to the pattern of adverse and ambivalent attachment behaviour in adulthood, with special reference to the development of a sense of self and how that influences relationships with others. Generally, it is important to focus on thoughts and feelings much more as opposed to the facts about the history. Specific relationship difficulties need to be explored, without omitting the protective factors such as good attachment experiences. History of trauma or abuse in the developmental period needs to be included in the formulation.

Assessment of personality disorder

We will now describe the most common methods for assessing personality disorder.

Unstructured clinical interview

A clinical interview, unstructured but following a diagnostic structure, for example the DSM-5. The person's behaviour over time is evaluated and attempts are made to establish the presence of traits characteristic of the diagnosis in a range of situations. In practice, this involves a thorough review of the available file information, an interview with the individual, a detailed developmental account, history of contact with mental health and criminal justice services, and information from third-party sources.

Psychometric questionnaires

A number of self-report questionnaires have been developed, including the Millon Clinical Multiaxial Inventory, 3rd edition (MCMI-III; Millon *et al*, 2009), the Personality Assessment Inventory (PAI; Morey, 1991), the Minnesota Multiphasic Personality Inventory-2 (MMPI-2; Butcher *et al*, 2001) and the Personality Diagnostic Questionnaire (PDQ-4; Hyler, 1994). These are primarily an assessment of traits, with the presence of a certain number leading to a categorical diagnosis. In settings such as probation, the Standardised Assessment of Personality – Abbreviated Scale (SAPAS) has just eight items and a cut-off score (Moran *et al*, 2003; Pluck *et al*, 2012). The overall value of the psychometric questionnaires is primarily for screening purposes, where brevity is an advantage.

Semi-structured interviews

The 'gold standard' approach to personality assessment makes use of semi-structured interviews such as the International Personality Disorder Examination (IPDE; Loranger *et al*, 1994), Structured Clinical Interview for DSM-IV Personality Disorders (SCID-II; Pfohl *et al*, 1997) or Personality Assessment Schedule (PAS; Tyrer *et al*, 1979). The Hare Psychopathy Checklist – Revised (PCL-R; Hare, 1991) is for identifying psychopathy, a subtype of antisocial personality disorder. These interviews require training, have a structured scoring system and direct the assessor to explore diagnostic symptoms relevant to each disorder.

The PCL-R has been re-cast as a more descriptive clinical tool through factor analysis by Cooke & Michie (2001), who have broken it down into three constituent factors, deleting seven of the 20 items primarily related to criminality and disapproved behaviours, namely:

- arrogant and deceitful interpersonal style
- deficient affective experience
- impulsive and irresponsible behavioural style.

In practice, people with personality disorder frequently are the higher-risk patients in a secure unit, being less predictable and there being fewer clear pathways of care, and potent therapeutic resources. Within the clinical setting, the assessment of personality pathology thus becomes particularly important. Developing a clear diagnostic formulation about the personality pathology can be combined with historical developmental and risk data to identify the characteristic patterns of behaviour that link personality to offending, to deteriorations in mental state during crises, and to factors that will escalate risk.

A formulation of risk should form an integral part of any assessment of personality disorder, particularly Cluster B disorders such as antisocial and borderline disorder (National Collaborating Centre for Mental Health, 2009*a*). Personality disorder features prominently in all violence risk assessment guides (Webster *et al*, 1997). There is strong evidence of a link between violent offending and a diagnosis of antisocial personality disorder, particularly psychopathy (Eronon *et al*, 1996; Hart *et al*, 2003; Coid *et al*, 2006; McMurran & Howard, 2009). Re-offending rates are higher within the personality disorder group, within both prison and hospital populations (Hemphill *et al*, 1998; Jamieson & Taylor, 2004). Borderline personality disorder is associated with a more general range of criminal activities, particularly intimate partner violence (Dutton, 2002; Critchfield *et al*, 2007). For other personality disorders, including those in Clusters A and C, there is insufficient evidence to robustly establish their link to violence (McMurran & Howard, 2009).

Management of personality disorders: the theory

With regard to the evidence base for the treatment of antisocial personality disorder, the UK Guideline Development Group for the National Institute for Health and Care Excellence (NICE) identified only five randomised controlled trials (RCTs), all of which examined substance misuse as an outcome variable rather than ameliorating specific traits of antisocial personality disorder (Duggan & Kane, 2010). There was only one RCT of cognitive–behavioural therapy (CBT) compared with treatment as usual (TAU) in 52 men, randomised to TAU plus CBT or TAU alone. At 12-month follow-up, both groups reported decrease in acts of verbal or physical aggression, but no other significant differences (Davidson *et al*, 2008).

For borderline personality disorder, dialectical behaviour therapy (DBT) was developed in the USA (Linehan, 1993) as a structured long-term treatment programme based on cognitive–behavioural principles to address the needs of women who self-harm. It is a combination of change and acceptance strategies, which forms the 'dialectic' from which it derives its name. Evidence from seven randomised controlled trials involving community patients showed significant improvement in symptoms of anxiety, depression and borderline personality disorder, as well as better engagement in treatment, compared to the TAU group. This evidence was used to recommend this method of treatment for women who self-harm (National Collaborating Centre for Mental Health, 2009*b*). It has also been used for male patients in forensic settings targeting anger and violence (Evershed *et al*, 2003), but lacks any RCT evidence for such use.

Another method of treatment with some evidence of efficacy is called mentalisation-based therapy (MBT), derived from psychodynamic psychotherapy and designed to increase self-reflective capacity. A total of 44 women with borderline personality disorder demonstrated statistically significant improvements in depressive symptoms, suicidal and self-mutilatory acts, in-patient days as well as improved social and interpersonal functioning in an MBT-based day-hospital treatment programme, maintained at 18-month and 5-year follow-ups (Bateman & Fonagy, 1999,

2001, 2008). A variant of MBT for out-patient treatment also produced good results (Bateman & Fonagy, 2009; Bateman, 2012).

Schema-focused therapy works on the basis that personality pathology develops from early maladaptive schema, assumptions about the self originating in childhood and self-perpetuating in adult life. Evidence of efficacy is from a multicentric trial carried out over a 4-year period in the Netherlands with 86 borderline patients randomised to schema or transference-focused psychotherapy, with 52% recovering in the schema group compared with 29% in the other group, a significant difference. It also had much lower dropout rates (Giesen-Bloo et al, 2006). These findings have subsequently been supported by results in other RCTs (Farrell et al, 2009).

There is recent evidence of the efficacy of cognitive analytic therapy (CAT), with an RCT comparing 24-session CAT with TAU at a specialist personality disorder out-patient clinic, showing significant improvement for the CAT group in psychological symptoms and interpersonal functioning (Clarke et al, 2013). Borderline self-harming patients were specifically excluded from the treatment group, which demonstrates that a structured therapy programme can be useful for all patients with a personality disorder, not just those with borderline personality disorder.

There is an evidence literature about efficacy of therapeutic community treatment for people with personality disorder, although this has to be treated with some caution given the difficulties of constructing robust research designs (Campbell, 2003). Evidence from the Henderson Hospital showed an improvement in measures such as impulsivity and other core features of personality disorder (Dolan et al, 1997; Davies et al, 1999; Warren et al, 2004). The research in HMP Grendon, a prison run on therapeutic community principles, for those who stayed in treatment for more than 18 months evidenced a 20% reduction in reconviction at 2 years compared with a matched waiting list control group, with some indication that this effect was sustained at 7 years; and a 60% reduction in the rate of recall for those released on licence during a life sentence (Taylor, 2000). These studies provide a degree of empirical support but they are not randomised, the effect size is weak and results are equivocal.

On current evidence, the management of personality disorder will generally be pragmatic. Needs may exist in multiple domains, including risk, experience of trauma, concurrent mental disorder and other factors. This formulation will inform the design and perhaps order of the treatment. The ingredients of a successful treatment plan might include a combination of group and individual treatment – enabling both focused individual support and challenge, and broader group-based social therapy.

In formulating a treatment plan, it is also important to be aware of all the special problems associated with assessment of these conditions:

- the high level of comorbidity (Tyrer et al, 1997)
- the fluctuating nature of personality status and level of acuity over time

- the need to have a long period of observation, preferably at least a year, before treatment can be said to be properly evaluated
- recognition that personality disorder is a multifaceted condition that can be influenced in many different ways and the interventions thus need to be by definition 'complex interventions' (Campbell *et al*, 2000).

Treatment maps under the three biopsychosocial headings: biological, psychological and social therapy.

1 *Biological treatment.* Medication has a role in the treatment of personality disorder (Tyrer & Bateman, 2004), focused on management of symptoms and comorbid conditions. NICE guidelines do not support the use of medication specifically for antisocial or borderline personality disorder, but there is evidence from a significant number of RCTs and systematic reviews that it helps in addressing specific difficulties, such as impulsivity, anger and self-harm. The evidence is stronger for borderline personality disorder in Cochrane review (Stoffers *et al*, 2010) than in antisocial personality disorder (Khalifa *et al*, 2010). Prescribing of psychotropic medication remains very high for patients with personality disorder in secure settings (Vollm *et al*, 2012); one of the commonest reasons cited by clinicians is the complex nature of patients in such settings and high levels of comorbidity. There is some recent evidence of the efficacy of clozapine (Frogley *et al*, 2013). However, none of these studies are based on evidence from RCTs, primarily used for formulation of NICE guidelines.

2 *Psychological treatment.* This is the primary mode of treatment for personality disorder. The evidence for the efficacy of various forms of psychological treatment has been described earlier in this section.

3 *Social therapy.* This would involve therapeutic activities, for example the provision of skills training, attendance at social skills groups, community meetings and anger management.

Measurement of outcomes is a complex area for any service treating personality disorder. Often, the development of a level of insight is the only valid parameter, including the acquisition of relapse prevention skills and the extent to which the patient has built on pre-existing strengths. It is very important to work out a treatment contract with the patient, which agrees the outcome measures in advance along with the formulation and a treatment plan to address them.

A specialist in-patient unit in practice

There is a large group of patients under the long-term hospital care of forensic psychiatrists in the UK, especially in high secure settings, whose mental illness improves to reveal an underlying personality disorder with associated risks that prevent easy rehabilitation: those stepping up from general psychiatric services and those transferred from prison, usually for extreme self-harm. Given the precarious evidence base and the fact that general units and wards treating this group can go badly wrong, one solution for the treatment of such patients is to refer them to more specialist treatment units.

The therapeutic community movement developed in the large asylums prior to the advent of community care. Over time one ward or unit would become the place to which people with mental disorder, but not psychosis, would gravitate. These were the forerunners of today's specialist personality disorder treatment wards. Many of them, by default, developed cultures similar to that described by Rapoport (1960) in his analysis of the social structure within the Henderson Hospital. In the absence of the foundation afforded by a clear positivist evidence base, 'expert' narrative accounts are influential. Livesley's (2003) principles have been widely cited: that a treatment has to be empathetic and validating; coherent and consistent; it should build and maintain motivation; and this within the frame of a collaborative relationship. We submit that the distinction between a specialist personality disorder unit and a ward that simply provides safe containment is the extent to which Livesley criteria are actively structured into the programme.

It is important for the staff group to be prepared to model personal accountability by tolerating their own decisions and behaviour being challenged. Such a treatment process enshrines a 'culture of enquiry' (Norton, 1992) which develops mentalisation by understanding ward events. The ward can be structured to unlock the therapeutic learning potential of the residential group by the facilitation and promotion of communication (Senge, 1993; Kennard, 1998) using the technique of regular and frequent community meetings attended regularly by all members of the multidisciplinary team, resulting in a social therapy milieu. Within this modified residential setting, patients are encouraged to participate in the more focused psychological cognitive skills programmes to build the frequently deficient core skills of thinking, communication and problem-solving; to develop motivation, and then to move on to more advanced, specifically offence-focused work, substance use, emotional management and so on.

At all times, the therapeutic focus is on the development of the patient's agency and responsibility; their recognition and active ownership of their risk profile; the development of their understanding of their trigger factors and risk situations; and an ability to manage themselves and these issues more effectively.

Conclusions

Personality disorders continue to cause uncertainty in psychiatrists owing to the conceptual challenges around diagnosis and lack of a good evidence relating to treatment and management. This is a rapidly developing area, where knowledge will continue to evolve with the progress of research. For services treating people with personality disorder it is important that good arrangements exist for training and supervision to enable them to manage the needs of this complex but interesting group of patients.

References

Alexander, R. & Cooray, S. (2003) Diagnosis of personality disorders in learning disability. *British Journal of Psychiatry*, **182** (suppl. 44), S28–S31.

American Psychiatric Association (2013) *Diagnostic and Statistical Manual of Mental Disorders Fifth Edition (DSM-5)*. APA.

Barrett, B., Byford, S., Sievewright, H., *et al* (2009) The assessment of dangerous and severe personality disorder: service use, cost, and consequences. *Journal of Forensic Psychiatry and Psychology*, **20**, 120–131.

Bateman, A. (2012) Treating BPD in clinical practice. *American Journal of Psychiatry*, **169**, 1–4.

Bateman, A. & Fonagy, P. (1999) The effectiveness of partial hospitalisation in the treatment of borderline personality disorder: a randomised controlled trial. *American Journal of Psychiatry*, **156**, 1563–1569.

Bateman, A. & Fonagy, P. (2001) The treatment of borderline personality disorder with psychoanalytically orientated partial hospitalization: an 18 month follow-up. *American Journal of Psychiatry*, **158**, 36–42.

Bateman, A. & Fonagy, P. (2008) 8-year follow-up of patients treated for borderline personality disorder: mentalization-based treatment versus treatment as usual. *American Journal of Psychiatry*, **165**, 631–638.

Bateman, A. & Fonagy, P. (2009) Randomized controlled trial of outpatient mentalization-based treatment versus structured clinical management for borderline personality disorder. *Americal Journal of Psychiatry*, **166**, 1355–1364.

Bender, D., Skodol, A., Dyck, I.R., *et al* (2007) Ethnicity and mental health utilization by patients with personality disorders. *Journal of Consulting and Clinical Psychology*, **75**, 992–999.

Blackburn, R. (2000) Treatment or incapacitation? Implications of research on personality disorders for the management of dangerous offenders. *Legal and Criminal Psychology*, **5**, 1–21.

Blais, M.A., Benedict, K.B. & Norman, D.K. (1998) Establishing the psychometric properties of the DSM-III-R personality disorders: implications for DSM-V. *Journal of Clinical Psychology*, **54**, 795–802.

Butcher, J.N., Dahlstrom, W.G., Graham, J.R., *et al* (2001) *Manual for the Restandarized Minnesota Multiphasic Personality Inventory: MMPI-2*. University of Minnesota Press.

Campbell, S. (2003) *The Feasibility of Conducting an RCT at HMP Grendon (Home Office Online Report 03/03)*. Home Office.

Campbell, M., Fitzpatrick, R., Haines, A., *et al* (2000) A framework for the design and evaluation of complex interventions which improve health. *BMJ*, **321**, 694–696.

Clark, L.A., & Harrison, J.A. (2001) Assessment instruments. In *Handbook of Personality Disorders: Theory, Research and Treatment* (ed. W.J. Livesley), pp. 277–306. Guilford Press.

Clarke, S., Thomas, P. & James, K. (2013) Cognitive analytic therapy for personality disorder: randomised controlled trial. *British Journal of Psychiatry*, **202**, 129–134.

Coid, J., Kahtan, N., Gault, S., *et al* (2000) Ethnic differences in admissions to secure forensic psychiatry services. *British Journal of Psychiatry*, **177**, 241–247.

Coid, J., Petruckevitch, A., Bebbington, P., *et al* (2002) Ethnic differences in prisoners. 1: Criminality and psychiatric morbidity. *British Journal of Psychiatry*, **181**, 473–480.

Coid J., Yang, M., Tyrer, P., *et al* (2006) Prevalence and correlates of personality disorder in Great Britain. *British Journal of Psychiatry*, **188**, 423–431.

Cooke, D. J. & Michie, C. (2001) Refining the construct of psychopathy: towards a hierarchical model. *Psychological Assessment*, **13**, 171–188.

Crawford, C., Rushwaya, T., Bajaj, P., *et al* (2012) The prevalence of personality disorder among ethnic minorities: findings from a national household survey. *Personality and Mental Health*, **6**, 175–182.

Critchfield, K.L., Levy, K.N. & Clarkin, J.F. (2007) The Personality Disorders Institute/Borderline Personality Disorder Research Foundation randomized control trial for borderline personality disorder: reliability of Axis 1 and 2 diagnoses. *Psychiatric Quarterly*, **78**, 15–24.

Davidson, K.M., Tyrer, P., Tata, P., *et al* (2008) Cognitive behaviour therapy for violent men with antisocial personality disorder in the community: an exploratory randomized controlled trial. *Psychological Medicine*, **39**, 569–577.

Davies, S., Campling, P. & Ryan, K. (1999) Therapeutic community provision at regional and district levels. *Psychiatric Bulletin*, **23**, 79–83.

de Bernier, G.-L., Kim, Y.-R. & Sen, P. (2014) A systematic review of the global prevalence of personality disorders in adult Asian populations. *Personality and Mental Health*, **8**, 264–275.

Dolan, B., Warren, F. & Norton, K. (1997) Change in borderline symptoms one year after therapeutic community treatment for severre borderline personality disorder. *British Journal of Psychiatry*, **171**, 274–279.

Duggan, C. (2011) Dangerous and severe personality disorder. *British Journal of Psychiatry*, **198**, 431–433.

Duggan, C. & Kane, E. (2010) Commentary: developing a national institute of clinical excellence and health guideline for antisocial personality disorder. *Personalty and Mental Health*, **4**, 3–8.

Dutton, D.G. (2002) Personality dynamics of intimate abusiveness. *Journal of Psychiatric Practice*, **8**, 216–228.

Eronon, M., Hakola, P. & Tiihonen, J. (1996) Mental disorder and homicidal behavior in Finland. *Archives of General Psychiatry*, **53**, 497–501.

Evershed, S., Tennant, A. & Boomer, D. (2003) Practice-based outcomes of dialectical behaviour therapy (DBT) targeting anger and violence, with male forensic patients: a pragmatic and non-contemporaneous comparison. *Criminal Behaviour and Mental Health*, **13**, 198–213.

Eysenck, H.J. (1990) Biological dimensions of personality. In *Handbook of Personality Theory and Research* (eds L.A. Pervin & O.P. John), pp. 244–276. Guilford Press.

Farrell, J.M., Shaw, I.A. & Webber, M.A. (2009) A schema-focused approach to group psychotherapy for outpatients with borderline personality disorder: a randomized controlled trial. *Journal of Behaviour Therapy and Experimental Psychiatry*, **40**, 317–328.

Ferguson, C.J. (2010) Genetic contributions to antisocial personality and behavior: a meta-analytic review from an evolutionary perspective. *Journal of Social Psychology*, **150**, 160–180.

First, M.B. (2005) Clinical utility: a prerequisite for the adoption of a dimensional approach to DSM. *Journal of Abnormal Psychology*, **114**, 560–564.

Frogley, C., Anagnostakis K., Mitchell, S., *et al* (2013) A case series of clozapine for borderline personality disorder. *Annals of Clinical Psychiatry*, **25**, 125–34.

Giesen-Bloo, J., van Dyck, R., Spinhoven, P., *et al* (2006) Outpatient psychotherapy for borderline personality disorder: randomized trial of schema-focused therapy vs transference-focused therapy. *Archives of General Psychiatry*, **63**, 649–658.

Hare, R.D. (1991) *The Hare Psychopathy Checklist – Revised*. Multi-Health Systems.

Hart, S.D., Kropp, P.K., Lawes, D.R., *et al* (2003) *The risk for sexual violence protocol; Structured professional guidelines for assessing risk of sexual violence*. Mental Health, Law and Policy Institute, Simon Fraser University.

Hemphill, J.F., Hare, R.D. & Wong, S. (1998) Psychopathy and recidivism: a review. *Legal and Criminological Psychology*, **3**, 139–170.

Hyler, S.E. (1994) Personality Diagnostic Questionnaire-4 (PDQ-4), New York Psychiatric Institute Illness. *American Journal of Psychiatry*, **143**, 279–289.

Jamieson, E. & Taylor, P.J. (2004) A re-conviction study of special (high security) hospital patients. *British Journal of Criminology*, **44**, 783–802.

Jang, K.L., Livesley, W.J., Vernon, P.A., *et al* (1996) Heritability of personality disorder traits: a twin study. *Acta Psychiatrica Scandinavica*, **94**, 438–444.

Kendler, K.S. & Eaves, L.J. (1986) Models for the joint effect of genotype and environment on liability to psychiatric illness. *American Journal of Psychiatry*, **143**, 279–289.

Kennard, D. (1998) *An Introduction to Therapeutic Communities*. Jessica Kingsley.

Khalifa, N., Duggan, C., Stoffers, J., *et al* (2010) Pharmacological interventions for antisocial personality disorder. *Cochrane Database of Systematic Reviews*, **8**, doi: 10.1002/14651858. CD007667.pub2.

Leese, M., Mulder, R.T. & Joyce, P.R. (1997) Temperament and the structure of personality disorder symptoms. *Psychological Medicine*, **27**, 1315–1325.

Linehan, M. (1993) *Cognitive–Behavioural Treatment of Borderline Personality Disorder*. Guilford Press.

Livesley, W.J. (2003) *Practical Management of Personality Disorder*. Guilford Press.

Livesley, W.J. (2007) A framework for integrating dimensional and categorical classifications of personality disorder. *Journal of Personality Disorders*, **21**, 199–224.

Livesley, W.J., Schroeder, M.L., Jackson, D.N., *et al* (1994) Categorical distinctions in the study of personality disorder: implications for classification. *Journal of Abnormal Psychology*, **103**, 6–17.

Loranger, A.W., Sartorius, N., Andreoli, A., *et al* (1994) The International Personality Disorder Examination: the World Health Organization/Alcohol, Drug Abuse, and Mental Health Administration international pilot study of personality disorders. *Archives of General Psychiatry*, **51**, 215–224.

Maden, T. (2007) Dangerous and severe personality disorder: antecedents and origins. *British Journal of Psychiatry*, **190** (suppl. 49), 8–11.

Markon, K.E., Krueger, R.F., Bouchard, T.J., *et al* (2002) Normal and abnormal personality traits: evidence for genetic and environmental relationships in the Minnesota Study of Twins Reared Apart. *Journal of Personality*, **70**, 661–693.

Markon, K.E., Krueger, R.F. & Watson, D. (2005) Delineating the structure of normal and abnormal personality: an integrative hierarchical approach. *Journal of Personality and Social Psychology*, **88**, 139–157.

McCrae, R.R. & Costa, P.T. (1987) Validation of the five-factor model of personality across instruments and obsevers. *Journal of Personality and Social Psychology*, **52**, 81–90.

McGilloway, A., Owen, R.A., Tennyson, L., *et al* (2010) A systematic review of personality disorder, race and ethnicity: prevalence, aetiology and treatment. *BMC Psychiatry*, **10**, 33.

McMurran, M. & Howard, R. (eds) (2009) *Personality, Personality Disorder and Violence*. Wiley-Blackwell.

Millon, T., Davis, R., Millon, C., *et al* (2009) *The Millon Clinical Multiaxial Inventory-III (MCMI-III)*. PsychCorp.

Moran, P. (2002) The epidemiology of personality disorders. *Psychiatry*, **1**, 8–11.

Moran, P., Leese, M., Lee, T., *et al* (2003) Standardised Assessment of Personality – Abbreviated Scale (SAPAS): preliminary validation of a brief screen for personality disorder. *British Journal of Psychiatry*, **183**, 228–232.

Morey, L.C. (1991) *Personality Assessment Inventory – Professional Manual*. Psychological Assessment Resources.

National Collaborating Centre for Mental Health (2009a) *Antisocial Personality Disorder: Treatment, Management and Prevention (CG77)*. National Institute for Health and Clinical Excellence.

National Collaborating Centre for Mental Health (2009b) *Borderline Personality Disorder: Treatment and Management (CG 78)*, p. 169. National Institute for Health and Clinical Excellence.

Norton, K. (1992) A culture of enquiry: its preservation or loss. *Therapeutic Communities*, **13**, 3–26.

O'Connor, B. (2002) The search for dimensional structure differences between normality and abnormality: a statistical review of published data on personality and psychopathology. *Journal of Personality and Social Psychology*, **83**, 962–982.

Paris, J. (1996) *Social Factors in Personality Disorder: A Biopsychosocial Approach to Etiology and Treatment*. Cambridge University Press.

Pfohl, B., Blum, N. & Zimmerman, M. (1997) *Structured Interview for DSM-IV Personality Disorders*. American Psychiatric Press.

Pluck, G., Sirdifield, C. & Brooker, C. (2012) Screening for personality disorder in probationers: validation of the Standardised Assessment of Personality – Abbreviated Scale (SAPAS). *Personality and Mental Health*, **6**, 61–68.

Probation Circular (2005) *Dangerous and Severe Personality Disorder Programme 40/2005*. TSO (The Stationery Office).

Rapoport, R. (1960) *The Community as Doctor: New Perspectives on a Therapeutic Community*. Tavistock Publications.

Reichborn-Kjennerud, T. (2010) The genetic epidemiology of personality disorders. *Dialogues in Clinical Neuroscience*, **12**, 103–114.

Rhee, S.H. & Waldman, I.D. (2002) Genetic and environmental influences on antisocial behaviour: a meta-analysis of twin and adoption studies. *Psychological Bulletin*, **128**, 420–529.

Rutter, M. (2007) Gene–environment interdependence. *Developmental Science*, **10**, 12–18.

Sarkar, J. & Duggan, C. (2012) Diagnosis and classification of personality disorder: difficulties, their resolution and implications for practice. In *Clinical Topics in Personality Disorder* (eds J. Sarkar & G. Adshead), pp. 156–171. RCPsych Publications.

Sarkar, S., Clark, B.S. & Deeley, Q. (2012) Differences between psychopathy and other personality disorders: evidence from neuroimaging. In *Clinical Topics in Personality Disorder* (eds J. Sarkar & G. Adshead), pp. 38–52. RCPsych Publications.

Sen, P. & Irons, A. (2010) Personality disorder and the Mental Health Act 1983 (amended). *Advances in Psychiatric Treatment*, **16**, 329–335.

Sen, P. & Ramaswamy, D. (2011) A balanced approach to race in the treatment of personality disorder. *Advances in Psychiatric Treatment*, **17**, 139–141.

Senge, P. (1993) *The Fifth Discipline: The Art and Practice of the Learning Organisation*. Random House.

Siever, L.J. (2005) Endophenotypes in the personality disorders. *Dialogues in Clinical Neuroscience*, **7**, 139–151.

Singleton, N., Meltzer, H, Gatward, R., *et al* (1998) *Psychiatric Morbidity Among Prisoners*. Office for National Statistics.

Skeem, J.L., Polaschek, D.L.L., Patrick, C.J., *et al* (2011) Psychopathic personality: bridging the gap between scientific evidence and public policy. *Psychological Science in the Public Interest*, **12**, 95–162.

Stevenson, J., Brodaty, H., Boyce, P., *et al* (2011) Personality disorder comorbidity and outcome: comparison of three age groups. *Australian and New Zealand Journal of Psychiatry*, **459**, 771–779.

Stoffers, J., Vollm, B.A., Rucker, G., *et al* (2010) Pharmacological interventions for borderline personality disorder. *Cochrane Database of Systematic Reviews*, **6**, Art. No.: CD005653.

Stuart, S., Pfohl, B., Battaglia, M., *et al* (1998) The co-occurrence of DSM-III-R personality disorders. *Journal of Personality Disorders*, **12**, 302–315.

Taylor, J., Loney, BR., Bobadilla, I., *et al* (2003) Genetic and environmental influences on psychopathy traits dimensions in a community sample of male twins. *Journal of Abnormal Child Psychology*, **31**, 633–645.

Taylor, R. (2000) *A Seven Year Reconviction Study of HMP Grendon Therapeutic Community*. Research Findings 115. Home Office Research, Development and Statistics Directorate.

Torgersen, S. (2000) Genetics of patients with borderline personality disorder. *Psychiatric Clinics of North America*, **23**, 1–9.

Tyrer, P. & Bateman, A.W. (2004) Drug treatment for personality disorders. *Advances in Psychiatric Treatment*, **10**, 389–398.

Tyrer, P., Alexander, M.S., Ciccheti, D., *et al* (1979) Reliability of a schedule for rating personality disorders. *British Journal of Psychiatry*, **135**, 168–174.

Tyrer, P., Gunderson, J., Lyons, M., *et al* (1997) Extent of comorbidity between mental state and personality disorders. *Journal of Personality Disorders*, **11**, 242–259.

Viding, E. (2005) Evidence for substantial genetic risk for psychopathy in 7-year-olds. *Journal of Child Psychology and Psychiatry*, **46**, 592–597.

Viding, E., Larsson, H. & Jones, A.P. (2008) Quantitative genetic studies of antisocial behaviour. *Philosophical Transactions of the Royal Society of London*, **363**, 2519–2527.

Vollm, B.A., Chadwick, K., Tarek, A., *et al* (2012) Prescribing of psychotropic medication for personality disordered patients in secure forensic settings. *Journal of Forensic Psychiatry and Psychology*, **23**, 200–216.

Waldman, I.D. & Rhee, S.H. (2007) Genetic and environmental influences on psychopathy and antisocial behaviour. In *Handbook of Psychopathy* (ed. C.J. Patrick), pp. 205–228. Guilford Press.

Warren, F., Evans, C. & Dolan, B. (2004) Impulsivity and self-damaging behaviour in severe personality disorder: the impact of democratic therapeutic community treatment. *Therapeutic Communities*, **25**, 55–71.

Webster, C., Douglas, K., Eaves, D., *et al* (1997) *HCR-20:Assessing Risk of Violence* (2nd edn). Mental Health, Law and Policy Institute, Simon Fraser University & British Columbia Forensic Psychiatric Services Commission.

Wilson, K., Juodis, M. & Porter, S. (2011) Fear and loathing in psychopaths: a meta-analytic investigation of the facial affect recognition deficit. *Criminal Justice and Behavior*, **38**, 659–668.

World Health Organization (2010) *International Classification of Diseases, 10th Revision (ICD-10)*. WHO.

CHAPTER 7

Women's mental health, aggression and offending

Katina Anagnostakis

Introduction

This chapter explores the relationship between mental disorder and offending behaviour in women, highlighting gender differences and considering how these have shaped the evolution of secure mental health services provision for women in the UK.

Prevalence of mental disorder in women

The relationship between female gender and mental disorder is far from straightforward, influenced in part by gender-specific social and cultural factors, and in part by genetic and environmental factors relating to mental disorders in both men and women. Generally speaking, the prevalence of severe mental illnesses such as schizophrenia and bipolar disorder is unrelated to gender and is broadly similar among men and women (Abel *et al*, 2010; Diflorio & Jones, 2010). However, some diagnoses can only be made in women as they relate specifically to a fundamental aspect of female gender, for example, postnatal depression and postpartum psychosis. Among other psychiatric conditions that occur in both genders there is a spectrum of relative prevalence between men and women. For example, conditions such as eating disorder predominate (over 90%) among women (Smink *et al*, 2012). Although interest in biological factors is growing, the social context of the lives of women and girls is believed to play a significant part in explaining this finding (Herpetz-Dahlmann *et al*, 2011).

The prevalence of non-psychotic disorders such as depression, anxiety disorder and post-traumatic stress disorder (PTSD) is higher among women than men (Angst *et al*, 2002; National Comorbidity Survey, 2005). Women have a longer average lifespan than men, rendering the prevalence, but not the incidence, of conditions such as dementia more common in women as they age (Schmidt *et al*, 2008). A similar explanatory model has been postulated to account for the higher prevalence of depression in women (Pilgrim, 2010). Historically, substance misuse has always been less common among women than men; however, this is a trend that has gradually been reversing, raising questions about changing social influences. Finally, certain psychiatric conditions are far less prevalent among women, most notably antisocial personality disorder. It is also notable that men complete suicide more commonly and via more violent means than women. This is in contrast to the higher prevalence of self-harming behaviour in women than in men (Canetto *et al*, 1998).

Biological factors

The consistency of data about gender differences in the prevalence, presentation and course of certain psychiatric disorders across cultures suggests that biological factors have a role to play. Several mechanisms implicating endocrine and, perhaps, genetic factors have been postulated.

The dynamic effect of ovarian sex steroid hormones on central nervous system development and function throughout the life cycle modulates many neurotransmitter systems implicated in affective and psychotic disorders (e.g. serotinergic, noradrenergic, dopaminergic and hypothalamic-pituitary adrenal axis) as well as the stress response, where gender differences exist in prevalence, presentation and course (Pau, 2000).

The early developmental organising/adult activating model predominates in our current understanding of how sex steroid central nervous system modulation produces differential effects on the male and female brain (Rubinow *et al*, 2002; Cook & Woolley, 2005). There is also a greater degree of fluctuation in the hormonal milieu across the lifespan in women, enhancing the potential for aberrant neurotransmission and stress response (Handa *et al*, 1994; Bangasser, 2013).

A good example of the impact of biological factors is the consistent finding of gender differences in the course of schizophrenia, namely a later age at onset in women and a second peak in incidence around the time of the menopause. These are thought in part to be attributable to the neuro-protective effect of oestrogen-enhancing presynaptic dopaminergic tone in women of reproductive age (Hayes *et al*, 2012).

Psychological factors

The link between disordered attachment and an increased risk of psycho-pathology has been well described in both men and women and has been heavily implicated in many psychiatric conditions where there is a female preponderance, for example anxiety disorder, chronic PTSD and dissociative symptoms (van der Kolk, 2005), borderline personality disorder and eating disorder (Clarkin & Posner, 2005; Tasca *et al*, 2011). Gender differences in other psychological factors exist, including stress response and emotional memory. However, attachment deserves particular attention due to its broad relevance to women's mental health. It is therefore understandable that attachment theory has influenced the high prevalence of attachment-based treatment models in mental health settings for women.

Sociocultural factors

There is some evidence that stigmatisation of women as vulnerable and less capable individuals can lead to pathologisation, over-diagnosis and over-medication (Wang *et al*, 2007). To compound matters, much psychiatric research, especially drug or treatment related, is biased towards the use of working-age male subjects and the results may not always generalise to women. Differences in help-seeking behaviour between men and women are also thought to bias many research findings (Judd *et al*, 2008).

Gender-based violence typically stems from the unequal power relationships that can exist between men and women. Such violence is typically directed against a woman because of her gender (United Nations Population Fund, 2005). There is a complex interrelationship between gender-based violence and psychiatric morbidity that further complicates our understanding of gender-related variations in psychiatric morbidity. Gender-based violence is a risk factor for mental illness, however, at the same time mental illness predisposes women to gender-based violence. The vicious cycle of violence and mental illness is not unique to women, but some of the literature suggests that women may be more vulnerable to this dynamic (Dillon *et al*, 2013).

A meta-analysis of women exposed to intimate partner violence revealed that 47.6% experienced depression, 17.9% suicidal behaviour, 63.8% PTSD, 18.5% alcohol misuse and 8.9% substance misuse (Golding, 1999). A dose-response relationship between the severity of violence and the risk for depression or PTSD suggested a causal association between intimate partner violence and mental illness in women, which in turn predisposed them to engaging in unhelpful coping mechanisms such as substance misuse (Golding, 1999). Further, the psychological sequelae of intimate partner violence such as low self-esteem, self-harm, chronic unhappiness and somatic complaints are well established. Intimate partner violence is also an independent risk factor for suicidal behaviour in women (Chowdhary & Patel, 2008).

Women are differentially affected by social stress, for example in terms of the likelihood of exposure. Generally speaking, across cultures, women are less affluent, carry a greater domestic labour burden and are more likely to be the victims of intra-familial sexual abuse. These factors may explain some gender differences in mental disorder.

The literature suggests that risk of psychological morbidity in women increases in association with social role revision. For example, young Asian women in the UK are at higher risk of self-harm (Mumford & Whitehouse, 1988), whereas eating disorders are emerging in non-Western cultures as women's social roles evolve and Western influences become more prominent. Further work is needed to tease out the relative contributions of gender and ethnicity, but there remains a broad consensus that women represent a higher mental health need group than men.

Female gender and offending

General population

Women are less likely to commit and be convicted of crime, especially sexual and violent crime, than men, with the result that women offenders are outnumbered by men within the general population by a factor of approximately four to one. Women are more likely to be the victims than the perpetrators of violent crime, with 38% of violent crime perpetrated against women (Ministry of Justice, 2007). Violence accounts for about 10% of convictions among women, with domestic violence predominating. Between 2006 and 2010 theft and handling stolen goods were consistently the most common indictable offence among women (Ministry of Justice, 2011a).

A minority of unlawful deaths are caused by women: 4% of murder, 12% of manslaughter and 20% of diminished responsibility verdicts in the UK (d'Orbán, 1991). A detailed examination of homicides committed by women illustrates most of the typical features of women offenders as a group, for example their victims are typically family relations and associations with personality pathology are strong.

The number of women arrested for domestic violence is rising (Magdol et al, 1997), with higher rates of personality disorder and mood disorder among female perpetrators of domestic violence compared with men (Henning et al, 2003). There are also associations with PTSD, generalised anxiety disorder and substance misuse (Stuart et al, 2006). Intimate partner violence in women is associated with Cluster B personality traits (Thornton et al, 2010), borderline personality disorder, communication and attachment problems and violence within other relationships (Bouchard et al, 2009).

Domestic violence, when perpetrated by women, is often a response to victimisation, but it is important to note that there are other significant risk factors. A study of violent female offenders in Finland revealed that they were typically single, unemployed, with a history of violence, comorbid personality disorder, substance misuse and mental illness. They had typically had adverse childhood experiences and adult relationship problems, had social skills deficits and possessed poor coping skills. Violence often resulted from interpersonal conflict, but not typically as a form of self-defence or a response to victimisation (Weizmann-Henelius, 2006).

As with men, women's antisocial behaviour usually emerges in adolescence, but then fluctuates more over time than in men, typically influenced by external circumstances such as peer group (Messer et al, 2004). For reasons as yet unclear, the age-related decline in offending rates tends to be slower among women than men.

Reoffending rates are lower among women at 18.3% v. 28.3% in men (Ministry of Justice, 2011b). It is evident that personality disorder in women is a better predictor of violent recidivism than mental illness (Putkonen et al, 2003).

Prison populations

Traditionally women have represented approximately 3–4% of the total prison population in the UK. The 10 years between 1996 and 2006 saw a disproportionate rise in the female prison population (94%) *v.* the male prison population (41%) (Ministry of Justice, 2007). Following a plateau of around 4500 women prisoners in 2006/2007, the numbers have very slowly declined over recent years. By February 2011, women accounted for 5% of the prison population and 16% of the probation case-load (Ministry of Justice, 2011*a*).

The social profile of women prisoners, in common with their male counterparts, is characterised by a high prevalence of childhood adversity, poor educational attainment and poor work record. However, in terms of social roles and networks, women prisoners have a distinct profile. Approximately 43% of women prisoners were living with children before being taken into custody, and of these approximately half were single parents. As a result, approximately 17 000 children per year in the UK are separated from their mothers through custody. Only 23% of these children are cared for by a partner, compared with 90% in the case of children of male prisoners. Furthermore, 80% of women prisoners lose the support of their partner while in prison (Department of Health, 2006). Also, as the female prison estate is smaller, women are generally held further away from their home area. Modern UK prisons cater increasingly well for the needs of new mothers, yet prison mother and baby units still exclude women with mental illness. Current models of custodial provision for women therefore further compound many of their existing social vulnerabilities. This can have significant implications not only for the children and families involved, but also for health and social care providers while women are in custody and on their release. In relation to mental health, women prisoners typically have far higher rates of psychiatric morbidity and more vulnerability factors than their male counterparts (Harris *et al*, 2007).

A consistent body of literature highlights the higher rates of drug dependence (Fazel *et al*, 2006) and lifetime incidence of trauma among women prisoners. Approximately half of women prisoners have suffered some form of abuse before imprisonment. Estimates of the proportion of those who have suffered sexual abuse range from 30 to 60%, in contrast with 10 to 14% of male prisoners (Malacova *et al*, 2012).

Women prisoners are characterised by greater behavioural disturbance than their male peers, with higher adjudication rates in custody (Ministry of Justice, 2007). They engage in more self-harm and aggression than male prisoners. O'Brien *et al* (2003) found that 26% of sentenced women prisoners had engaged in self-harm or suicidal behaviour during the previous year, approximately four times higher than the rates in male prisoners.

In addition to the higher prevalence of mental disorder, women in prison experience comorbid mental health problems more frequently than their male counterparts, typically borderline personality disorder, mental illness

103

such as affective disorder and alcohol or substance misuse. They are also more likely than men to have undergone previous psychiatric treatment, either in the community or within a prison setting (Bartlett, 2007). Women offenders have approximately double the rate of Mental Health Act 1983 disposals as male offenders. This may reflect their profile as a group with greater mental health need, but is also likely to be indicative of traditionally different approaches towards male and female offenders in the courts and in secure mental health services.

The higher suicide rate in women's prisons between 1999 and 2004 formed part of the motivation for the Corston review (Corston, 2007). It found that women prisoners presented with levels of psychiatric morbidity five times higher than rates in the general population and called for a number of reforms to the women's prison estate, particularly identification of alternatives to custody for all but the most dangerous women offenders. Some progress has been made, but services to bridge the gap between community and custodial settings remain underdeveloped.

Secure hospital populations

The profile of women in secure hospital settings mirrors their counterparts in criminal justice settings, with a few exceptions. The majority of women are under 30 years old and early adversity is common, including abuse and educational difficulties. Women in secure mental health services are less likely to be mothers than those in the prison population.

Women in secure hospital settings typically present with complex comorbidities involving major mental illness, personality disorder, PTSD and substance misuse (Bartlett, 1993). It is therefore no surprise that interpersonal problems characterised by extreme projections and acting out are a typical feature of this patient group.

Women in secure mental health settings present less of a threat to the public than their male counterparts (Bartlett, 1993); however, their behaviour in hospital tends to be more challenging than that of the males, with a disproportionate number of assaults on staff, seclusions and self-harm. The prevalence of self-harm has exceeded 80% in some samples (Bland *et al*, 1999; Uppal & McMurran, 2009).

Transfers between hospitals are more common than among males in secure hospital settings, and previous convictions are less frequent, despite the fact that violent behaviour is typical (Bartlett, 1993). The past 8–10 years has seen a general trend for more admissions from prison as well as certain changes in the offending profile of women in secure services: lower IQ, younger age and predominance of arson and aggression (Long *et al*, 2008).

Estimates of the prevalence of personality disorder among women offenders range from 20 to 70%, while it appears that personality disorder may be more of a risk factor for offending in women than in men (Eronen *et al*, 1996). Poor impulse control and affect regulation as well as narcissism and paranoid personality style have been implicated as key personality dimensions mediating violent behaviour in women (Nestor, 2002). However, it is important to recognise that, in reality, there is a high degree of comorbidity with different subtypes of personality disorder among female samples in prison settings or among women offenders. It is likely that a combination of traits such as rule-breaking and volatile behaviour, as well as distorted and odd perceptions, rather than a particular personality disorder diagnosis itself may be a high-risk combination for women: one that also carries a worse prognosis for progress within institutions (Warren et al, 2002). Other social and developmental vulnerability may aggravate this relationship. These findings in part reflect the sometimes unsatisfactory categorical personality disorder classification system.

The prevalence of antisocial personality disorder is far lower among women than men, but recent work suggests that its incidence may have been underestimated (Dolan & Vollm, 2009). The condition may increase the risk of violence by women over 50 times v. a factor of 10 for males (Eronen et al, 1996). Some suggest that the most serious female offenders are similar to male violent offenders in their history of conduct disorders, substance misuse and antisocial personality disorder (Lewis, 2010).

Substance misuse has become increasingly important as a factor determining risk of violence and aggression in women over recent years, replicating the trend seen in men. Whereas once substance use was thought to be far more prevalent among male than female offenders, this gap is narrowing. The rates in younger women are of particular concern (GENACIS, 2005). One study comparing intoxicated and non-intoxicated female offenders in Finland found that those who had been intoxicated typically had low cognitive ability and a more antisocial personality profile (Weizmann-Henelius et al, 2009).

Finally, reoffending rates are 15% for women discharged from medium secure psychiatric care in the UK; of these, 6% are grave and 5% are violent offences (Coid, 2007).

Trauma

An understanding of the effects of trauma and victimisation on women is central to understanding the presentation of women in secure mental health settings as a significant proportion of such women have histories of trauma and victimisation. In many cases women have suffered early and prolonged physical, sexual and emotional trauma. Therefore, features of chronic PTSD such as interpersonal difficulties, impulsivity, re-enactment and self-mutilation, dissociative symptoms and unstable mood are common in this group. There is a well-established link in both genders between the experience of violence or victimisation and later assaultive behaviour (Flannery, 2002).

Many psychological theories have been proposed to underpin female violence, for instance it may be that it reflects an unconscious mechanism recreating the abuse suffered or that the traumatised woman becomes more 'dangerous' by virtue of her status as a survivor (Adshead, 1998). Victims are prone to develop persecutory attributions and find it difficult to appreciate their own contribution to problems (van der Kolk *et al*, 1996). Some develop a heightened sensitivity to threat or impaired stimulus discrimination and social development, all possible sequelae of trauma. Furthermore, traumatised women often lack the skills to resolve problems and especially interpersonal conflicts, making anger, threats or bullying more likely responses.

Attachment

Attachment theory and an understanding of reflective function provide a possible means of understanding and linking the mental processes involved in forming early attachment and those involved in offending. The original link between offending and attachment difficulties hypothesised by Bowlby (1978) has been supported by more recent work which found that only 5% of serious offenders had a secure attachment style (van Ijzendoorn *et al*, 1997). Violent offenders thus typically have higher rates of insecure attachment and lower rates of reflective capacity. This, in turn, is associated with a reduced sense of responsibility and understanding of consequences of actions, as well as an over-reliance on a punitive and less flexible range of internal working models. The evidence suggests that the link is complex and subject to other factors, but it has been replicated in many different samples. Attachment theory also provides a very useful model for understanding institutional aggression, which is typically more prevalent among women in secure environments (Adshead, 1998).

There is relatively little gender-specific research that helps us to understand the links between offending and mental disorder among women.

In terms of hormonal factors, there is evidence for increased rates of aggression in the para-menstruum, but this is not correlated in the literature with self-reported pre-menstrual tension (d'Orbán & Dalton, 1980). What evidence there is suggests that hormonal changes may be a trigger for violence in vulnerable women.

Evolution of secure mental health services for women

Traditionally the needs of women, who have always represented a minority in prison and secure hospital settings, tended to be overlooked. The 1970s was characterised by a narrow focus on psychopathology, whereas more recent policy recognises that the mental health needs of women in relation to their offending must be addressed in tandem with their broader mental health needs. Women offenders typically serve shorter sentences than men, therefore bridging the gap between custodial settings and the community presents a challenge that requires flexibility from services in terms of responsivity and liaison. *Into the Mainstream* (Department of Health, 2000) highlighted the failure of services to recognise and address the mental health needs of female offenders.

Historically, women in secure mental health services were treated within predominantly male services, yet recent service developments have been far more focused on meeting the specific needs of women. The contraction of the UK high secure estate in the early 2000s, including the creation of a single national women's high secure service at Rampton Hospital, gave rise to the development of women's enhanced medium secure services in London, Leicester and Manchester and an expansion in the women's medium secure estate. This segregation of services gave rise to an ongoing debate about whether single-gender provision of this kind reduces the risk of victimisation of women by peers in hospital in addition to providing for their other specific needs (Mezey *et al*, 2005).

The profile of women within secure mental health services remains such that they are a significant minority, approximately 15% of all individuals; still, their numbers have been steadily rising. It is also notable that length of stay for women in secure services has typically been 3 times longer than for their male counterparts and 4 times longer than for other women in prison (Long *et al*, 2008; Blattner & Dolan, 2009).

Treatment models for women in secure mental health services have developed greatly during recent years, recognising the importance of several key principles. The need for privacy, a safe place to receive treatment and recover and a need to take account of women's diverse roles are important considerations in the planning of secure services. The work of organisations such as the Royal College of Psychiatrists' Quality Network has ensured that gender-informed standards for secure services for women have been mandated within medium security for some years. Similar initiatives have more recently emerged to guide the development of low secure services.

Practical aspects of secure care provision for women

A coherent philosophy of care is important, with attachment-focused models predominating, recognising the diagnostic profile of this group. Women typically require lower levels of perimeter security but higher levels of relational security than men. On the whole, psychological treatment models and nursing care must therefore be designed to enhance relational security within such settings for women and to take account of their histories of trauma, personality difficulties and substance misuse.

The gender make-up of the staff team, staff training and awareness are crucial in terms of providing a therapeutic environment. Care pathways are of fundamental importance to women in terms of their recovery, especially considering the challenges presented by their sociocultural vulnerability.

The role of the social worker as part of the multidisciplinary team, thus supporting women in maintaining their many roles and facilitating child visiting is important, as is growing expertise in gender-informed risk assessment, for example with the advent of HCR-20 for women (de Vogel *et al*, 2012).

Perhaps unsurprisingly given the high levels of comorbidity, the use of medication tends to be high in this group. One study estimated that 97% of women in secure settings were prescribed antipsychotics and 91% antidepressants (Bland *et al*, 1999). Gender issues in prescribing must be taken into account. Our own research findings confirm that women in secure services as a high-risk group in terms of self-harm and aggression benefit from a problem-based approach whereby pharmacotherapy is targeted at symptom clusters. A degree of emotional and behavioural stability achieved in this way allows women to engage in the psychosocial treatment necessary for their recovery. In some cases, novel approaches such as the use of clozapine in borderline personality disorder allow the most risky and complex groups of women with high levels of need and challenging behaviour, who have often experienced repeated placement failures, to progress therapeutically (Frogley *et al*, 2013).

A structured therapeutic environment, where boundaries and expectations are clear, addresses attachment issues and facilitates the necessary relational security. Extra-care and low-stimulus areas can provide a very helpful alternative to seclusion for women in secure settings.

Dialectical behaviour therapy (DBT) and cognitive–behavioural therapy (CBT) or cognitive analytic therapy (CAT) form the basis of psychological treatment approaches in many secure services for women. This reflects the high rates of comorbid personality disorder in this population. Replacing maladaptive patterns of cognition, affective response and behaviour with helpful and adaptive coping skills allows women to progress to less secure settings where the therapeutic focus can place an increasing emphasis on supporting women in their efforts to be more responsible and self-reliant as they rehabilitate.

Specific offence-related therapeutic work tends to be integrated with psychosocial treatment as a whole, recognising the fact that as a group women's mental health needs are often a fundamental part of their offending patterns, rather than always a necessary focus for separate therapeutic endeavours. Having said this, ever more sophisticated gender-specific risk assessment tools now allow us to specifically identify risk factors for future offending and address these.

Conclusions

Despite all of the positive developments, many based on sound evidence relating to the needs of mentally disordered women offenders, it remains the case that there are some significant ongoing gaps in provision which hamper the progress of women. Notably, provision of good in-reach services to women's prisons remains patchy geographically and suicides within the women's prison estate remain a regular occurrence. The gap between prison and community-based services continues to allow a significant proportion of women to become 'revolving-door' inmates. Geographic inequalities persist in the provision of medium and low secure services. This is further complicated by the existing commissioning arrangements for secure care for women, which create an artificial barrier between high, medium and low secure provision. As a result, there is widespread disparity in the outcomes for women in secure services around the country. Also, the development of step-down services from secure care has not kept pace with other service developments in this sector, giving rise to a silting up of secure services and excessive lengths of stay for too many women in secure settings. Finally, until more of an emphasis is placed by policy makers on the psychosocial antecedents of mental disorder and offending among women, they are likely to remain a disproportionately complex and challenging group within secure mental health services.

References

Abel, K.M., Drake, R. & Goldstein, J.M. (2010) Sex differences in schizophrenia. *International Review of Psychiatry*, **22**, 417–28.

Adshead, G. (1998) Psychiatric staff as attachment figures: understanding management problems in psychiatric services in the light of attachment theory. *British Journal of Psychiatry*, **172**, 64–69.

Angst, J., Gamma, A., Gastpar, M., *et al* (2002) Gender differences in depression: epidemiological findings from the European Depression I and II Studies. *European Archives of Psychiatry and Clinical Neuroscience*, **252**, 201–209.

Bangasser, D.A. (2013) Sex differences in stress-related receptors: 'micro' differences with 'macro' implications for mood and anxiety disorders. *Biological Sex Differences*, **4**, 2.

Bartlett, A. (1993) Rhetoric and reality: what do we know about English special hospitals? *International Journal of Law and Psychiatry*, **16**, 27–51.

Bartlett, A. (2007) Women in prison: concepts, clinical issues and care delivery. *Psychiatry*, **6**, 444–448.

Bland, J., Mezey, G.C. & Dolan, B. (1999) Special women, special needs: a descriptive study of female special hospital patients. *Journal of Forensic Psychiatry*, **10**, 34–45.

Blattner, R. & Dolan, M. (2009) Outcome of high security patients admitted to a medium secure unit: the Edenfield Centre study. *Medicine Science and the Law*, **49**, 247–256.

Bouchard, S., Sabourin, S., Lussier, Y., *et al* (2009) Relationship quality and stability in couples when one partner suffers from borderline personality disorder. *Journal of Marital and Family Therapy*, **35**, 446–455.

Bowlby, J. (1978) Attachment theory and its therapeutic implications. *Adolescent Psychiatry*, **6**, 5–33.

Canetto, S.S. & Sakinofsky, I. (1998) The gender paradox in suicide. *Suicide and Life Threatening Behaviour*, **28**, 1–23.

Chowdhary, N. & Patel, V. (2008) The effect of spousal violence on women's health: findings from the Stree Arogya Shodh in Goa, India. *Journal of Postgraduate Medicine*, **54**, 306–312.

Clarkin, J.F. & Posner, M. (2005) Defining the mechanisms of borderline personality disorder. *Psychopathology*, **38**, 56–63.

Coid, J. (2007) A third of men and 15% of women discharged from medium secure forensic psychiatry services in the UK re-offend. *Evidence-Based Mental Health*, **10**, 128.

Cook, B.M. & Woolley, C.S. (2005) Gonadal hormone modulation of dendrites in the mammalian CNS. *Journal of Neurobiology*, **64**, 34–46.

Corston, J. (2007) *The Corston Report: A Report by Baroness Jean Corston of a Review of Women with Particular Vulnerabilities in the Criminal Justice System*. Home Office.

Department of Health (2000) *Women's Mental Health: Into the Mainstream*. Department of Health.

Department of Health (2006) *Women at Risk: The Mental Health of Women in Contact with the Criminal Justice System*. Department of Health.

de Vogel, V., de Vries Robbe, M., van Kalmhout, W., *et al* (2012) Risicotaxatie van geweld bij vrouwen: ontwikkeling van de 'Female Additional Manual' (FAM) [Risk assessment of violent women: development of the 'Female Additional Manual' (FAM)]. *Tijdschrift voor Psychiatrie*, **54**, 329–338.

Diflorio, A. & Jones, I. (2010) Is sex important? Gender differences in bipolar disorder. *International Review of Psychiatry*, **22**, 437–452.

Dillon G., Hussain, R., Loxton, D., *et al* (2013) Mental and physical health and intimate partner violence against women: a review of the literature. *International Journal of Family Medicine*, article ID: 313909.

Dolan, M. & Vollm, B. (2009) Antisocial personality disorder and psychopathy in women: a literature review on the reliability and validity of assessment instruments. *International Journal of Law and Psychiatry*, **32**, 2–9.

d'Orbán, P.T. (1991) Women, violent crime and the menstrual cycle. *Medicine, Science and the Law*, **31**, 183.

d'Orbán, P.T. & Dalton, J. (1980) Violent crime and the menstrual cycle. *Psychological Medicine*, **10**, 353–359.

Eronen, M., Hakola, P. & Tiihonen, J. (1996) Mental disorders and homicidal behavior in Finland. *Archives of General Psychiatry*, **53**, 497–501.

Fazel S., Bains, P. & Doll, H. (2006) Substance abuse and dependence in prisoners: a systematic review. *Addiction*, **101**, 181–191.

Flannery, R.B. Jr. (2002) Repetitively assaultive psychiatric patients: review of published findings, 1978–2001. *Psychiatry Questions*, **73**, 229–237.

Frogley, C., Anagnostakis, K., Mitchell, S., *et al* (2013) Retrospective study of clozapine in borderline personality disorder. *Annals of Clinical Psychiatry*, **25**, 125–134.

GENACIS Project Final Report (2005) *Gender, Culture and Alcohol Problems: A Multinational Study*. Berlin Institute of Medical Informatics.

Golding, J.M. (1999) Intimate partner violence is a risk factor for mental disorders: a meta-analysis. *Journal of Family Violence*, **14**, 99–132.

Handa, R.J., Burgess, L.H., Kerr, J.E., *et al* (1994) Gonadal steroid hormone receptors and sex differences in the hypothalamo-pituitary adrenal axis. *Hormones and Behaviour*, **28**, 464–476.

Harris, F., Hek, G. & Condon, l. (2007) Health needs of prisoners in England and Wales: the implications for prison healthcare of gender, age and ethnicity. *Health and Social Care in the Community*, **15**, 56–66.

Hayes, E., Gavrilidis, E. & Kulkarni, J. (2012) The role of oestrogen and other hormones in the pathophysiology and treatment of schizophrenia. *Schizophrenia Research Treatment*, article ID: 540273.

Henning, K., Jones, A. & Holdford, R. (2003) Treatment needs of women arrested for domestic violence: a comparison with male offenders. *Journal of Interpersonal Violence*, **18**, 839–856.

Herpertz-Dahlmann, B., Seitz, J. & Konrad, K. (2011) Aetiology of anorexia nervosa: from a 'psychosomatic family model' to a neuropsychiatric disorder? *European Archives of Psychiatry and Clinical Neuroscience*, **261** (suppl. 2), S177–181.

Judd, F., Komiti, A. & Jackson, H. (2008) How does being female assist help seeking for mental health problems? *Australian and New Zealand Journal of Psychiatry*, **42**, 24–29.

Lewis, C.F. (2010) Childhood antecedents of adult violent offending in a group of female felons. *Behaviour Science and Law*, **28**, 224–234.

Long, C., Fulton, B. & Hollin, C. (2008) The development of a 'best practice' service for women in a medium-secure psychiatric setting: treatment components and evaluation. *Clinical Psychology and Psychotherapy*, **15**, 304–319.

Magdol, L., Moffitt, T.E., Caspi, A., *et al* (1997) Gender differences in partner violence in a birth cohort of 21-year-olds: bridging the gap between clinical and epidemiological approaches. *Journal of Consultation in Clinical Psychology*, **65**, 68–78.

Malacova, E., Butler, T., Yap, L., *et al* (2012) Sexual coercion prior to imprisonment: prevalence, demographic and behavioural correlates. *International Journal of STD and AIDS*, **23**, 533–539.

Messer, J., Maughan, B., Quinton, D., *et al* (2004) Precursors and correlates of criminal behaviour in women. *Criminal Behaviour and Mental Health*, **14**, 82–107.

Mezey, G., Hassell, Y. & Bartlett, A. (2005) Safety of women in mixed-sex and single-sex medium secure units: staff and patient perceptions. *British Journal of Psychiatry*, **187**, 579–582.

Ministry of Justice (2007) *Criminal Statistics 2006: England and Wales*. Ministry of Justice.

Ministry of Justice (2011*a*) *Criminal Justice Statistics: England and Wales 2010 (Sentencing Tables A5.5)*. Ministry of Justice.

Ministry of Justice (2011*b*) *Proven Reoffending Statistics*. Quarterly Bulletin, January to December 2009, England and Wales, p. 17. Ministry of Justice.

Mumford, D.B. & Whitehouse, A.M. (1988) Increased prevalence of bulimia nervosa among Asian schoolgirls. *BMJ*, **297**, 718.

National Comorbidity Survey (2005) *Lifetime Prevalence of DSM-IV/WMH-CIDI Disorders by Sex and Cohort*. NCS-R Update July 2007. Available at http://www.hcp.med.harvard.edu/ncs/ (accessed 30 March 2015).

Nestor, P.G. (2002) Mental disorder and violence: personality dimensions and clinical features. *American Journal of Psychiatry*, **159**, 1973–1978.

O'Brien, M., Mortimer, L., Singleton, N., *et al* (2003) Psychiatric morbidity among women prisoners in England and Wales. *International Review of Psychiatry*, **15**, 153–157.

Pau, K.Y. (2000) Oestrogen upregulates noradrenalin release in the mediobasal hypothalamus and tyrosine hydroxylase gene expression in the brain stem of ovariectomized rhesus macaques. *Journal of Neuroendocrinology*, **12**, 899–909.

Pilgrim, D. (2010) Mind the gender gap: mental health in a post feminist context. In *Oxford Textbook of Women and Mental Health* (ed. D. Kohen), pp. 7–16. Oxford University Press.

Putkonen, H., Komulainen, E.J., Virkkunen, M., *et al* (2003) Risk of repeat offending among violent female offenders with psychotic and personality disorders. *American Journal of Psychiatry*, **160**, 947–951.

Rubinow, D.R., Schmidt, P.J., Roca, C.A., *et al* (2002) Gonadal hormones and behavior in women: concentrations vs context. In *Hormones, Brain and Behavior* (ed. D.W. Pfaff), pp. 37–73. Academic Press.

Schmidt, R., Kienbacher, E., Benke, T., *et al* (2008) Sex differences in Alzheimer's disease. *Neuropsychiatry*, **22**, 1–15.

Smink, F.R., van Hoeken, D. & Hoek, H.W. (2012) Epidemiology of eating disorders: incidence, prevalence and mortality rates. *Current Psychiatry Reports*, **14**, 406–414.

Stuart, G.L., Moore, T.M., Gordon, K.C., *et al* (2006) Psychopathology in women arrested for domestic violence. *Journal of Interpersonal Violence*, **21**, 376–389.

Tasca, G. A., Ritchie, K. & Balfour, L. (2011) Implications of attachment theory and research for the assessment and treatment of eating disorders. *Psychotherapy (Chic)*, **48**, 249–259.

Thornton, A.J.V., Graham-Kevan, N. & Archer, J. (2010) Adaptive and maladaptive personality traits as predictors of violent and nonviolent offending behavior in men and women. *Aggressive Behaviour*, **36**, 177–186.

United Nations Population Fund (2005) *State of the World Population 2005: The Promise of Equality: Gender Equity*. Reproductive Health and the Millenium Development Goals. UNFPA.

Uppal, G. & McMurran, M. (2009) Recorded incidents in a high-secure hospital: a descriptive analysis. *Criminal Behaviour and Mental Health*, **19**, 265–276.

van der Kolk, B.A. (2005) Disorders of extreme stress: the empirical foundations of a complex adaptation to trauma. *Journal of Traumatic Stress*, **18**, 389.

van der Kolk, B.A., Pelcovitz, D., Roth, S., *et al* (1996) Dissociation, somatization, and affect dysregulation: the complexity of adaptation of trauma. *American Journal of Psychiatry*, **153** (suppl. 7), S83–93.

van IJzendoorn, M.H., Feldbrugge, J.T. & Derks, F.C. (1997) Attachment representations of personality-disordered criminal offenders. *American Journal of Orthopsychiatry*, **67**, 449–459.

Wang, J., Fick, G., Adair, C., *et al* (2007) Gender specific correlates of stigma toward depression in a Canadian general population sample. *Journal of Affective Disorders*, **103**, 91–97.

Warren, J.I., Burnette, M., South, S.C., *et al* (2002) Personality disorders and violence among female prison inmates. *Journal of the American Academy of Psychiatry & the Law*, **30**, 502–509.

Weizmann-Henelius, G. (2006) Violent female perpetrators in finland: personality and life events. *Nordic Psychology*, **58**, 280–297.

Weizmann-Henelius, G., Putkonen, H., Naukkarinen, H., *et al* (2009) Intoxication and violent women. *Archives of Women's Mental Health*, **12**, 15–25.

CHAPTER 8

Offenders with intellectual disability in secure services and the criminal justice system

Eddie Chaplin and Jane McCarthy

Introduction

This chapter provides an introduction to and offers an overview of the current evidence base relating to offenders with intellectual disability. In particular, it discusses clinical presentation, risk assessment, clinical interventions and service provision for this group.

Definition and terminology

Although the term 'mental retardation' is still used as a diagnostic term in the *International Classification of Diseases* (ICD-10; World Health Organization, 1992), it is perceived to be offensive to people with intellectual disability and has been replaced in policy, administrative and legislative forums in many countries by 'intellectual disability' (Salvador-Carulla *et al*, 2011). The term mental retardation will be updated to intellectual developmental disorders in the ICD-11 manual currently being revised. Often terminology to describe this group changes according to the context. For example, intellectual disability is still often substituted for learning disabilities in the UK by both services and user groups and is the term used in the Mental Health Act. This chapter will use the term intellectual disability, which is defined as impairments in social and intellectual functioning that occur during the developmental period (Department of Health, 2001).

The Mental Health Act 1983 for England and Wales sets out the law for the assessment and treatment of people with mental disorder and the criteria for compulsory action to be taken where the person is a risk to themselves or others, while safeguarding the individual. This includes civil detention and disposal or transfer to healthcare via the courts as a sentence or pre-sentencing assessment. The Act also legislates on appropriate aftercare, treatment and consent, safeguards, advocacy and appeals. The definition of mental disorder under the Act has been updated and replaced by a wider definition in the 2007 amendments to 'any disorder or disability of the mind'. This does not include intellectual disability *per se*. The Act is clear that people with intellectual disability shall not be considered 'to be suffering from mental disorder' and therefore cannot be considered for detention for assessment and/or treatment under the Act simply as a result of their intellectual disability, unless the disability is associated with abnormally aggressive or seriously irresponsible conduct.

Epidemiology of intellectual disability and offending

The World Health Organization (WHO) estimates the worldwide prevalence of intellectual disability at around 3% (World Health Organization, 2001). In England, the figure is 1.2 million for mild to moderate intellectual disability and 210 000 for severe to profound intellectual disability using a population estimate of 2.5% (Department of Health, 2001). Severe and profound intellectual disability is uniformly distributed geographically, irrespective of socioeconomic status, whereas mild intellectual disability is influenced by socioeconomic disadvantage and increases in urban areas (Department of Health, 2001).

The prevalence rates of offending reported for people with intellectual disability are often contradictory. In the early 20th century there was a view that lower cognitive ability led to criminal behaviour. Early positivist theory aimed to offer a scientific rationale for criminality by studying a person's physical, genetic and psychological presentation. The assumption was that individuals who committed offences were thought to be biologically different to non-offenders (Goddard, 1912, 1914, 1920; Goring, 1913 reprinted 1972; Beirne, 1988). This early research was hugely confounded by the measures of cognitive ability used and limited access to education of those studied.

In modern times, studies of offenders with intellectual disability have often been limited by their methodology, for example inconsistent definitions of offending behaviour, challenging behaviour, antisocial behaviour, the definition of impaired intellectual functioning and the research setting. However, there have been wider population studies which have provided an insight into the role of impaired cognitive ability as a risk factor for offending behaviour. A prospective follow-up study of 411 working-class boys born in 1953 and living in south London, examined the cognitive abilities, personal attainment and a number of other variables to offending. Of the 30% of boys convicted of a criminal offence before the age of 32, those convicted were more likely to have a number of characteristics, including intellectual impairment, poorer backgrounds, poorer schooling and lower academic achievement. This group also showed signs of neurodevelopmental disability, with more symptoms of hyperactivity and impulsivity. They were also more likely to come from homes where the parents had a history of conviction, especially the father. The characteristics of future 'chronic offenders' enabled the prediction of future criminality in the boys from the age of 8–10 years (West & Farrington, 1973; Farrington, 1995).

Hodgins (1992), having conducted a retrospective analysis of the 1953 Swedish birth cohort study of 15 117 people, of which 192 had intellectual disability, reported that men with intellectual disability were three times more likely to offend, while women were four times more likely to offend. In terms of violent offences the rates for men increased to 5.5, with females nearly 25 times more likely to offend, although this was lower than for women with a mental disorder (nearly 28 times more likely) or those with substance misuse (nearly 55 times more likely).

In both the studies by West & Farrington (1973) and Hodgins (1992), the groups with impaired cognitive abilities would not necessarily meet current diagnostic criteria for intellectual disability using international classification systems, but the studies do illustrate that the link between IQ and offending is robust. Impaired cognitive ability is one of many biopsychosocial factors linked to offending behaviour; more overt environmental ones include familial influences such as poor child rearing and social influences such as socioeconomic deprivation, peer and community factors (Farrington, 1995).

Reported rates of offending behaviour by people with intellectual disability vary between 40 and 70%. This variation is seen in offence-specific estimates; for example, Gross (1985) found that between 21 and 50% of offenders with intellectual disability had committed a sex offence. The belief that sex offences are over-represented in people with intellectual disability has been a point of debate and was challenged by Gilby et al (1989), who found no evidence to suggest either under- or over-representation of people with intellectual disability as sex offenders. Hayes (1991) reported that in a New South Wales prison population, 3.7% of offenders with intellectual disability had committed a sexual offence, compared with 4% of offenders without. In a study of 2286 male sex offenders and paraphiliacs and 241 non-sex offender controls from a university psychiatric hospital and private clinic database, it was reported that intellectual disability was not over-represented among sex offenders and paraphiliacs in either general or offence-specific subgroups (Langevin & Curnoe, 2008). With a lack of prevalence studies it is likely that biased samples have contributed to the assumption that people with intellectual disability are often reported as over-represented as sex offenders.

Prevalence rates of violence for people with intellectual disability have been reported as between 20 and 60% across community and in-patient settings (Taylor, 2002). Prevalence rates can also be examined from another perspective: 'which offenders have intellectual disability and which people will offend' (McBrien, 2003). However, a lack of controlled studies involving offenders with and without intellectual disability make this direct comparison difficult (Taylor & Lindsay, 2010). Gray et al (2007) compared a group with intellectual disability comprising 118 (81.4%) men and 27 (18.6%) women, and a group without intellectual disability comprising 843 (85.6%) men and 153 (15.4%) women. The first group was reconvicted at a significantly lower rate, with a reconviction rate for violent offences after

2 years at 4.8%, compared with 11.2% in the second group, whereas for general offences the rate of reconviction was 9.7% for the first and 18.7% for the second group.

Community populations

There is a geographical disparity in the rates of reported offending behaviour in people with intellectual disability. For example, in Cambridge, UK, in a community sample of 385 individuals with intellectual disability in residential homes or attending day services, 2% (7 people) had police involvement in the preceding year, although none were prosecuted and only one person was cautioned (Lyall et al, 1995). Whereas in London, UK it was reported that from 180 people with intellectual disability identified from two service providers, 9% (17 people) were involved with the police in the past 12 months, more than half of whom (9 people) had been arrested, received a caution, appeared in court or been convicted (McNulty et al, 1995). Of 1326 adults known to intellectual disability services in south-west England, McBrien et al (2003) found that 7% came into contact with the criminal justice system, with 3% having a conviction and 0.8% serving a current sentence.

In many areas of the UK, community services are still poorly developed for violent offenders with intellectual disability. Wheeler et al (2009) undertook a study of 237 people referred to community intellectual disability services (CLDT): 49 had prior contact with the criminal justice system, while the other 188 were referred to the CLDT due to antisocial behaviour and had no criminal justice system contact. The referral rates represented 3.8% of the known adult intellectual disability population. Although most of the offender group had mild intellectual disability, this was not a statistically significant predictor of contact with the criminal justice system.

Prison population

In a review of 12 000 prisoners with intellectual disability in studies from England, Wales, Australia, New Zealand and Dubai, prevalence rates for intellectual disability ranged from 0 to 2.9%, with most studies reporting between 0.5 and 1.5%. In two studies where basic screening techniques were used, rates increased from 2.6 to 11.2%, with a pooled prevalence of screen positive cases of 6.1% (Fazel et al, 2008). In line with No One Knows (a UK-wide programme led by the Prison Reform Trust designed to explore the prevalence, needs and experiences of people with learning difficulties and intellectual disability), Talbot and colleagues (Talbot & Riley, 2007; Talbot, 2009) reported 7% of prisoners having an IQ of less than 70, with a further 25% having an IQ of less than 80. It is worth remembering that screening studies by nature are over-inclusive and report inflated rates of a disorder (Fazel et al, 2008). The majority of those screened not meeting the diagnostic criteria for intellectual disability but reaching the screening threshold will still have a degree of cognitive and social impairment and are classified as having a borderline intellectual functioning. This group is often characterised by similar unrecognised or unmet needs and vulnerability, but will often not meet eligibility criteria for health and social care services in the wider community.

An estimated 3% of prisoners who die by suicide have a primary diagnosis of intellectual disability (Shaw *et al*, 2003). In Victoria, Australia, a sample of 102 prisoners with intellectual disability was compared with a random sample of 244 prisoners. Both groups had been released from custody over the same time period. The study reported that intellectual disability was not overrepresented but prisoners with intellectual disability experienced difficulties relating to future release, for example moving to a minimum security setting, with the majority being classified as 'medium security' or getting parole on the date they were first eligible to apply (Holland & Persson, 2011). They were less likely than prisoners without intellectual disability to be sentenced on reception to prison (45% *v.* 56% respectively), although they were also more likely to have prior involvement with the criminal justice system and were said to have a higher risk of reoffending.

The true prevalence from these studies is therefore very difficult to determine for a number of reasons. These range from the definition of intellectual disability, as those with borderline intellectual functioning are often included, how crime and alleged crime is reported and managed, and geographical and individual variation in service provision and referral criteria. Issues of social deprivation, lack of employment, poverty, isolation and other factors, independently associated with intellectual disability and criminality, serve only to make any association or correlation between the two even less clear (Harding *et al*, 2009).

In summary, people with intellectual disability have lower rates of reconviction than those without. They form a small proportion of the prison population, but when individuals with borderline intellectual functioning are included they account for nearly a quarter of prisoners. When looking at community samples of adults in contact with intellectual disability services the prevalence rate for offending behaviour is between 2 and 7%.

Assessment and clinical presentation of intellectual disability and offending

The assessment of people with intellectual disability must be undertaken with the aim of reaching a multidisciplinary diagnostic formulation to include management of risk behaviours and therapeutic need. Diagnosis of intellectual disability should be confirmed by standardised assessments of IQ and adaptive functioning. People with intellectual disability who offend may present with a number of comorbid conditions such as mental illness and autism spectrum disorders. Offending by people with autism spectrum disorder is an under-researched area in spite of feelings that it should be given a higher priority for some time (O'Brien, 2002). For further details on the assessment of people with an autism spectrum disorder please refer to Chapter 10, 'Secure care for people with autism spectrum disorder'.

To assist the identification of mental illness, the Royal College of Psychiatrists developed the *Diagnostic Criteria for Psychiatric Disorders for Use with Adults with Learning Disabilities/Mental Retardation* (DC-LD) (Royal College of Psychiatrists, 2001), and Fletcher *et al* (2007) the *Diagnostic Manual – Intellectual Disability* (DM-ID). This was considered necessary owing to the often complex picture of mental illness in people with intellectual disability linked to atypical presentation and symptomatic heterogeneity (Kerker *et al*, 2004). Any link between diagnoses, symptoms, psychopathology and offending is poorly understood, with studies only recently looking at the link, for example, between attention-deficit hyperactivity disorder (ADHD) and conduct disorder and offending (Lindsay *et al*, 2010). There is a lack of matched studies that contrast offender and non-offender intellectual disability groups with mental health needs. A short review of comorbid mental illness in those with intellectual disability across settings (Hobson & Rose, 2008) and a study on substance misuse in a prison setting (Klimecki *et al*, 1994) both suggest that those with comorbid conditions may be at increased risk of offending. In a random sample of 3563 prisoners in England and Wales (total prison population 61944), 170 (4%) of the sample had intellectual disability as defined by an estimated IQ of less than 65, using the Quick Test (Ammons & Ammons, 1962) and an education level below GCSE. The intellectual disability group showed a significantly higher prevalence of probable psychosis, attempted suicide and cannabis use. The group were also characterised as more likely to be on remand, while those not on remand were more likely to receive shorter sentences (Hassiotis *et al*, 2011).

Offenders with intellectual disability share psychosocial characteristics with offenders without intellectual disability, such as being young, male, with high rates of substance misuse, antisocial behaviour, higher unemployment, poorer socioeconomic status and history of abuse (Day, 1988; Murphy *et al*, 1995; Barron *et al*, 2002). In a study of 477 people with intellectual disability referred across forensic service pathways for antisocial or offending behaviour, 35% (165 individuals), reported a history of abuse or neglect as a child and had displayed the same index behaviour previously, although for many it had not resulted in police involvement or action. Of the sample, 180 (38%) had previously been charged with at least one criminal offence, often with their first incident at a relatively young age (mean 15.1 years, s.d. 10.8 years).

A study by Holland *et al* (2002) described two groups of offenders. The first group were socially disadvantaged with mental health and substance misuse problems, not known to intellectual disability services, whereas the second group were more likely to be known to intellectual disability services and have challenging behaviour. The distinction between challenging behaviour and offending is not clear, such that criminal justice pathways allow professional discretion but risk inconsistent approaches to diversion, prosecution and sentencing.

Risk assessment

Risk assessment for mentally disordered offenders has developed over the past 40 years and the reported applicability/accuracy of using the established generic guides, such as the HCR-20 (Webster *et al*, 1997), has lessened the pressure to modify them for intellectual disability populations. Historically the introduction of risk assessment measures to support decision-making in clinical practice has been delayed because of worries over the role that cognitive impairments might play in the reliability and validity of results. In any case, the initial assessment must include developmental history, including childhood trauma, psychiatric assessment, history of substance misuse, assessment of the level of functioning, and history of offending and challenging behaviour, to both inform the assessment and to corroborate information.

There are now an increasing number of studies that have used risk assessment measures validated in general forensic samples (without intellectual disability) and that have demonstrated positive results. These include the Violence Risk Appraisal Guide (VRAG), applied in a community sample of 58 people with intellectual disability and a history of antisocial behaviour, where it was a good predictor of risk over an average follow-up of just over 15 months (Quinsey *et al*, 2004). In another study (Gray *et al*, 2007), using a case note analysis, it was reported that the HCR-20, at the point of discharge from medium secure services, was an effective predictor of violence in people with intellectual disability in spite of the longer spells between offending reported for this group. Lindsay *et al* (2008) evaluated the HCR-20, VRAG and Static-99 (www.static99.org), across three levels of in-patient security (high, medium and low) and community forensic services. Their case note review, supplemented by key workers' information, reported that the HCR-20 was a significant predictor across all levels of security, whereas the VRAG achieved significance in high security and community services. The Static-99 was predictive of sexual risk.

In a study of 73 offenders with intellectual disability with comorbidity (54.8% personality disorder, 28.8% psychotic disorder and 8% mood disorder) in the national high-secure hospital for England and Wales, 60 people were followed up for a year (Morrissey *et al*, 2007). The study found that the HCR-20 performed better than the Psychopathy Checklist – Revised (PCL-R; Hare, 2003) in predicting institutional aggression in people with intellectual disability during the 12 months following assessment. Previous research in an English medium secure unit had reported that the Psychopathy Checklist Screening Version (PCL-SV; Hart *et al*, 1995) was a good predictor of in-patient violence and added to the predictive validity of the VRAG and the historical scale of HCR-20 (Doyle *et al*, 2002). In their evaluation of the Rapid Risk Assessment for Sex Offence Recidivism (RRASOR; Hanson, 1997), Harris & Tough (2004) reported that the RRASORs predictors were equally valid for people with intellectual disability as for other offender populations. The literature thus far seems to suggest that the key to using these measures in practice is to beware of the limitations that they, not having been validated for people with intellectual disability *per se*, have (McGrath *et al*, 2007). However, it seems that those risk assessment guides that have at least moderate predictive accuracy with some intellectual disability offender groups, can be woven into existing assessment protocols in clinical settings to give a more reliable estimate of risk. There is little in the way of prospective or longitudinal studies for people with intellectual disability and the use of the risk assessment tools.

In terms of specialist sexual offending risk assessment in people with intellectual disability, Wilcox *et al* (2009) examined sexual recidivism using three sex offending-specific risk assessment instruments: the Static-99, Risk Matrix 2000 (RM 2000; Hanson & Thornton, 2000) and the RRASOR. From a sample of 27 sex offenders with intellectual disability, 30% (8 individuals) were reconvicted and the remainder were reported as offence free at 76-month follow-up, with the Static-99 outperforming the RM 2000 and the RRASOR in predicting sexual recidivism. An intellectual disability-specific sexual risk assessment instrument – the Assessment of Risk and Manageability of Intellectually Disabled Individuals who Offend – Sexually (ARMIDILO-S; Lofthouse *et al*, 2013) – has shown promising early results. A sample of 88 sex offenders was divided into two groups: those with special needs as defined with intellectual disability to borderline intellectual functioning (IQ 70–80) and those without. Both groups were reported to be convicted at the same rate. The ARMIDILO-S was the best predictor for sexual reconviction among the special needs group compared with the RRASOR, Risk Matrix 2000 – Sexual Violence (RM 2000-SV; Thornton *et al*, 2003), Sexual Violence Risk-20 (SVR-20; Boer *et al*, 1997), with the first two measures reported to be no better than chance for the special needs group (Blacker *et al*, 2011).

In spite of a growing evidence base there is variation in the use of these structured risk assessment tools but probably the most widely used in the intellectual disability population is the HCR-20 for prediction of violence.

Treatment programmes and secure care

In treating mentally disordered offenders with intellectual disability, the first stage is to address any mental health issues and how functioning deficits affect the individual in terms of behaviour and coping strategies. Best practice for the assessment and management of mental illness, such as psychosis, mood disorders and neurodevelopmental conditions (e.g. autism and attention-deficit hyperactivity disorder) is synthesised within current National Institute for Health and Care Excellence (NICE) guidelines in the UK. These are mostly developed with the general population in mind but in some cases offer specific comment about people with intellectual disability, as in the depression, personality disorder and autism guidelines. There is also national guidance on the management of challenging behaviour (Royal College of Psychiatrists *et al*, 2007). As well as the specific offence interventions for people with intellectual disability in secure care there are also a number of specific care models that offer broader therapeutic approaches. Morrissey *et al* (2012) describe the evaluation of a therapeutic community intervention for men with intellectual disability and personality disorder at a high secure hospital and noted an improvement in psychological functioning and reduction in seclusion hours in this interim 1-year follow-up study.

There are still questions of the long-term effectiveness of many of the treatment models used. For example, current specific interventions commonly delivered for offenders with intellectual disability include anger treatment, which assumes that anger is often an antecedent to violence. Thus interventions aimed at reducing anger form a theoretical basis for the treatment of violence (Taylor, 2002). Although the evidence is still limited, over 18 sessions of individual anger treatment participants achieved significantly lower anger scores on a number of measures compared with waiting list controls (Taylor *et al*, 2005). More recently, the SOTSEC-ID project (Sex Offender Treatment Services Collaborative – Intellectual Disabilities, 2010) reported on 13 groups, containing in total 46 men with mild to borderline intellectual disability with 'sexually abusive behaviour', who took part in a 1-year cognitive–behavioural therapy (CBT) group. Over the duration of the programme and 6 months post-intervention there were no non-sex offences committed by anyone in the group. Three men (6.5%) recorded 8 incidents of non-contact sexually abusive behaviour during the project or at 6-month follow-up, 8.7% ($n=4$ men) were responsible for 9 incidents of non-contact sexually abusive behaviours recorded and there were 2 incidents of contact sexually abusive behaviour recorded. Three of the four men who were involved in sexually abusive incidents at follow-up had a diagnosis of autism spectrum disorder as opposed to intellectual disability, which may suggest different treatment and monitoring needs between some of these diagnostic groups.

Firesetting

The risk of firesetting behaviour among people with intellectual disability is unclear. Like with sex offending, there is a historical assumption that it is overrepresented in people with intellectual disability. A study by (Lindsay *et al*, 2006) reported that arson was not overrepresented in people with intellectual disability during a 12-year follow-up of a community forensic service. There is little in the way of empirical research into firesetting in people with intellectual disability. In a study across three levels of security (community, low/medium and high), arson as an index offence ranged from 2.9% (2/69) to 21.4% (15/70), while a history of arson ranged from 11% (8/73) to 27.1% (19/70) (Hogue, 2006). In terms of treatment, there are a limited number of studies, most of which are not recent. The introduction of social skills training was compared with a control treatment designed to control for attention and expectancy of change on two groups of five male arsonists in a maximum security hospital. The second group contained people with borderline and mild intellectual disability, four of whom had comorbid mental disorder. Both groups received eight sessions of both treatments. The social skills training saw significant improvements not replicated by the control treatment, with no evidence of firesetting behaviour at 1-year follow-up (Rice & Chaplin, 1979). Other published works on treatment have been based on CBT. Clare *et al* (1992) reported a single case study of a young man's assessment and treatment of firesetting using a CBT model. This is an approach that has since been modified for use within group programmes and has been reported in a case series of six female firesetters, which have reported good responses in terms of general improvement in clinical measures related to motivations for firesetting behaviour and no reports of firesetting 2 years following completion of the programme (Taylor *et al*, 2006). Using a similar approach in a mixed-gender group of 14 firesetters in low secure services aimed to reduce fire interest and attitudes, significant improvements were noted on the fire-specific measures (Taylor *et al*, 2002).

Services and outcomes

Service provision for people with intellectual disability who offend or have challenging behaviour varies both nationally and internationally and is influenced by a number of complex factors. In the UK, the 'Butler report' (Home Office & Department of Health, 1975) introduced medium secure services, although their development for people with intellectual disability was slow. The 'Reed report' (Department of Health & Home Office, 1992), which reviewed health and social services for mentally disordered offenders, highlighted the needs of the intellectual disability group and advocated a philosophy of least restrictive practice, as do the two Mansell reports (1992, 2007), which also outline best practice guidance for developing and managing services for people with intellectual disability and challenging behaviour. Both Mansell reports advocated care within community settings wherever possible, with the development and expansion of person-centred services. Services nationally have developed but all too often have been in the context of disjointed or non-existent care pathways. A number of services characterised by poor and unacceptable standards have been highlighted by recent inquiries (Commision for Healthcare Audit and Inspection, 2006; Healthcare Commission, 2007; Department of Health, 2012).

Mental healthcare for people with intellectual disability in the UK is provided through generic adult and specialist intellectual disability services. Specialist in-patient units will generally offer open and locked beds, although the inappropriate use and overuse of assessment and treatment services, instead of structured and supportive community services, is an issue highlighted in the inquiries referenced above. Secure in-patient services for people with intellectual disability are divided into three levels of security in the UK. High secure care for people with intellectual disability is provided at the national centre at Rampton Hospital, with medium and low secure care provided throughout the country by both National Health Service (NHS) and independent sector providers. Low secure services for people with intellectual disability in practice accept both offenders and non-offenders, whereas medium and high secure services will typically be dominated by offenders. There are no records of current total numbers using secure intellectual disability provision. A scoping exercise of secure services in 2009 (Alexander *et al*, 2011) estimated the number of people with intellectual disability in England in secure accommodation provided by the NHS and the independent sector to be: high secure 48 (NHS 100%), medium secure 414 (NHS 210 (50.7%), independent sector 204 (49.3%)) and low secure 1356 (NHS 342 (25.2%), independent sector 1014 (74.8%)). People with intellectual disability who need high security are characterised by higher treatment needs, younger age, recent violent conduct and high-profile index offence (Thomas *et al*, 2004).

Alexander *et al* (2006) examined outcomes from an English regional medium secure unit during two phases over a 12-year period, 1987 to 1993 and 1994 to 2000. They found that the patient characteristics of the two cohorts differed over time. This included higher rates of a number of historical factors for cohort 1: higher rates of previous hospital admissions (93% *v.* 79%), forensic history (74% *v.* 31%) and admission from prison (37% *v.* 19%). In cohort 2, a higher proportion were admitted on civil sections (53% *v.* 26%), in spite of a reported pattern of similar index offences between the two cohorts. Personality disorder, a history of theft or burglary, and young age increased the risk of reconviction. Re-admissions were associated with offending-type behaviours rather than any clinical diagnosis.

A survey of mental health and intellectual disability in low secure units in England (20 low secure services, 12 mental health units and 8 intellectual disability units) found that intellectual disability units tended to be less secure, used older buildings, had fewer beds and had a greater proportion of female staff than mental health units. This lack of purpose-built provision for people with intellectual disability gave rise to a number of concerns over observation and security (Beer *et al*, 2005). The same study found from staff interviews that a third of the patients detained were felt to be in the wrong level of security, with the vast majority in conditions of greater security than perceived necessary.

A 14-year evaluation of a UK national low secure mixed-gender service in south-east London (Reed *et al*, 2004) contrasted offenders (45 individuals) with non-offenders (41 individuals) who had been admitted and discharged from the service. The offender group was defined as those detained under criminal sections of the Mental Health Act or on probation order during the admission, whereas the non-offender group was detained under civil sections and lacked a history of custodial sentences or high secure admission. The demographic and clinical profiles between the two groups did not differ apart from a higher rate of personality disorder in the offender group. There were no significant differences between the groups for incidents of challenging behaviour, violence towards property, sexual assault and firesetting during the study. While in-patients, the study reported that the non-offenders showed increased 'challenging behaviour' in terms of assaults on staff and other patients and used objects as weapons significantly more frequently, whereas the offender group had a higher rate of self-injurious behaviour. The study also noted that non-offenders were more often restrained and relocated, although seclusion rates did not differ. The offender group was less likely to be admitted from the community and subsequently more likely to be discharged to non-community placements.

A lack of local or regional specialist services offering a high degree of structure and secure services for people with intellectual disability in some areas of the country has given rise to out-of-area placements (Chaplin *et al*, 2010; Hall *et al*, 2011). Chaplin and colleagues contrasted the characteristics of 44 people with intellectual disability placed out of area with those placed locally. They suggested that what precipitated and then maintained these placements were violence against the person and persistent aggressiveness by the patient with intellectual disability aimed towards others and the environment at the obvious cost of greater isolation from their families and distance from home.

In terms of community outcomes, Lindsay *et al* (2006) reported a 12-year follow-up of a community forensic intellectual disability service in Scotland. The study focused on three groups: 121 male sex offenders, 105 other male offenders and 21 female offenders. Average IQ for the groups was between 64.9 and 67.5. The sex offenders were more likely to be older than the other groups and characterised by relationship and daily living skills problems. A demographic shift was found over time, as people who were recruited later into the study tended to be younger than those in earlier cohorts. There were significant differences in the rates of reoffending between groups (59% for male offenders, compared with 23% for male sex offenders and 19% for female offenders) over 12 years.

Services for women with intellectual disability

Women's secure services have developed from mainstream forensic and intellectual disability service models (Beber, 2012). Female intellectual disability offending rates are comparable with those of the general population (Lindsay *et al*, 2006). However, Wheeler *et al* (2009) found the rate of referrals for women with intellectual disability for offending and antisocial behaviour at nearly 40%, which was nearer to the rate of male referrals at just over 60% and greater than in the general offending literature relating to women. The sample was unusual in that it uncovered women with intellectual disability and offences/convictions against children such as neglect and cruelty. The reasons for this are unclear and there is a danger that a group of women with intellectual disability are being criminalised as a result of their poor reactions to stress and being unable to cope with a dependant without adequate support and/or monitoring. A review of female admissions to one of three national high secure hospitals over a 6-month period in 1994 reported that 26% had borderline intellectual disability (Bland *et al*, 1999). Since then women's high secure services have evolved principally to what is now termed enhanced medium secure facilities, and so like the remainder of women who offend, women with intellectual disability are generally managed at lower levels of security than men.

Conclusions

The move towards treatment and care for people with intellectual disability being delivered in the least restrictive environments and the closure of long-term institutions has seen the development of more community provision for this group, albeit inconsistent and fragmented in many areas. A recent report of abuse in secure services has again questioned the appropriateness of such services for people with intellectual disability (Department of Health, 2012). Research into offenders with intellectual disability has suffered from wide methodological disparities, making generalisation difficult, but there is emerging evidence on the prevalence across the criminal justice pathway. The emphasis of future service research is likely to focus on recognising people with intellectual disability earlier in the criminal justice pathway and diverting them to more appropriate treatment and cost-effective services thought to be beneficial to the patients' treatment needs and recovery. The provision of basic community forensic intellectual disability services is still underdeveloped across the country, as it is in prisons and the entire criminal justice system. There is a growing evidence base on risk assessments in intellectual disability and specific offence-related interventions, such as sex offending treatment programmes that have shown promise and have been adopted into clinical practice.

Improvements in clinical practice will be underpinned by developing care pathways across secure services and the criminal justice system based on the latest evidence on multidisciplinary assessments, formulation and interventions for those with intellectual disability. This chapter has focused on research to date across secure services, risk assessment tools and offence-related interventions for those with intellectual disability. In the future offender intellectual disability research will focus much more on outcomes and subgroups, such as those with autism spectrum disorder in secure pathways, and the cost-effectiveness of services from a public health perspective.

References

Alexander, R., Hiremath, A., Chester, V., *et al* (2011) Evaluation of treatment outcomes from a medium secure unit for people with intellectual disability. *Advances in Mental Health and Intellectual Disabilites*, **5**, 22–32.

Alexander, R.T., Crouch, K., Halstead, S., *et al* (2006) Long-term outcome from a medium secure service for people with intellectual disability. *Journal of Intellectual Disability Research*, **50**, 305–315.

Ammons, R.B. & Ammons, C.H. (1962) *The Quick Test (QT)*. Psychological Test Specialists.

Barron, P., Hassiotis, A. & Banes, J. (2002) Offenders with intellectual disability: the size of the problem and therapeutic outcomes. *Journal of Intellectual Disability Research*, **46**, 454–463.

Beber, E. (2012) Women with intellectual disability in secure settings and their mental health needs. *Advances in Mental Health and Intellectual Disabilities*, **6**, 151–158.

Beer, D., Turk, V., McGovern, P., *et al* (2005) Characteristics of low secure units in an English region: audit of twenty mental health and learning disabilities units for patients with severe challenging behaviour. *Journal of Psychiatric Intensive Care*, **1**, 25.

Beirne, P. (1988) Heredity versus environment: a reconsideration of Charles Goring's The English Convict (1913). *British Journal of Criminology*, **28**, 315–339.

Blacker, J., Beech, A., Wolcox, D., *et al* (2011) The assessment of dynamic risk and recidivism in a sample of special needs sexual offenders. *Psychology, Crime & Law*, **17**, 75–92.

Bland, J., Mezey, G. & Dolan, B. (1999) Special women, special needs: a descriptive study of female special hospital patients. *Journal of Forensic Psychiatry*, **10**, 34–45.

Boer, D.P., Hart, S.D., Kropp, P.R., *et al* (1997) *Manual for the Sexual Violence Risk – 20: Professional Guidelines for Assessing Risk of Sexual Violence*. The Mental Health, Law & Policy Institute, Vancouver.

Chaplin, E., Kelesidi, K., Emery, H., *et al* (2010) People with learning disabilities placed out of area: the South London experience. *Journal of Learning Disabilities and Offending Behaviour*, **1**, 5–14.

Clare, I.C.H., Murphy, G.H., Cox, D., *et al* (1992) Assessment and treatment of fire setting: a single case investigation using a cognitive behavioural model. *Criminal Behaviour and Mental Health*, **2**, 253–268.

Commission for Healthcare Audit and Inspection (2006) *Investigation into the Provision of Services for People with Learning Disabilities at Cornwall Partnership NHS Trust*. Commission of Healthcare Audit and Inspection.

Day, K. (1988) A hospital-based treatment programme for male mentally handicapped offenders. *British Journal of Psychiatry*, **153**, 635–644.

Department of Health (2001) *Valuing People: A New Strategy for Learning Disability for the 21st Century*. Department of Health.

Department of Health (2012) *Department of Health Transforming Care: A National Response to Winterbourne View Hospital: Department of Health Review Final Report*. Department of Health.

Department of Health & Home Office (1992) *Review of Health and Social Services for Mentally Disordered Offenders and Others Requiring Similar Services (Cm 2088)*. HMSO.

Doyle, M., Dolan, M. & McGovern, J. (2002) The validity of North American risk assessment tools in predicting in-patient violent behaviour in England. *Legal and Criminological Psychology*, **7**, 141–154.

Farrington, D.P. (1995) The Twelfth Jack Tizard Memorial Lecture. *Journal of Child Psychology and Psychiatry*, **36**, 929–964.

Fazel, S., Xenitidis, K. & Powell, J. (2008) The prevalence of intellectual disabilities among 12,000 prisoners – a systematic review. *International Journal of Law and Psychiatry*, **31**, 369–373.

Fletcher, R., Loschen, E., Stavrakaki, C., *et al* (eds) *(2007) Diagnostic Manual – Intellectual Disability (DM-ID): A Textbook of Diagnosis of Mental Disorders in Persons with Intellectual Disability.* NADD Press.

Gilby, R., Wolf, L. & Goldberg, B. (1989) Mentally retarded adolescent sex offenders: a survey and pilot study. *Canadian Journal of Psychiatry*, **34**, 542–548.

Goddard, H.H. (1912) *The Kallikak Family: A Study in the Heredity of Feeble-Mindedness.* Macmillan.

Goddard, H.H. (1914) *Feeble-Mindedness: Its Causes and Consequences.* Macmillan.

Goddard, H.H. (1920) *Human Efficiency and Levels of Intelligence.* Princeton University Press.

Goring, C. (1913) (reprinted 1972) *The English Convict: A Statistical Study.* HMSO.

Gray, N.S., Fitzgerald, S., Taylor, J., *et al* (2007) Predicting future reconviction in offenders with intellectual disabilities: the predictive efficacy of VRAG, PCL-SV, and the HCR-20. *Psychological Assessment*, **19**, 474–479.

Gross, G. (1985) *Activities of the Developmental Disabilities Adult Offender Project.* Washington State Developmental Disability Planning Council.

Hall, I., Yacoub, E. & Babur, Y. (2011) Secure inpatient services for people with intellectual disability: lessons from developing a new service. *Advances in Mental Health and Intellectual Disabilites*, **4**, 15–24.

Hanson, R.K. (1997) *The Development of a Brief Actuarial Risk Scale for Sexual Offence Recidivism (User Report 97-04).* Department of the Solicitor General of Canada.

Hanson R.K. & Thornton, D. (2000) Improving risk assessments for sex offenders: a comparison of three actuarial scales. *Law and Human Behaviour*, **24**, 119–136.

Harding, D., Deeley, Q. & Robertson, D. (2009) History, epidemiology and offending. In *Working with People with Learning Disabilities and Offending Behaviour: A Handbook* (eds E. Chaplin, J. Henry & S. Hardy). Pavilion.

Hare, R. (2003) *The Hare Psychopathy Checklist-Revised (PCL-R)*, 2nd edn. Multi-Health Systems.

Harris, A.J.R. & Tough, S. (2004) Should actuarial risk assessments be used with sex offenders who are intellectually disabled? *Journal of Applied Research in Intellectual Disabilities*, **17**, 235–241.

Hart, S.D., Cox, D.N. & Hare, R.D. (1995) *The Hare Psychopathy Checklist: Screening Version (PCL:SV).* Multi-Health Systems.

Hassiotis, A., Gazizova, D., Akinlonu, L., *et al* (2011) Psychiatric morbidity in prisoners with intellectual disabilities: analysis of prison survey data for England and Wales. *British Journal of Psychiatry*, **199**, 156–157.

Hayes, S. (1991) Sex offenders. *Journal of Intellectual and Developmental Disability*, **17**, 221–227.

Healthcare Commission (2007) *Investigation into the Service for People with Learning Disabilities Provided by Sutton and Merton Primary Care Trust.* Healthcare Commission.

Hobson, B. & Rose, J.L. (2008) The mental health of people with intellectual disabilities who offend. *Open Criminology Journal*, **1**, 12–18.

Hodgins, S. (1992) Mental disorder, intellectual deficiency and crime: evidence from a birth cohort. *Archives of General Psychiatry*, **49**, 476–483.

Hogue, T., Steptoe, L., Taylor, J.L., *et al* (2006) A comparison of offenders with intellectual disability across three levels of security. *Criminal Behaviour and Mental Health*, **16**, 13–28.

Holland, S. & Persson, P. (2011) Intellectual disability in the Victorian prison system: characteristics of prisoners with an intellectual disability released from prison in 2003–2006. *Psychology, Crime & Law*, **17**, 25–41.

Holland, T., Clare, I.C.H. & Mukhopadhay, T. (2002) Prevalence of 'criminal offending' by men and women with intellectual disability and the characteristics of 'offenders': implications for research and service development. *Journal of Intellectual Disability Research*, **46**, 6–20.

Home Office & Department of Health (1975) *Report of the Committee on Mentally Abnormal Offenders*. HMSO.

Kerker, B.D., Owens, P.L., Zigler, E., *et al* (2004) Mental health disorders among individuals with mental retardation: challenges to accurate prevalence estimates. *Public Health Reports*, **119**, 409–417.

Klimecki, M.R., Jenkinson, J. & Wilson, L. (1994) A study of recidivism among offenders with an intellectual disability. *Australia & New Zealand Journal of Developmental Disabilities*, **19**, 209–219.

Langevin, R. & Curnoe, S. (2008) Are the mentally retarded and learning disordered overrepresented among sex offenders and paraphilics? *International Journal of Offender Therapy and Comparative Criminology*, **52**, 401–415.

Lindsay, W.R., Steele, L., Smith, A.H.W., *et al* (2006) A community forensic intellectual disability service: twelve year follow up of referrals, analysis of referral patterns and assessment of harm reduction. *Legal and Criminological Psychology*, **11**, 113–130.

Lindsay, W.R., Hogue, T.E., Taylor, J.L., *et al* (2008) Risk assessment in offenders with intellectual disability: a comparison across three levels of security. *International Journal of Offender Therapy and Comparative Criminology*, **52**, 90-111.

Lindsay, W.R., Holland, T., Wheeler, J.R., *et al* (2010) Pathways through services for offenders with intellectual disability: a one- and two-year follow-up study. *American Journal on Intellectual and Developmental Disabilities*, **115**, 250–262.

Lofthouse, R.E., Lindsay, W.R., Totsika, V., *et al* (2013) Prospective dynamic assessment of risk of sexual reoffending in individuals with an intellectual disability and a history of sexual offending behaviour. *Journal of Applied Research in Intellectual Disabilities*, **26**, 394–403.

Lyall, I., Holland, A.J. & Collins, S. (1995) Offending by adults with learning disabilities and the attitudes of staff to offending behaviour: implications for service development. *Journal of Intellectual Disability Research*, **39**, 501–508.

Mansell, J.L. (1992) *Services for People with Learning Disabilities and Challenging Behaviour or Mental Health Needs: Report of a Project Group*. Department of Health.

Mansell, J.L. (2007) *Services for People with Learning Disabilities and Challenging Behaviour or Mental Health Needs: Report of a Project Group (Revised Edition)*. Department of Health.

McBrien, J. (2003) The intellectually disabled offender: methodological problems in identification. *Journal of Applied Research in Intellectual Disabilities*, **16**, 95–105.

McBrien, J., Hodgetts, A. & Gregory, J. (2003) Offending and risky behaviour in community services for people with intellectual disabilities in one local authority. *Journal of Forensic Psychiatry & Psychology*, **14**, 280–297.

McGrath, R.J., Livingston, J.A. & Falk, G. (2007) A structured method of assessing dynamic risk factors among sexual abusers with intellectual disabilities. *American Journal of Mental Retardation*, **112**, 221–229.

McNulty, C., Kissi-Deborah, R. & Newsom-Davies, I. (1995) Police involvement with clients having intellectual disabilites: a pilot study in South London. *Mental Handicap Research*, **8**, 129–136.

Morrissey, C., Mooney, P., Hogue, T.E., *et al* (2007) Predictive validity of the PCL-R for offenders with intellectual disability in a high security hospital: treatment progress. *Journal of Intellectual and Developmental Disability*, **32**, 125–133.

Morrissey, C., Taylor, J. & Bennett, C. (2012) Evaluation of a therapeutic community intervention for men with intellectual disability and personality disorder. *Journal of Learning Disabilities and Offending Behaviour*, **3**, 52–60.

Murphy, G., Harnett, H. & Holland, A. (1995) A survey of intellctual disabilites amongst men on remand in prison. *Mental Handicap Research*, **8**, 81–98.

O'Brien, G. (2002) Dual diagnosis in offenders with intellectual disability: setting research priorities: a review of research findings concerning psychiatric disorder (excluding personality disorder) among offenders with intellectual disability. *Journal of Intellectual Disability Research*, **46** (suppl. 1), 21–30.

Quinsey, V.L., Book, A. & Skilling, T.A. (2004) A follow-up of deinstitutionalized men with intellectual disabilities and histories of antisocial behaviour. *Journal of Applied Research in Intellectual Disabilities*, **17**, 243–253.

Reed, S., Russell, A., Xenitidis, K., *et al* (2004) People with learning disabilities in a low secure in-patient unit: comparison of offenders and non-offenders. *British Journal of Psychiatry*, **185**, 499–504.

Rice, M.E. & Chaplin, T.C. (1979) Social skills training for hospitalised male arsonists. *Journal of Behaviour Therapy and Experimental Psychiatry*, **10**, 105–108.

Royal College of Psychiatrists (2001) *DC-LD: Diagnostic Criteria for Psychiatric Disorders for Use with Adults with Learning Disabilities/Mental Retardation (OP48)*. Gaskell.

Royal College of Psychiatrists, British Psychological Society & Royal College of Speech and Language Therapists (2007) *Challenging Behaviour – A Unified Approach: Clinical and Service Guidelines for Supporting People with Learning Disabilities Who Are at Risk of Receiving Abusive or Restrictive Practices*. RCPsych.

Salvador-Carulla, L., Reed, G., Vaez-Azizi, L., *et al* (2011) Intellectual developmental disorders: towards a new name, definition and framework for 'mental retardation/intellectual disability' in ICD-11. *World Psychiatry*, **10**, 175–180.

Sex Offender Treatment Services Collaborative – Intellectual Disabilities (SOTSEC-ID) (2010) Effectiveness of group cognitive-behavioural treatment for men with intellectual disabilities at risk of sexual offending. *Journal of Applied Research in Intellectual Disabilities*, **23**, 537–551.

Shaw, J., Appleby, L. & Baker, D. (2003) *Safer Prisons: A National Study of Prison Suicides 1999–2000 by the National Confidential Inquiry into Suicides and Homicides by People with Mental Illness*. National Confidential Inquiry.

Talbot, J. (2009) No One Knows: offenders with learning disabilities and learning difficulties. *International Journal of Prisoner Health*, **5**, 141–152.

Talbot, J. & Riley, C. (2007) No One Knows: offenders with learning difficulties and learning disabilities. *British Journal of Learning Disabilities*, **35**, 154–161.

Taylor, J.L. (2002) A review of the assessment and treatment of anger and aggression in offenders with intellectual disability. *Journal of Intellectual Disability Research*, **46** (suppl. 1), 57–73.

Taylor, J.L. & Lindsay, W.R. (2010) Understanding and treating offenders with learning disabilities: a review of recent developments. *Journal of Learning Disabilities and Offending Behaviour*, **1**, 5–16.

Taylor, J.L., Thorne, I., Robertson, A., *et al* (2002) Evaluation of a group intervention for convicted arsonists with mild and borderline intellectual disabilities. *Criminal Behaviour and Mental Health*, **12**, 282–293.

Taylor, J.L., Novaco, R.W., Gillmer, B.T., *et al* (2005) Individual cognitive-behavioural anger treatment for people with mild-borderline intellectual disabilities and histories of aggression: a controlled trial. *British Journal of Clinical Psychology*, **44**, 367–382.

Taylor, J.L., Robertson, A., Thorne, I., *et al* (2006) Responses of female fire-setters with mild and borderline intellectual disabilities to a group intervention. *Journal of Applied Research in Intellectual Disabilities*, **19**, 179–190.

Thomas, S.D., Dolan, M., Johnston, S., *et al* (2004) Defining the needs of patients with intellectual disabilities in the high security psychiatric hospitals in England. *Journal of Intellectual Disability Research*, **48**, 603–610.

Thornton, D., Mann, R., Webster, S., *et al* (2003) Distinguishing and combining risks for sexual and violent recidivism. In *Understanding and Managing Sexually Coercive Behavior*

129

(eds R. Prentky, E. Janus, M. Seto, *et al*), Annals of the New York Academy of Sciences, vol. 989, pp. 225–235. New York Academy of Sciences.

Webster, C.D., Douglas, K.S., Eaves, D., *et al* (1997) *HCR-20: Assessing the Risk of Violence (Version 2)*. Simon Fraser University & Forensic Psychiatric Services Commission of British Columbia.

West, D.J. & Farrington, D.P. (1973) *Who Becomes Delinquent? Second Report of the Cambridge Study in Delinquent Development*. Heinemann Educational for the Cambridge Institute of Criminology.

Wheeler, J.R., Holland, A.J., Bambrick, M., *et al* (2009) Community services and people with intellectual disabilities who engage in anti-social or offending behaviour: referral rates, characteristics, and care pathways. *Journal of Forensic Psychiatry & Psychology*, **20**, 717–740.

Wilcox, D., Beech, A., Markall, H.F., *et al* (2009) Actuarial risk assessment and recidivism in a sample of UK intellectually disabled sexual offenders. *Journal of Sexual Aggression*, **15**, 97–106.

World Health Organization (1992) *The ICD-10 Classification of Mental and Behavioural Disorders: Clinical Descriptions and Diagnostic Guidelines*. WHO.

World Health Organization (2001) *The World Health Organisation Report 2001 – Mental Health: New Understanding, New Hope*. WHO.

CHAPTER 9

Secure mental healthcare for young people

Enys Delmage and Ernest Gralton

Introduction

Mentally disordered young offenders are a complex group in whom multiple comorbidities, elements of social and educational disability, high rates of physical health problems and frequent drug and alcohol problems are present. The risk factors associated with both offending behaviour and mental disorder in young people are well established and include social disadvantage, parental loss, broken homes, poverty, abusive and neglectful experiences and abandonment (Junger-Tas, 1994; Kazdin, 1995; Rutter & Smith, 1995; Rutter *et al*, 1998; Rutter, 2000). Management challenges for mental health professionals include the highly nomadic lifestyle of the young person and his or her family, poor previous experiences with mental health and social services and subsequent resistance to support, complex comorbid psychopathology and a lack of community resources to aid reintegration following an in-patient admission. In recent years both the 'Bradley report' (Department of Health, 2009) and the *Breaking the Cycle* report (Ministry of Justice, 2010) have placed an emphasis on diversion from custody and early treatment of mental disorder in young offenders. The National Service Framework for Children (Department of Health, 2004) has also been influential in increasing early intervention for mentally disordered young offenders and diverting them from young offender institutions. This chapter explores the background context to these objectives and the role played by secure in-patient mental health services for young people. Initially, we focus on the prevalence of mental disorder in young offenders and the available specialist treatment resources in England and Wales. There follows a description of the secure provision for young people and the management challenges associated with this group, the available models of care and specific elements of treatment packages. The chapter concludes with a discussion of the management of transitions for young people to their next placement following a period of secure care.

The chapter focuses largely on mentally disordered young offenders. However, secure mental health services do manage other groups of young people to be deemed at high risk of harm to themselves (for instance, through self-harming or suicidal behaviour) or others, who have not been diverted from the criminal justice system. The chapter content is also relevant to these groups and we therefore use the term secure child and adolescent mental health services ('secure CAMHS') rather than 'forensic services' to refer to the range of provision.

Offending in young people

Self-report survey data indicate that 26% of young people aged 10 to 17 years have committed one of twenty core offences in the past 12 months (Roe & Ashe, 2008). Property offences were committed by 14% of respondents and violent offences by 19%. In 2009/2010 young people aged 10–17 years accounted for 17% of all arrests in England and Wales but for only 11% of the population of individuals of offending age and are therefore overrepresented in terms of arrest rates (Ministry of Justice, 2012). In 2010/2011, the average number of young people aged under 18 years in custody in England and Wales was 2040. Of those detained in 2011, about a quarter (26%) were held on remand, while 55% were serving a detention and training order (DTO; maximum length 24 months), with the remaining 19% serving long-term sentences. Most (95%) young people in custodial care were male and a similar proportion were aged 15 to 17 years. Young people from a Black and minority ethnic background are also overrepresented in custodial settings, accounting for 36% of detainees, but only represent 14% of the general 10- to 17-year-old population. The total cost to the country of youth offending in terms of police and related justice costs has been estimated at £4 billion annually (Police Foundation, 2010).

Mental disorder in looked after children and young offenders

Mental disorder is a prominent feature in young people in institutional care. The point prevalence of mental disorder among looked after children aged 5 to 17 years was examined in a nationally representative sample of British children (Ford et al, 2007). Young people in local authority accommodation were more likely to have any mental disorder (46%) than a matched age control group living in the most socioeconomically disadvantaged private households (15%) or in non-disadvantaged private households (9%).The most common condition was conduct disorder, with 27% of looked after children and 5.3% of disadvantaged population controls meeting diagnostic criteria. Further, 11% of looked after children had an anxiety disorder (6% in disadvantaged private households) and 3% had depression (1% in disadvantaged households). Further, 9% were hyperactive (compared with 1%) and 3% had autism spectrum conditions (compared with 0.1%). In other analyses, children in England with a mental disorder were more than five times as likely to have been in trouble with the police as their general population counterparts (26% v. 5%; Meltzer et al, 2003).

The rate of mental health problems is even higher among young offenders. A review of 30 years of international literature on mental health problems in young people in contact with the criminal justice system found prevalence reports of between 25 and 81% (Rutter et al, 1998). This wide variation may result from different diagnostic criteria and the varying stages at which individuals enter research studies, for example on admission to secure facilities, pre-conviction and post-conviction. One large representative US study of 1829 detained young people made efforts to circumnavigate this variability and found that two-thirds of males and about three-quarters of females met the diagnostic criteria for one or more psychiatric disorders (Teplin et al, 2002). Most males (61%) and females (70%) met criteria for at least one disorder other than conduct disorder, notably affective disorders (19% and 28% for males and females respectively), anxiety disorders (21% and 31%), attention-deficit hyperactivity disorder (ADHD; 17% and 21%) and substance use disorder (51% and 47%). Mental health problems among young people in secure care are three times higher than in age-matched controls in the community (Jacobson et al, 2010). A history of childhood abuse and neglect are common features of both young male and female offenders (McManus et al, 1984). Young people who have experienced abuse are 11 times more likely to be arrested for a violent crime than non-abused peers (Swanston et al, 2003).

Personality disorder prevalence estimates using the Structured Clinical Interview for DSM-IV Axis II Personality Disorder (SCID-II; First et al, 1997) for antisocial, paranoid and borderline disorders were 76%, 26% and 24% respectively among male remand young offenders in England and Wales and 81%, 22% and 17% among male sentenced young offenders (aged under 21 years) (Lader et al, 2000). These figures are, however, substantially higher than estimates from other countries and in older prisoners.

Research commissioned by the Youth Justice Board found a 5% point prevalence of psychosis in 13- to 18-year-olds in custody (Chitsabesan et al, 2006), high prevalence of self-harm and suicidal thoughts (Table 9.1).

Drug dependence has also been identified in 57% of male remand young offenders, 70% of male sentenced young offenders, and 51% of female sentenced young offenders (Lader et al, 1998; Singleton et al, 1998), with rates of up to 85% use of drugs and alcohol in the community (Hammersley et al, 2003).

Research indicates high levels of need in a number of areas of functioning among young people in custody, including mental health (31%), education or work (36%) and social relationships (48%) (Chitsabesan et al, 2006). Young offenders in the community have been found to have significantly more needs than those in secure care and their needs are often unmet. The same study highlighted that one in five young offenders had an intellectual

Table 9.1 Prevalence of self-harm and mental disorders among young offenders (aged 13 to 18 years)

	Male remand offenders	Male sentenced offenders	Female sentenced offenders
Post-traumatic stress disorder	4%	4%	7%
Suicidal thoughts (lifetime prevalence)	38%	28%	51%
Suicide attempt (lifetime history)	20%	16%	32%
Non-suicidal self-harm during detention	7%	9%	11%

Source: Chitsabesan *et al* (2006).

disability (IQ<70). Despite high levels of need, mental health service use has been reported as low, particularly among young offenders in the community (Barrett *et al*, 2006).

The financial cost of mental disorder to society is high. Scott *et al* (2001, 2006) showed that public costs incurred by children with conduct disorder amounted to £70000 per person (of which the cost to health services was only 3%) from age 10 to age 28 v. £7000 for a person without conduct disorder. Barrett *et al* (2006) report that the average cost of providing mental health services to young offenders in custody was £40000 per year (excluding the societal cost of crime), with greater costs being incurred by those of younger age and with depressed mood.

Specialist provision for mentally disordered young offenders

Secure in-patient child and adolescent mental health services

The adolescent secure in-patient estate in England and Wales differs markedly from adult secure services and the categories of low, medium and high security are not mirrored. There is no high secure provision for adolescents, but in very rare cases young people have been transferred before their eighteenth birthday to one of the high secure hospitals. The majority of secure CAMHS meet medium secure standards, but it is perhaps more intuitive to think of the adolescent forensic estate as 'secure CAMHS in-patient provision' rather than focusing on the level of security. Individual units in the UK are tasked with managing young people ranging from those who as adults may have required high security, through to young people who are ready for a transition into community services. Secure CAMHS units must therefore provide the equivalent of high, medium and low secure-type services for their patients.

While each region does not require its own secure CAMHS in-patient service, units are not distributed evenly around the country and most are located in the south of England (O'Herlihy *et al*, 2003). The resulting lack of local provision can create some challenges since young people may have to be placed in a location geographically remote from their home address.

Community adolescent forensic services

The recommendations of Lord Bradley's review of people with mental health problems or intellectual disabilities in the criminal justice system (Department of Health, 2009) specified a need for locality services. Currently, there are two models of provision for community adolescent forensic services. Both aim to meet regional need in terms of assessment and treatment.

1   Community-based forensic teams: provide specialist, peripatetic consultation, liaison, assessment and treatment for generic CAMHS teams and other services. They provide 'in-reach' services to local authority secure children's homes and young offender institutions, as well as having links with youth offending teams (YOTs), multi-agency public protection panels (MAPPPs) and adult forensic and generic mental health services. These teams have emerged as part of community services rather than from adult medium secure in-patient services.

2   Forensic adolescent consultation and treatment service (FACTS) teams, conversely, have developed largely from services providing medium secure care. They can provide assessment (including detailed risk assessment) and sometimes treatment – these models can provide input regionally, nationally or in combination.

The secure CAMHS hospital setting

Young people up to the age of 18 years who are considered to be a risk to themselves or others can be detained in secure children's homes, secure training centres or young offender institutions on secure accommodation orders (Children Act 1989). Admission to a secure child and adolescent mental health setting is indicated where the young person has mental health needs, can be detained under the Mental Health Act 1983 and is displaying behaviour which poses a serious risk to others. Alternatively, admission is indicated for young people in custodial care who present a serious risk of suicide and/or severe self-harm. The National In-patient Child and Adolescent Psychiatry Study (NICAPS; O'Herlihy *et al*, 2003) established that the most common principal diagnoses of young people admitted to forensic and secure adolescent services were schizophrenia, delusional or psychotic disorder (49%), personality disorders (23%) and affective disorders (7%). One study of the characteristics of 80 adolescents referred for specialist secure in-patient care (Wheatley *et al*, 2004) revealed that almost all (92%) were identified as at risk for physical aggression and over half (53%) had been charged with at least one offence. Most were at risk for self-harm (71%), while other common risks were self-neglect (49%), firesetting (32%) and victimisation (31%). Almost half (45%) of individuals referred were receiving constant observation at the time of assessment. This study also suggested that a significant degree of traumatisation existed among the patient group, with 19% holding a principal diagnosis of post-traumatic stress disorder. The international literature suggests very high levels of psychiatric comorbidity (Vermeiren *et al*, 2006; Colins *et al*, 2010).

Route of admission into secure CAMHS

Young people can be admitted to secure CAMHS from a variety of settings, including:

- home
- local authority children's home
- hospital orders from courts (sections 35–38 of the Mental Health Act 1983)
- transfer from young offenders' institutions, secure training centres or local authority secure children's homes (sections 47 or 48 of the Mental Health Act 1983)
- other hospital placement.

The legal frameworks which most frequently apply in terms of admission are either the civil or the criminal procedure sections of the Mental Health Act 1983. It is rare for a young person to be voluntarily admitted to a secure CAMHS, and use of the Mental Capacity Act 2005 would usually be precluded since 16- and 17-year-olds cannot be admitted under the Act to conditions amounting to a deprivation of liberty.

Management challenges in secure CAMHS

Multiple psychiatric comorbidity

A specific challenge for secure CAMHS is that multiple diagnoses often coexist within one individual. Concurrent comorbidities can include substance misuse associated with psychosis, conduct disorder or mixed disorders of conduct and emotions, attachment difficulties, hyperkinetic disorders and intellectual disability. A further challenge is that, in comparison with other mentally disordered young people, the disorders in this group have often gone unrecognised throughout childhood owing to poor engagement with local health services, school and Social Services. Frequent geographical transitions which do not facilitate protracted assessment, and a lack of clarity regarding who is responsible for the young person, may also exacerbate the situation. Multiple mental disorders linked with offending behaviour are often associated with polypharmacy. This can represent an attempt to ameliorate the aggressive and/or self-injurious aspects of the young person's presentation, but unfortunately it is often only possible to remove these medications for clarity in terms of psychopathology once the young person is in a secure mental health facility.

Peer susceptibility

Young people have a heightened susceptibility to be influenced by peers (Steinberg, 2008) probably related to lack of ventral striatum brain maturity (Pfeifer *et al*, 2011), combined with a phase of increased impulsivity, sensation-seeking and risk-taking behaviour (van Leijenhorst *et al*, 2010). Collusion in antisocial activities can be especially prevalent among mentally disordered young offenders. For these reasons, high staff/patient ratios are likely to be effective in breaking down some of the most unhelpful interactions and in facilitation of information-gathering to help avoid any challenges before they materialise. Collusion does need serious consideration since it is therapeutically unhelpful, can lead to victimisation of other young people and can also lead to assaults on staff, serious damage to property and even the evacuation and closure of secure adolescent units. Smaller unit size can aid in the management of collusion. Units of 8–10 beds are preferable, with some capacity for transitions along a care pathway when it becomes unsafe for a young person to remain in a specified unit.

Models of care

Given that adolescents are a different population to adults, the question is how should secure in-patient services for adolescents differ from adult secure in-patient units? Many of the issues around procedural and environmental security will be very similar but there may be some important differences. Any model for the care of adolescents must be grounded in developmental principles. A developmental perspective includes an understanding of three core elements: brain maturation, the environmental interface and the mastery of key developmental tasks (Harris, 2000). Because neurodevelopmental disorders are by their very nature complex and interrelated, single treatments in isolation are very unlikely in themselves to produce significant and sustained effects. Treatment will be informed by thorough assessment processes following admission which typically take up to 12 weeks. Length of stay is typically between 12 and 18 months. Multiple modalities of treatment (including remedial education) must be combined through multidisciplinary working. This produces a complex treatment system with varying professional perspectives, relationship priorities and goals.

Solution-focused principles

The demands made by adolescent populations on staff teams are significantly higher than those made by adult populations and they require a high level of structured activity and routine (Rose, 2004). Adolescents, and particularly those with offending histories, are a difficult to engage population and solution-focused principles which help provide young people with a range of prosocial options for dealing with stressful situations can be particularly helpful in promoting good relationships with staff (Gralton *et al*, 2006).

Nutrition

Nutrition is rarely discussed as an issue in models of secure care for young people. This is surprising as nutritional deficits have been implicated in the development of behavioural disturbance, antisocial personality disorder, hyperactivity and impaired cognitive function (Raine *et al*, 2003; Liu *et al*, 2004; Dani *et al*, 2005; Walker *et al*, 2007). Long-chain Omega 3 fatty acids are essential building blocks for brain development and can only be obtained from specific dietary sources, most notably oily fish; the current Western diet is very low in these essential nutrients (Richardson, 2006). Mammals fed diets low in Omega 3 fatty acids have impaired brain repair (Bourre *et al*, 1989) and there is already strong evidence that these essential nutrients can reduce aggression in adolescent offenders whose brains are still developing and have the chance of repairing neurological deficits (Gesch *et al*, 2002). Adolescents in secure in-patient settings should therefore be offered a diet high in Omega 3 fatty acids and other essential nutrients or should have these supplemented (Hibbeln *et al*, 2006).

Physical activity

Exercise is an effective treatment in disruptive behaviour disorders and has few side-effects (Allison *et al*, 1995). Exercise increases neural plasticity and brain repair probably by the up-regulation of brain-derived neurotrophic factor (Vaynman & Gomez-Pinilla, 2005). Sports and exercise programmes are important for a range of reasons, including weight control, teaching leadership and social interaction, to reduce overall arousal and to promote brain recovery in adolescents.

Physical touch

Secure services are likely to have policies that limit physical touch for two main reasons: first, because there are many patients who have existing histories of inappropriate sexual behaviour, and second, to try to prevent staff themselves being accused of inappropriate physical contact. However, touch is a requirement for normal brain development in children. It has been established that primates who are deprived of touch develop a range of abnormal and aggressive behaviours (Harlow & Suomi, 1971). Many young people who come into secure settings have histories of abuse and neglect. This may be complicated by histories of sexual offending and inappropriate patterns of sexual arousal. Later in this chapter we discuss a sensory integration approach which can offer the opportunity to meet sensory deficits in a safe and appropriate manner.

Pathway approach

One important message for the young person in an adolescent secure in-patient setting is that the service will not effect a transition to a different service simply because highly aggressive or severely self-injurious behaviour is shown. While the risks to the individual and other young people must be managed, these challenges are dealt with in situ, which aids to the sense of security and safe containment for the mentally disordered young offender. From this juncture, a pathway approach can be adopted whereby the young person can develop, with the aid of the therapeutic regime, appropriate coping skills to be able to manage in conditions of reduced security, and therefore make a transition to a ward where the onus is on giving the young person incremental increases in personal responsibility while testing risk. On these transition and continuing care wards the young people spend more time in community settings and are supported by staff to engage in vocational activities, which can include attendance at local colleges and so forth.

Specific treatment packages

Treatment in secure adolescent in-patient settings consists of highly specialised therapeutic input in all of the modalities that would be expected in generic in-patient CAMHS, including education, therapeutic social work, psychology, psychiatry, occupational therapy, art psychotherapy, vocational work and nursing input. The highly specialised treatments are numerous and can include:

- offence-specific work such as sex offender treatment groups and firesetting work adapted for younger people
- moral reasoning group and individual work
- drug and alcohol education and treatment
- aggression management
- Treatment and Education of Autistic and related Communication handicapped Children (TEACCH) approaches in education (Mesibov et al, 2005)
- a focus on child protection and police liaison, often facilitated by a therapeutic social work team
- tailored family therapy
- dialectical behaviour therapy.

Cognitive and behavioural interventions

Group-based cognitive and behavioural interventions are recommended in the National Institute for Health and Care Excellence (NICE) guideline related to adolescents with emerging personality difficulties (National Institute for Health and Clinical Excellence, 2009). The NICE guidelines also highlight that positive and reinforcing strategies are more successful than negative or punitive sanctions. Family work, problem-solving skills training, generation of alternative coping strategies and target-setting, anger management work and treatment of psychiatric comorbidity are recommended.

Risk assessment

Best practice involves the use of recognised structured clinical and risk assessment tools. For example, the Psychopathy Checklist – Youth Version (Hare *et al*, 2006), the Structured Assessment of Violence Risk in Youth (SAVRY; Borum, 2006) and the Estimate of Risk of Adolescent Sexual Offence Recidivism (ERASOR; Worling, 2004).

Education

Educational interventions form a key element of treatment. Engagement while in secure CAMHS care is likely to have longer-term benefits primarily because the young person's post-discharge trajectory is likely to fail unless it includes aspects of education or vocational work. Often young people in secure care have had very negative experiences of home and community education and gravitate towards antisocial activities and identities. Secure CAMHS hospitals provide the flexibility for smaller class sizes, including one-to-one sessions and a gradual introduction to larger groups. This offers an adaptive approach that assists the young person in engaging in educational opportunities. The full timetable affords the young person the same opportunities that would be usual for their counterparts in the community. With encouragement, their success can build confidence and self-esteem, as well as enhancing their identity.

Occupational therapy

The use of activity to build motivation and confidence in personal effectiveness forms one of the core components of the occupational therapy treatment approach. Occupational therapy interventions assist in supporting individuals to perform their daily occupational activities and roles to a satisfying and effective level. Through a range of activities, the occupational therapy timetable assists in developing a young person's responsibility, motivation, positive social roles, routines, interactions and life skills to improve occupational functioning. Occupational therapy interventions within a secure CAMHS hospital setting focus on increasingly challenging activities and skill-building, with personal responsibility for behaviour being a fundamental part of this challenge. The young person is subsequently able to have regular and meaningful vocational, leisure and educational commitments on discharge, and these activities can be helpful in relapse prevention and avoiding recourse to antisocial coping mechanisms.

Sensory integration approach

Many young people in secure in-patient CAMHS have sensory needs as a result both of neglect of these needs as children and of not having developed more sophisticated coping mechanisms through normal development. Unmet sensory needs can result in the young person accessing stimulation through unhelpful routes including inappropriate touch of others or through hostility and aggression. This may include seeking out restraint situations to meet motion (vestibular) and touch (haptic) needs. Highly sensitive children, on the other hand, may require low-stimulus approaches which aid in anxiety reduction and subsequent reductions in aggression as a default coping mechanism.

The sensory integration approach can include the use of tactile objects that the young person can manipulate, exercise equipment including swings and trampolines, as well as stress balls and weighted blankets, which are selected and utilised by the young person to either stimulate in states of low energy or help to calm in situations of over-arousal. This has the added benefit of teaching the young person that they can manage their needs themselves in a constructive way rather than having recourse to self-harm or aggression.

Dialectical behaviour therapy

This therapeutic approach combines elements of cognitive–behavioural therapy (CBT) in relation to emotional regulation with principles of mindfulness and meditation (Linehan *et al*, 1991, 1993). It involves a combination of individual and group work approaches with commitment from the patient to be involved in the process. The components can be helpful with emerging personality disorder, and specifically for work on self-injurious and aggressive behaviour (Rathus & Miller, 2000, 2002), although the weight of the evidence base is currently in adults with borderline personality disorder (Bloom *et al*, 2012). These include the facilitation and support of the development of stress tolerance skills and a consideration of the interpersonal dynamics involved in a series of relationships with different individuals. There are numerous ways in which the principles of dialectical behaviour therapy can be applied both formally and informally, from routine community meetings to direct individual sessions over a period of time.

Medication

It is important to treat comorbidity where it occurs in secure in-patient CAMHS settings. Common mental disorders can interact with underlying personality difficulties to detrimental effect. For example, irritability associated with depression or overactivity in mania may amplify aggressive behaviour in those with conduct disorder. Given the frequency of comorbidity, it is important to have a clear picture of these interactions and to treat each disorder appropriately.

Pharmacological treatments, however, tend to have a less prominent role in the direct treatment of the disorder of conduct and emotions. This is in part due to the lack of evidence to support the use of medication – currently only risperidone is licensed in the UK for the short-term (maximum 6 weeks) symptomatic treatment of persistent aggression in adolescents. There is emerging evidence that risperidone is also useful in the treatment of behavioural disorders associated with autism (Canitano & Scandurra, 2008) and intellectual disabilities (Bezuidenhout *et al*, 2012) in children and adolescents. Further, sodium valproate may have utility in treatment of conduct disorder (Steiner *et al*, 2003) and clozapine may have a place in the treatment of emotionally unstable personality traits associated with comorbidity (Fajumi *et al*, 2012). Further analysis of the available evidence can be found in the 2013 NICE guideline *Antisocial Behaviour and Conduct Disorders in Children and Young People*. The widespread use of medication in this group remains limited owing to the lack of available evidence.

Discharge from secure CAMHS: transition challenges

One of the major challenges in relation to secure in-patient CAMHS care is managing young people who have had, for myriad reasons, to make numerous changes of residence in their lives and who find attachment and trust very difficult to achieve safely. It is not uncommon to work with young people who have had more than 50 Social Services placements before hospital admission and who may have scant support from their families. Ongoing involvement from key workers in the community, notably social workers, is therefore crucial during the in-patient stay. There is also a need for the transition from secure in-patient CAMHS to be managed very carefully.

Both the relatively long length of stay and the intensity of treatments offered in secure in-patient CAMHS mean that close alliances will have developed between the young person and both staff and other service users. The NICE guideline for antisocial personality disorder (National Institute for Health and Clinical Excellence, 2009) highlights the importance of avoiding unnecessary transfer of care between institutions whenever possible. Failure to manage transitions is not uncommon in mentally disordered young offenders, with the result that many have histories of intermittent short periods in community placements interspersed with longer stays in a variety of units offering varying levels of security. High recidivism rates in this population can result in frequent stays in young offender institutions or secure training centres as well as in an early history of frequent readmission to local authority secure children's homes. Young people with autism spectrum disorders may require even fewer transitions owing to their difficulties in managing change. Single, well-planned transitions from secure services to highly structured community settings may be the best option.

The transition from the secure CAMHS in-patient setting to the next placement must be dealt with very carefully if it is not to replicate the young person's previous abandonment experiences. Ideally, a decision to discharge should be based on completion of therapeutic work and clinical and risk-related readiness rather than on financial demands. This can be a particular challenge for the management of transition for young people reaching 18 years of age because responsibility for funding often changes at this time.

Some individuals can make a transition to independent living or adult hospital services easily at the point of their eighteenth birthday, but others remain vulnerable, developmentally immature or remain at risk due to the nature of their mental disorder. For these individuals, continuing care after the eighteenth birthday in a secure CAMHS setting can be beneficial and can reduce the level of security that they will ultimately require or reduce their overall length of hospital stay.

Ideally, where a community placement is being sought, the next move from hospital should be to a step-down service that has continued in-reach from the secure CAMHS clinical team and which itself employs appropriately trained clinical staff. Such a placement represents the first stage towards independent living while maintaining the continuity of care. Aftercare packages should be multidisciplinary and multi-agency – a wide variety of professionals from a number of different agencies are required to make independent living possible and to circumnavigate some of the difficulties of the past. The aftercare package frequently involves the structure of community treatment orders, section 117 aftercare, guardianship orders and conditional discharges as part of the service delivered by Social Services, mental health, education/vocation and various other agencies that can add to the prerequisite scaffolding needed to support the young person.

Unfortunately, not all circumstances allow for a pathway approach to care that results in independent living. This may be the case in the context of young people with developmental disability or an acquired brain injury. However, the focus should remain on allowing the individual to have the maximum degree of freedom and independence possible in the context of the associated risks.

Conclusions

In summary, mental disorders are common in young offenders who have frequently experienced mistreatment in early life. The group displays high levels of unmet need related to their mental health, education and social functioning and the cost to society is significant. Secure CAMHS in-patient care is indicated for mentally disordered young offenders and for others who present a high risk of harm to others or to themselves. Secure CAMHS care requires the application of specific developmental knowledge to intervention and an integrated multidisciplinary approach will facilitate effective treatment. For those able to move towards independent living, early discharge planning with multi-agency involvement is likely to maximise the chances of long-term success.

References

Allison, D., Faith, M. & Franklin, R. (1995) Antecedent exercise in the treatment of disruptive behaviour: a meta-analytic review. *Clinical Psychology: Science and Practice*, **2**, 279–303.

Barrett, B., Byford, S., Chitsbesan, P., *et al* (2006) Mental health provision for young offenders: service use and cost. *British Journal of Psychiatry*, **188**, 541–546.

Bezuidenhout, H., Wiysonge, C. & Bentley, J. (2012) Risperidone for disruptive behaviour disorders in children with intellectual disabilities (Protocol). *Cochrane Database of Systematic Reviews*, **7**, CD009988.

Bloom, J.M., Woodward, E.N., Susmaras, T., *et al* (2012) Use of dialectical behavior therapy in inpatient treatment of borderline personality disorder: a systematic review. *Psychiatric Services*, **63**, doi: 10.1176/appi.ps.201100311.

Borum, R. (2006) *Manual for the Structured Assessment of Violence Risk in Youth (SAVRY)*. Psychological Assessment Resources.

Bourre. J., Durrand, G., Pascal, G., *et al* (1989) Brain cell and tissue recovery in rats made deficient in n-3 fatty acids by alteration of dietary fat. *Journal of Nutrition*, **119**, 15–22.

Canitano, R. & Scandurra, V. (2008) Risperidone in the treatment of behavioural disorders associated with autism in children and adolescents. *Neuropsychiatric Disease and Treatment*, **4**, 723–730.

Chitsabesan, P., Kroll, L., Bailey, S., *et al* (2006) Mental health needs of young offenders in custody and the community. *British Journal of Psychiatry*, **188**, 534–540.

Colins, O., Vermeiren, R., Vreugdenhil, C., *et al* (2010) Psychiatric disorders in detained male adolescents: a systematic literature review. *Canadian Journal of Psychiatry*, **55**, 255–263.

Dani, J., Burrill, C. & Demmig-Adams, B. (2005) The remarkable role of nutrition in learning and behaviour. *Nutrition and Food Science*, **35**, 258–263.

Department of Health (2004) *National Service Framework for Children, Young People and Maternity Services*. Department of Health.

Department of Health (2009) *The Bradley Report: Lord Bradley's Review of People with Mental Health Problems or Learning Disabilities in the Criminal Justice System*. Department of Health.

Fajumi, T., Manzoor, M. & Carpenter, K. (2012) Clozapine use in women with borderline personality disorder and co-morbid learning disability. *Journal of Learning Disabilities and Offending Behaviour*, **3**, 6–11.

First, M.B., Gibbon, M., Spitzer, R.L., *et al* (1997) *Structured Clinical Interview for DSM-IV Axis II Personality Disorders (SCID-II)*. American Psychiatric Press.

Ford, T., Vostanis, P., Meltzer, H., *et al* (2007) Psychiatric disorder among British children looked after by local authorities: comparison with children living in private households. *British Journal of Psychiatry*, **190**, 319–325.

Gesch, C., Hammond, S., Hampson, S., *et al* (2002) Influence of supplementary vitamins, minerals and essential fatty acids on the antisocial behaviour of young adult prisoners: a randomised placebo-controlled trial. *British Journal of Psychiatry*, **181**, 22–28.

Gralton, E., Udu, V. & Ranasinghe, S. (2006) A solution-focused model and inpatient secure settings. *British Journal of Forensic Practice*, **8**, 24–30.

Hammersley, R., Marsland, L. & Reid, M. (2003) *Substance Use by Young Offenders*. Research, Development and Statistics Directorate of the Home Office.

Hare, R., Neumann, C., Kosson, D., *et al* (2006) Factor structure of the Hare Psychopathy Checklist: Youth Version (PCL: YV) in incarcerated adolescents. *Psychological Assessment*, **18**, 142–154.

Harlow, H. & Suomi, S. (1971) Social recovery by isolation-reared monkeys. *Proceedings of the National Academy of Sciences of the United States of America*, **68**, 1534–1538.

Harris, J. (2000) Multimodal interventions for developmental neuropsychiatric disorders. In *Developmental Disability and Behaviour* (eds. C. Gillberg & G. O'Brien). Mac Keith Press.

Hibbeln, J., Ferguson, T. & Blasbalg, T. (2006) Omega-3 fatty acid deficiencies in neurodevelopment, aggression and autonomic dysregulation: opportunities for intervention. *International Review of Psychiatry*, **18**, 107–118.

Jacobson, J., Bhardwa, B., Gyateng, T., *et al* (2010) *Punishing Disadvantage: A Profile of Children in Custody*. Prison Reform Trust Publications.

Junger-Tas, J. (1994) *Delinquent Behavior Among Young People in the Western World*. Kugler Publications

Kazdin, A. (1995) *Conduct Disorders in Childhood and Adolescence*. Sage Publications.

Lader, D., Singleton, N. & Meltzer, H. (1998) *Psychiatric Morbidity among Young Offenders in England and Wales (Office for National Statistics)*. TSO (The Stationery Office).

Lader, D., Singleton, N. & Meltzer, H. (2000) *Psychiatric Morbidity among Young Offenders in England and Wales*. Office for National Statistics.

Linehan, M.M., Armstrong, H.E., Suarez, A., *et al* (1991) Cognitive-behavioral treatment of chronically parasuicidal borderline patients. *Archives of General Psychiatry*, **48**, 1060–1064.

Linehan, M.M., Heard, H.L. & Armstrong, H.E. (1993) Naturalistic follow-up of a behavioural treatment of chronically parasuicidal borderline patients. *Archives of General Psychiatry*, **50**, 971–974.

Liu, J., Raine, A., Venables, P.H., *et al* (2004) Malnutrition at age 3 years and externalizing behavior problems at ages 8, 11, and 17 years. *American Journal of Psychiatry*, **161**, 2005–2013.

McManus, M., Alessi, N., Grapentine, W., *et al* (1984) Psychiatric disturbance in serious delinquents. *Journal of the American Academy of Child Psychiatry*, **23**, 602–615.

Meltzer, H., Gatward, R., Corbin, T., *et al* (2003) *The Mental Health of Young People Looked After by Local Authorities in England: Summary Report*. The Stationery Office (TSO).

Mesibov, G.B., Shea, V. & Schopler, E. (2005) *The TEACCH Approach to Autism Spectrum Disorders*. Springer.

Ministry of Justice (2010) *Breaking the Cycle: Effective Punishment, Rehabilitation and Sentencing of Young Offenders*. TSO (The Stationery Office).

Ministry of Justice (2012) *Youth Justice Statistics 2010/11*. England and Wales: Youth Justice Board/Ministry of Justice Statistics Bulletin. Ministry of Justice.

National Institute for Health and Clinical Excellence (2009) *Antisocial Personality Disorder (CG77)*. NICE.

National Institute for Health and Clinical Excellence (2013) *Antisocial Behaviour and Conduct Disorders in Children and Young People: Recognition, Intervention and Management (CG158)*. NICE.

O'Herlihy, A., Worrall, A., Lelliott, P., *et al* (2003) Distribution and characteristics of in-patient child and adolescent mental health services in England and Wales. *British Journal of Psychiatry*, **183**, 547–551.

Pfeifer, J., Masten, C., Moore, W., *et al* (2011) Entering adolescence: resistance to peer influence, risky behavior, and neural changes in emotion reactivity. *Neuron*, **69**, 1029–1036.

Police Foundation (2010) *Time for a Fresh Start: The Report of the Independent Commission on Youth Crime and Antisocial Behaviour*. The Police Foundation (http://www.police-foundation.org.uk/uploads/catalogerfiles/independent-commission-on-youth-crime-and-antisocial-behaviour/fresh_start.pdf).

Raine, A., Mellingen, K., Liu, J., *et al* (2003) Effects of environmental enrichment at ages 3–5 years on schizotypal personality and antisocial behavior at ages 17 and 23 years. *American Journal of Psychiatry*, **160**, 1627–1635.

Rathus, J. & Miller, A. (2000) DBT for adolescents: dialectical dilemmas and secondary treatment targets. *Cognitive and Behavioral Practice*, **4**, 425–434.

Rathus, J. & Miller, A. (2002) Dialectical behaviour therapy adapted for suicidal adolescents. *Suicide and Life-Threatening Behavior*, **32**, 146–157.

Richardson, A. (2006) Omega 3 fatty acids in ADHD and related neurodevelopmental disorders. *International Review of Psychiatry*, **18**, 155–172.

Roe, S. & Ashe, J. (2008) *Young people and crime: findings from the 2006 Offending, Crime and Justice Survey*. Home Office Statistical Bulletin, 15 July (http://dera.ioe.ac.uk/9140/1/hosb0908.pdf).

Rose, J. (2004) The residential care and treatment of adolescents. In *From Toxic Institutions to Therapeutic Environments* (eds. P. Campling, S. Davies & G. Farquharson). Royal College of Psychiatrists.

Rutter, M., Giller, H. & Hagell, A. (1998) *Antisocial Behavior by Young People*. Cambridge University Press.

Rutter, M. & Smith, D. (1995) *Psychosocial Disorders in Young People: Time Trends and Their Causes*. Academia Europaea Publications.

Rutter, M. (2000) *Resilience Reconsidered: Conceptual Considerations, Empirical Findings, and Policy Implications. Handbook of Early Childhood Intervention*. Cambridge University Press.

Scott, S., Knapp, M. & Henderson, J. (2001) Financial cost of social exclusion: follow up study of antisocial children into adulthood. *BMJ*, **323**, 1–5.

Scott, S., Knapp, M. & Romeo, R. (2006) Economic cost of severe antisocial behaviour in children – and who pays it. *British Journal of Psychiatry*, **188**, 547–553.

Singleton, N., Meltzer, H. & Gatward, R. (1998) *Psychiatric Morbidity among Prisoners in England and Wales*. TSO (The Stationery Office).

Steinberg, L. (2008) A social neuroscience perspective on adolescent risk-taking. *Developmental Review*, **28**, 78–106.

Steiner, H., Petersen, M., Saxena, K., *et al* (2003) Divalproex sodium for the treatment of conduct disorder: a randomized controlled clinical trial. *Journal of Clinical Psychiatry*, **64**, 1183–1191.

Swanston, H., Parkinson, P., O'Toole, B., *et al* (2003) Juvenile crime, agression and delinquency after sexual abuse. *British Journal of Criminology*, **43**, 729–749.

Teplin, A., Abram, K., McClelland, G., *et al* (2002) Psychiatric disorders in youth in juvenile detention. *Archives of General Psychiatry*, **59**,1133–1143.

van Leijenhorst, L., Moor, B., Op de Macks, Z., *et al* (2010) Adolescent risky decision making: neurocognitive development of reward and control regions. *Neuroimage*, **51**, 345–355.

Vaynman, S. & Gomez-Pinilla, F. (2005) License to run: exercise impacts functional plasticity in the intact and injured central nervous system by using neurotrophins. *Neurorehabilitation and Neural Repair*, **19**, 283–295.

Vermeiren, R., Jespers, I. & Moffitt, T. (2006) Mental problems in juvenile justice populations. *Child Psychiatric Clinics of North-America*, **15**, 333–351.

Walker, S., Chang, S., Powell, C., *et al* (2007) Early childhood stunting is associated with poor psychological functioning in late adolescence and effects are reduced by psychosocial stimulation. *Journal of Nutrition*, **137**, 2464–2469.

Wheatley, M., Waine, J., Spence, K., *et al* (2004) Characteristics of 80 adolescents referred to secure inpatient care. *Clinical Psychology and Psychotherapy Journal*, **11**, 83–89.

Worling, J. (2004) The Estimate of Risk of Adolescent Sexual Offense Recidivism (ERASOR): preliminary psychometric data. *Sexual Abuse: A Journal of Research and Treatment*, **16**, 235–254.

CHAPTER 10

Secure care for people with autism spectrum disorder

Jane Radley and Huw Thomas

Introduction

Historically, relatively little attention has been paid to the specialist needs of people with autism spectrum disorders (ASDs) within forensic hospital services. This is partly because it was seen as a condition affecting children, and partly because the relationship between the condition and offending and challenging behaviour has only been recognised relatively recently. In the UK a high-profile campaign by the National Autistic Society led to the Autism Act 2009 and a national strategy (Department of Health, 2010), which has increased awareness of the condition among psychiatrists and other health professionals. This has been followed by the publication of a National Institute for Health and Care Excellence (NICE) guideline on the recognition, referral, diagnosis and management of adults on the autism spectrum (National Institute for Health and Clinical Excellence, 2012).

Whereas in the UK psychiatric training has, in the past, paid insufficient regard to the existence of ASD in adults without an intellectual disability, the demand for services for people with ASD is now too great to be met by specialist teams alone. This was recognised by the Royal College of Psychiatrists, which published recommendations on diagnosis and assessment, management, service provision, research and training (Royal College of Psychiatrists, 2014) and which has developed teaching programmes aimed at equipping general psychiatrists with the necessary skills to recognise and treat this group of patients (Royal College of Psychiatrists, 2011).

All psychiatrists should have a basic knowledge of autism spectrum disorders. However, the more complex or high-risk cases are likely to require specialist services.

In this chapter we examine the history, definition and classification of ASD. We describe the epidemiology of the condition, its relation to offending and challenging behaviours and its treatment and management in secure care.

Definition and classification of ASD

We use the term autism spectrum disorder, although it is recognised that some prefer the term autism spectrum condition. Pervasive developmental disorder is also used; it encompasses ASD and the rare and severe Rett's syndrome and childhood disintegrative disorder. The conditions included within the autism spectrum are classified as childhood autism, atypical autism and Asperger's syndrome in the *International Classification of Diseases* (ICD-10; World Health Organization, 2008). In the *Diagnostic and Statistical Manual* (DSM-IV-TR; American Psychiatric Association, 2000) the classification included autism, Asperger's syndrome and pervasive developmental disorder not otherwise specified (PDD-NOS). However, DSM-5 has reduced these categories to one category of autism spectrum disorder and created a new condition of social communication disorder (American Psychiatric Association, 2013).

Autism

The term autism was first used by the Swiss psychiatrist Eugene Bleuler to describe the emotional deficits characteristic of patients with schizophrenia. He derived it from the Greek word for self (*auto-*), meaning a person living in their own world (Bleuler, 1911). Leo Kanner (1943) then used the term 'early infantile autism' to describe the difficulties of social interaction in a series of 11 patients he had seen, noting that their symptoms were lifelong. The characteristics of the condition were further elucidated by Lorna Wing and Judith Gould (Wing & Gould, 1979). They described a 'triad of impairments' comprising deficits in social communication, social interaction and social imagination. They considered the condition as a spectrum because of the marked variations in severity and symptomatology seen across the three domains in different individuals. This heterogeneity can make diagnosis and classification difficult.

Social communication deficits range from a complete absence of verbal communication in severely affected individuals to subtle abnormalities in the use of language in some patients with Asperger's syndrome. Common difficulties include a very literal use of language with an inability to understand idiom and allegory, or a formal and stilted manner of speaking. Non-verbal communication is also commonly affected, with poor use of eye contact and limited use of gesture being characteristic features. Difficulties in reciprocal social interaction result from an inability to understand others' thoughts and feelings, sometimes described as a lack of 'theory of mind' or 'mind blindness' (Baron-Cohen, 1995). This leads to individuals being unable to develop or maintain friendships, and many experience bullying and isolation at school and in the workplace. Deficits in social imagination are demonstrated by stereotyped and repetitive patterns of behaviour, such as a liking for routine, and intense and circumscribed interests. Sensory perceptual abnormalities are also common in people with ASD but do not form part of the diagnostic criteria (O'Neill & Jones, 1997).

149

Asperger's syndrome

The term Asperger's syndrome was coined by Lorna Wing to refer to people with ASD who do not have an intellectual disability and who have good verbal skills (Wing, 1981). She had read the paper by Hans Asperger (1944) which described four children who had 'severe and characteristic difficulties of social integration'. Although in all his cases the children's language was fluent, their style of communication was unusual, for example, the choice of words was often pedantic and formal and non-verbal communication was largely absent. In addition, patients with Asperger's often became obsessed with unusual subjects, such as historical coats of arms, poisons or complex machinery. He also noted that his patients were markedly clumsy; the presence of coordination disorders is now recognised as a common comorbidity with ASD rather than a core feature of the disorder. Wing described a series of children with similar symptoms. Asperger's paper was later translated into English by Uta Frith (1991), leading to further recognition of the disorder. The term Asperger's syndrome is now falling out of use as it is recognised that the distinction between it and other forms of ASD cannot be clearly defined. It is absent from DSM-5 and is likely to disappear from ICD-11.

There is an important distinction between individuals on the autism spectrum who also have an intellectual disability often described as having 'classic' or 'Kanner's' autism, and more able people with autism who may be described as having Asperger's syndrome or 'high functioning ASD' in relation to secure services. The first group may present frequent challenging behaviour in the form of physical assaults on family and carers, sexually inappropriate behaviour or destruction of property, but they are unlikely to have received a criminal conviction as their obvious disability leads to their early diversion from the criminal justice system into the healthcare system. The second group, on the other hand, are more likely to have been convicted of a criminal offence and to have been sent to hospital via the courts (Langstrom *et al*, 2009). People with a mild intellectual disability (IQ 50–70) may fall into either group, depending on the pattern of their cognitive impairments, the level of their communication skills and their adaptive living skills.

Epidemiology

The accepted prevalence of ASD has steadily increased over the years since it was first described. It was initially thought to be a rare disorder and in the 1960s and 70s rates as low as 0.7 per 1000 were reported (Wing & Potter, 2002). However, these figures were rates for Kanner's autism in children, as Asperger's syndrome was not widely recognised at that time. Ehlers & Gilberg (1993) reported a rate of 7 per 1000 in children aged 7–16 if children with Asperger's syndrome were included. Suggestions of an 'epidemic of autism', however, appear to be unfounded and the likely causes of the increase in prevalence are changes in diagnostic criteria (Fombonne *et al*, 2011), increasing awareness of the existence of the disorder, recognition that it can be associated with other conditions and development of specialist services (Wing & Potter, 2002).

There has been little prevalence research in adults, but a representative survey of more than 7000 individuals aged 16 years and over living in England (National Centre for Social Research, 2009; Brugha *et al*, 2011) found that 1.0% of the adult population had ASD, using the threshold of a score of 10 or more on the Autism Diagnostic Observation Schedule (Lord *et al*, 1989), with rates of 1.8% for men and 0.2% for women. It has always been recognised that rates of ASD were higher in males than females. Kanner (1943) reported a ratio of 4:1, as did Ehlers & Gillberg (1993), whereas Wing (1981) thought the rate was 15 times more in males than in females.

Offending in ASD

Studies of the prevalence of ASD in secure services have shown higher rates than the 1% now thought to be found in the general population. Scragg & Shah (1994) reported a prevalence of 1.5 to 3% in the high secure hospitals in the UK. However, this finding probably does not indicate an increased rate of offending in people with ASD, rather that people with ASD in the UK who offend are more likely to be admitted to secure psychiatric services than to enter the prison system. It has proved difficult to assess the prevalence of ASD in prisons because of the lack of a suitable screening tool; a recent study in Scottish prisons failed to identify any cases of ASD among 2458 prisoners screened (Robinson *et al*, 2012). In a UK community sample, Woodbury-Smith *et al* (2006) found lower rates of offending in people with ASD than in the general population, and established that offenders with ASD were less likely to have used drugs, but more likely to have committed criminal damage or violent offences.

Although the prevalence of offending in people with ASD probably does not differ significantly from that in the general population, there is evidence that the pattern of offending is different. Firesetting offences are more frequent than would be expected in the general population or in mentally disordered offenders (Hare *et al*, 1999; Mouridsen *et al*, 2008), as is violence (Woodbury-Smith *et al*, 2006). Stalking may also be more common (Stokes *et al*, 2007). However, sexual offences and acquisitive offences are relatively less common. Both alcohol and drug misuse and drug offences (Allen *et al*, 2007) have been reported in this population but appear to be less common than in the general population.

In general, the risk factors for offending in individuals with ASD appear to be the same as those in the general population (Langstrom *et al*, 2009). These include male gender, comorbid mental illness and drug use. However, the clinical features of ASD contribute to offending in some people, and where this occurs it is important to understand the link between the disorder and the offence in order that appropriate treatment can be provided within secure services.

Lack of theory of mind is a common factor in offending in these individuals. People with ASD can lack the skills to avoid conflict such as reading, and responding to, the non-verbal communication of others. People who are poor at reading non-verbal cues can misread changes in tone of voice or facial expression that indicate anger and provide a warning that an escalation of the conflict may ensue.

Many people with ASD have little experience of friendship and may crave acceptance and belonging, particularly as they enter adolescence. This can make them vulnerable to exploitation, particularly as they may lack the social skills to exercise good judgement about the motives of others. Individuals with ASD may also be drawn towards friendships and sexual relationships with people who, even though they are much younger than them, are their emotional peers. This leads to a risk of offending against minors. Difficulty finding appropriate sexual partners because of poor social communication, social isolation and lack of confidence may lead to sexual frustration and related offending behaviour such as stalking or sexual assault. The risk of stalking may be compounded by the somewhat obsessive nature of the condition.

Special interests may lead people into offending in a variety of ways. An intense desire to obtain items related to special interests may lead to acquisitive crimes such as shoplifting or other straightforward offences such as riding on trains without a ticket. It is possible that an intense interest in violent fantasies, films or computer games may contribute to the risk of violent offending, although there is as yet no published evidence to support this conjecture for individuals with ASD, nor indeed in the general population (Sherry, 2001). A special interest in fires or fire engines may contribute to the risk of arson, although the evidence for this currently relies on case reports (e.g. Radley & Shaherbano, 2011).

Diagnosis and assessment

Diagnosis of ASD, especially if not detected in childhood, can be difficult. Assessment of people suspected of having an ASD in secure services should include, as well as a standard clinical psychiatric assessment, a formal diagnostic assessment using a recognised assessment tool, neuropsychological testing and sensory screening. Even in cases where the diagnosis might be considered obvious from the history and mental state examination, such assessments provide detailed information about the individual which can help with the planning and delivery of further interventions.

A variety of assessment tools are available, each with advantages and disadvantages. The Autism Diagnostic Interview, Revised (ADI-R; Lord *et al*, 1994) is a structured interview with a parent or carer which focuses on the person's behaviour at the age of 4 or 5. It is administered by a trained professional and consists of 93 questions covering the person's social interaction, communication and patterns of behaviour. The Autism Diagnostic Observation Schedule (ADOS; Lord *et al*, 1989) is a series of structured and semi-structured tasks that enable the examiner to assess the patient's current social and communication skills. It is complementary to the ADI-R and together they provide a very reliable diagnostic assessment. However, if it is not possible to complete the ADI-R because of the absence of a suitable informant, the DISCO (Diagnostic Interview for Social and Communication Disorders; Wing *et al*, 2002) may be useful. This is an interview with a relative or carer, but does not focus on a specific period in the patient's life.

The Autism Spectrum Quotient (AQ; Baron-Cohen *et al*, 2001a; Woodbury-Smith *et al*, 2005) and the Empathy Quotient (EQ; Baron-Cohen & Wheelwright, 2004) are self-report questionnaires that can be useful in highlighting the areas of difficulty in which patients have insight with regard to their ASD. They have been combined with other information to form the Adult Asperger Assessment (AAA; Baron-Cohen *et al*, 2005) which can be used for diagnostic assessments. The Developmental, Dimensional and Diagnostic Interview (3di; Skuse *et al*, 2004) is a computerised parent interview which is relatively quick to administer and easy to use.

Further assessments that may be useful include the 'Reading the Mind in the Eyes' test (Baron-Cohen *et al*, 2001b), which provides a measure of a person's ability to correctly recognise and interpret facial expressions, often impaired in individuals with ASD, and the Awareness of Social Inference Test (TASIT; McDonald *et al*, 2003), which provides a systematic examination of social perception.

Obtaining a cognitive profile using IQ tests such as the WAIS-IV (Wechsler Adult Intelligence Scale, fourth edition; Wechsler, 2010) and tests of executive function such as the BADS (Behavioural Assessment of Dysexecutive Syndrome; Wilson *et al*, 1998) often provides useful information. Patients with ASD often have variable performance on the subtests of the WAIS, with verbal IQ frequently but not inevitably lower than performance IQ (Siegel & Minshew, 1996). An awareness of a particular individual's pattern of deficits, while not aiding diagnosis, can aid the delivery of information and psychological therapy.

Following the confirmation or otherwise of the diagnosis of ASD, it is important to correctly identify any comorbid psychiatric disorders (see below), which can also contribute to offending behaviour such as psychosis, ADHD and anxiety disorders. Initial assessments will also include assessing any sensory issues, identifying occupational and educational skills deficits and identifying the nature and extent of the communication and social skills deficits.

Psychiatric comorbidity

As the clinical manifestations of Asperger's syndrome are heterogeneous, comorbid psychiatric disturbances may obscure the symptoms and consequently the diagnosis of ASD may be missed (Sverd, 2003). Equally, in patients with ASD, symptoms of psychiatric disorders may be misinterpreted as manifestations of the ASD and therefore remain untreated. The combination of mental illness or other developmental disorders with ASD can increase the risk of offending in a number of ways.

Attention deficit disorder, with or without hyperactivity, is very commonly comorbid with ASD (Goldstein & Schwebach, 2004). The impulsivity associated with this condition, combined with difficulty coping with changes in environment or routine, or misunderstandings of social situations, can result in impulsive violent outbursts. High levels of anxiety are common in people with ASD. When under stress some individuals may decompensate, which can manifest as an explosion of indiscriminate anger and aggression. Stressors are many and varied and include things which most people might be expected to cope with relatively easily, such as changes of routine, as well as experiences which are stressful for anyone, but much more common for people with ASD, such as sensory overload and bullying. Individuals with ASD may develop psychotic symptoms (Hutton *et al*, 2008) which may be acute, transient and stress-related, or may be expressions of an underlying psychotic illness such as schizophrenia or bipolar disorder. In some cases, people with ASD commit violent offences during an episode of psychosis in response to paranoid delusions or because of command hallucinations. People with ASD are not immune to developing personality disorders and the combination of ASD and psychopathy may lead to an increased risk of violent offending (Murphy, 2007).

Treatment and management

There is very little research on treatment specifically for offenders with ASD. It is reasonable to assume that approaches which benefit people with ASD who are not in a secure setting will also be of benefit in the forensic population. Approaches commonly used in secure services can be adapted to meet the particular needs of people with ASD. Common strategies include use of a therapeutic milieu, treatment of mental and physical health problems, explanation of the diagnosis, social skills training, empathy skills training, cognitive–behavioural therapy (CBT), education and preparation for employment (Dein & Woodbury-Smith, 2010).

A small number of specialist low and medium secure services for adults with ASD have been developed in the UK in recent years, mainly in the independent sector. In general, they cater for people with ASD who do not have significant intellectual disabilities, as this group can usually be effectively managed within secure intellectual disability services. These specialist services may have advantages over mainstream services in that they can provide an appropriate physical environment, specialist professionals, a therapeutic milieu and specific treatment programmes.

Environment, therapeutic milieu and activity

There are no existing guidelines on how to provide the optimal secure hospital environment for people with ASD and little relevant published research. The following observations are based on clinical experience from running specialist ASD wards. Ward size is important, as bringing together a group of people with social communication disorders inevitably brings with it the potential for various problems. Many people with ASD have little understanding, or interest in the needs, of others owing to what has been called poor theory of mind or 'mind blindness' (Baron-Cohen, 1995). This inability to see things from another person's perspective can make communal living particularly difficult. Before admission to hospital many people with ASD will have lived alone, with limited social contacts, or they have continued to be cared for by their families who have learnt how to accommodate their routines and idiosyncrasies. They often struggle to adapt to a living situation where the needs of other patients are paid equal attention to their own. Problems related to this increase with numbers of patients and experience suggests that patient numbers above 12 to 15, depending on various factors such as IQ range and level of challenging behaviours, are unmanageable.

Physical environment is also important. Provision of multiple living areas to allow patients to have time apart from the main group is helpful as are seating arrangements which allow individuals sufficient personal space. Some patients will have a particular need for special dining arrangements owing to high anxiety about eating with others. This can be achieved by allowing the patients to eat in separate rooms away from the main dining area or having a second sitting after most patients had finished eating. Access to cooking facilities on the ward can be invaluable for those patients who, owing to sensory sensitivities, have a restricted diet and cannot tolerate hospital food even when this is of a generally good standard and acceptable to most people. Such patients can be supported to cook their own meals as much as is possible.

Access to exercise facilities is important not only for maintaining fitness and a healthy bodyweight in hospital, but people with ASD may use exercise to manage anxiety and promote sleep. They may have developed their own fixed exercise routines, without which they will struggle to settle into a new environment. Opportunity to exercise can be provided by running exercise programmes on the ward or providing a garden or courtyard area where patients can run around or play sports. There are obvious advantages in having access to more expensive facilities such as a multi-gym, sports hall and swimming pool, which are increasingly available in modern secure hospitals. Having activities available on the ward may benefit particular patients who are too anxious to attend sessions in other parts of the hospital or in the community where they may have to encounter unfamiliar faces.

Access to computers and a sensory room (with the usual safeguards and individual risk assessments) are particularly recommended. The use of computers appeals to many patients with ASD as it allows them to pursue a very wide range of interests without having to make ordinary social contact. However, access to the internet can present particular problems, so procedures for monitoring and restricting the type of information patients are accessing and who they are communicating with should be in place. This is particularly important when managing patients who have been involved in antisocial or criminal activity related to computers and the internet such as hacking and cyber-stalking.

Sensory sensitivities are an important issue for many people with ASD. Each person has an individual 'sensory profile' and can be hypo- or hypersensitive in any sensory modality. This has implications for building design, particularly with regard to noise and temperature. Complaints about the noise level in hospital wards are common in people with ASD who may have hypersensitive hearing. Sources of noise include doors closing or being locked and unlocked, staff carrying out observations and alarms going off. These are all difficult to avoid, even in modern well-designed secure services, but the aim should be to have awareness and to minimise disturbance where this is possible. Patients who are sensitive to noise may find it helpful to wear earplugs or earphones/ headphones and listen to their own noise (music or relaxing sounds) to block out other people's noise which they cannot control. Staff should also be aware that some people with ASD are hypersensitive to touch. A gently placed guiding hand may be very uncomfortable for someone with this type of hypersensitivity and may provoke an unexpectedly extreme reaction. There are also implications for catering departments, as patients who are hypersensitive to taste or texture may only be able to eat certain foods or drink certain liquids. Some people with ASD who have olfactory hypersensitivity may find the body odour of staff or other patients in hospital unpleasant, but this has not been a common problem in our experience. Although important to some individuals with ASD, lighting levels and colours are not a common source of problems in secure units.

Sensory rooms (which deliver sensory stimuli in a distraction-free area using lighting effects, music, scents and so on) are popular with some patients with ASD (with or without an associated intellectual disability) for relaxation and recreation. However, there has not been sufficient research to establish these as an evidence-based treatment.

Many patients with ASD will have 'special interests', which can be essential to their well-being. Many will be unable to cope and will suffer significant distress if unable to pursue an interest. Supporting special interests where possible and appropriate is likely to aid engagement with treatment. If special interests are very time-consuming and are thought to be interfering with engagement in therapy, limits may need to be introduced. In this case the limits are best set through a process of negotiation, where possible. In many cases, activities related to special interests can be used as an incentive for participating in therapy or making progress in reducing undesirable behaviours.

Structure and a predictable routine are considered beneficial for most people with ASD, and are part of the 'SPELL' framework recommended by the National Autistic Society (Siddles *et al*, 1997). SPELL stands for Structure, Positive (approaches and expectations), Empathy, Low arousal and Links. This approach emphasises the benefits of providing predictable structured routines, improving confidence and self-esteem, developing insight into how the person with ASD thinks and feels, minimising distraction and over-stimulation in the environment, and creating links with other individuals and organisations. The importance of providing genuine, meaningful routines is probably better understood in services for people with intellectual disability than in general psychiatric wards, and is one of the hallmarks of a good-quality ASD service. Without sufficient structure and routine patients can decompensate in various ways, including violent outbursts.

Anxiety management is of crucial importance when someone with an ASD is placed in secure care. For a person losing their freedom, coming into an unfamiliar closed environment and having to associate with strangers and follow externally imposed rules is likely to be stressful. For someone with ASD it combines a multitude of challenges that they are particularly ill equipped to cope with.

Medication

Comorbid psychiatric disorders should be treated pharmacologically in the same way as for any other patient. Severe anxiety, which is very common in patients with ASD, often responds well to a selective serotonin reuptake inhibitor (SSRI). There is not a great deal of evidence for the effectiveness of pharmacological treatments in ASD in the absence of comorbid disorders (Williams *et al*, 2011), but a systematic review of the antipsychotic drug risperidone (Jesner *et al*, 2007) found that it was helpful in reducing irritability, repetition and social withdrawal in autism. Comorbid medical conditions should also be appropriately treated. Epilepsy is more common in people with ASD than in the general population, although this is largely due to the increased incidence of this disorder in people with intellectual disability (Tuchman & Rapin, 2002).

Risk assessment can be informed by using standard tools such as the HCR-20 (Webster *et al*, 1997) and PCL-R (Hare, 2003). Although there is no specific research regarding their use in ASD, the evidence that the factors underlying violent offending are similar in this group (Langstrom *et al*, 2009) supports their use, and there is some evidence of their value from case reports (Murphy, 2007)

Specialist therapies

A formal psychoeducation programme for people on the autism spectrum entitled 'Being Me' has been produced by the National Autistic Society (2008). It uses video clips and written exercises which some patients find useful. Many patients with ASD resist attending group-based therapies because of social anxiety, and therefore therapy may be best conducted individually, at least initially. Attending less challenging groups such as discussion groups or ward meetings may also help prepare the patient for the challenges of group therapy. With appropriate preparation and support the majority of people with ASD can be successfully included in treatment groups and this can aid the development of social and communication skills.

There is some evidence that social skills can be improved in children and adolescents with ASD through social skills training, although the benefits may be limited by lack of generalisation to other settings (Laugeson *et al*, 2009; Charman, 2011). Poor social skills can be a common contributory factor to offending in adults with ASD and social skills training may be beneficial for ASD patients in secure settings.

The Treatment and Education of Autistic and related Children with a Communication Handicap (TEACCH) programme was originally developed for children with autism without language. It includes techniques such as using shapes as visual cues to identify things. This may be applied to adults in secure settings by using visual aids to the identification of places or objects on the hospital ward.

Social Stories™ (Gray, 1998) have been found to be effective in improving social understanding and behaviour in children with ASD and no associated intellectual disability and can be adapted for use with adults. Developed by a school psychologist, they describe specific situations or concepts and provide information using a defined format about what to expect in that situation and how to respond.

Speech and Language Therapy (SaLT) is not always available in psychiatric services but is a particularly important component of most specialist ASD services. People with ASD, even those who have good verbal skills and a high IQ, typically have a range of communication and social skills deficits which speech and language therapists are particularly well placed to address. These may include failure to modulate the volume of speech, poor skills at turn-taking in conversation and lack of confidence in initiating conversation. SaLT also pays attention to non-verbal communication and wider social skills, such as teaching people to use and recognise gestures, paying attention to their proximity to the person they are addressing and modifying abnormal levels of eye contact. Specialist services often include speech and language therapists with experience of working with adults with ASD.

Non-specialist services

Not all people with ASD who require secure hospital care will be admitted to specialist services. Owing to the difficulties of diagnosing these conditions in adults it is likely that a proportion of these will be unrecognised. Consideration should be given to an ASD diagnosis in patients who isolate themselves, appear to have difficulty with social interaction, who do not make friends and who exhibit repetitive behaviours or a strong preference for rigid routines. Further pointers towards the diagnosis can be obtained by exploring the patient's history, paying particular attention to how long such traits appear to have been present. Information from a parent or other informant who has known the person since childhood is invaluable in this respect. There are aids to diagnosis available for non-specialists (Royal College of Psychiatrists, 2011), which do not require any training. In more complex cases a specialist opinion may be sought.

Although many of the features of a specialist service cannot be easily replicated in a non-specialist service, there are various approaches which may be beneficial. Providing predictability by using timetables and sticking to appointment times is likely to be helpful. Verbal communication can be augmented by simple techniques such as providing written summaries of meetings or directing the patient to other written information which is relevant to their diagnosis and treatment. An awareness of their needs may allow some flexibility in the way ward rules are applied, for example allowing the person to use ear plugs to manage sensitivity to ward noise and allowing them to pursue their special interests where possible.

Conclusions

Autism spectrum disorders are a heterogeneous group of conditions that include characteristics which may lead to offending. People with ASD in secure services require a detailed assessment to distinguish the factors leading to offending, whether they are aspects of the ASD, intellectual disability or comorbid mental illness or personality disorder. Treatment approaches may need to be adapted to allow for the particular difficulties of those with ASD and for some individuals specialist secure services are the most helpful.

References

Allen, D., Evans, C., Hider, A., *et al* (2007) Offending behaviour in adults with Asperger syndrome. *Journal of Autism and Developmental Disorders*, **38**, 748–758.

American Psychiatric Association (2000) *Diagnostic and Statistical Manual of Mental Disorders, Fourth Edition, Text Revision (DSM-IV-TR)*. APA.

American Psychiatric Association (2013) *Diagnostic and Statistical Manual of Mental Disorders (5th edn) (DSM-5)*. APA.

Asperger, H. (1944) Die 'Autistichen Psychopathen' im Kinder- salter. *Archiv für Psychiatrie und Nervenkrankheiten*, **117**, 76–113.

Baron-Cohen, S. (1995) *Mind Blindness: An Essay on Autism and Theory of Mind*. MIT Press.

Baron-Cohen, S. & Wheelwright, S. (2004) The Empathy Quotient: an investigation of adults with Asperger's syndrome or high functioning autism and normal sex differences. *Journal of Autism and Developmental Disorders*, **34**, 163–175.

Baron-Cohen, S., Wheelwright, S., Skinner, R., *et al* (2001*a*) The Autism Spectrum Quotient (AQ): evidence from Asperger syndrome/high-functioning autism, males and females, scientists and mathematicians. *Journal of Autism and Developmental Disorders*, **31**, 5–17.

Baron-Cohen, S., Wheelwright, S., Hill, J., *et al* (2001*b*) The 'Reading the Mind in the Eyes' Test, revised version: a study with normal adults with Asperger syndrome or high-functioning autism. *Journal of Child Psychology and Psychiatry*, **42**, 241–251.

Baron-Cohen, S., Wheelwright, S., Robinson, J., *et al* (2005) The Adult Asperger Assessment: a diagnostic method. *Journal of Autism and Developmental Disorders*, **35**, 807–819.

Bleuler, E. (1911) *Dementia Praecox oder Gruppen der Schizophrenien*. Franz Deuticke.

Brugha, T.S., McManus, S., Smith, J., *et al* (2011) Validating two survey methods for identifying cases of autism spectrum disorder among adults in the community. *Psychological Medicine*, 29 July, 1–10.

Charman, T. (2011) Commentary: glass half full or half empty? Testing social communication interventions for young children with autism – reflections on Landa, Holman, O'Neill, and Stuart. *Journal of Child Psychology and Psychiatry*, **52**, 22–23.

Dein, K. & Woodbury-Smith, M. (2010) Asperger Syndrome and criminal behaviour. *Advances in Psychiatric Treatment*, **16**, 37–43.

Department of Health (2010) *Fulfilling and Rewarding Lives: The Strategy for Adults with Autism in England*. Department of Health.

Ehlers, S. & Gilberg, C. (1993) The epidemiology of Asperger's syndrome. *Journal of Child Psychology and Psychiatry*, **34**, 1327–1350.

Frith, U. (1991) *Autism and Asperger Syndrome*. Cambridge University Press.

Fombonne, E., Quirke, S. & Hagen, A. (2011) Epidemiology of pervasive developmental disorders. In *Autism Spectrum Disorders* (eds D.G. Amaral, G. Dawson & D.H. Geschwind), pp. 90–111. Oxford University Press.

Goldstein, S. & Schwebach, A. (2004) The comorbidity of pervasive developmental disorder and attention deficit hyperactivity disorder. *Journal of Autism and Developmental Disorders*, **34**, 329–339.

Gray, C.A. (1998) Social stories and comic strip conversations with students with Asperger syndrome and high functioning autism. In *Asperger's Syndrome or High-Functioning Autism?* (eds E. Schopler, G.B. Mesibov & L.J. Kunce), pp. 167–198. Plenum Press.

Hare, D., Gould, J., Mills, R., *et al* (1999) *A Preliminary Study of Individuals with Autistic Spectrum Disorders in Three Special Hospitals in England*. National Autistic Society.

Hare, R.D. (2003) *Hare Psychopathy Checklist-Revised (PCL-R)*. Pearson.

Hutton J., Goode S., Murphy M., *et al* (2008) New-onset psychiatric disorders in individuals with autism. *Autism*, **12**, 373–390.

Jesner, O., Aref-Adib, M., Coren, E. (2007) Risperidone for autism spectrum disorder. *Cochrane Database of Systematic Reviews*, **1**, CD005040.

Kanner, L. (1943) Autistic disturbances of affective contact. *Nervous Child*, **2**, 217–250.

Langstrom, A., Grann, M., Ruchkin V., *et al* (2009) Risk factors for violent offending in autism spectrum disorder: a national study of hospitalized individuals. *Journal of Interpersonal Violence*, **24**, 1358–1370.

Laugeson, E.A., Frankel, F., Mogil, C.E., *et al* (2009) Parent-assisted social skills training to improve friendships in teens with autism spectrum disorders. *Journal of Autism and Developmental Disorders*, **39**, 596–606.

Lord, C., Rutter, M., Goode, S., *et al* (1989) Autism Diagnostic Observation Schedule: a standardized observation of communicative and social behavior. *Journal of Autism and Developmental Disorders*, **19**, 185–212.

Lord, C., Rutter, M. & Le Couteur, A. (1994) Autism Diagnostic Interview-Revised: a revised version of a diagnostic interview for caregivers of individuals with possible pervasive developmental disorders. *Journal of Autism and Developmental Disorders*, **24**, 695–685.

McDonald, S., Flanagan, S., Rollins, J., *et al* (2003) TASIT: a new clinical tool for assessing social perception after traumatic brain injury. *Journal of Head Trauma Rehabilitation*, **18**, 219–238.

Mouridsen, S., Bente, R., Isager, T., *et al* (2008) Pervasive developmental disorders and criminal behaviour: a case control study. *International Journal of Offender Therapy and Comparative Criminology*, **52**, 196–205.

Murphy, D. (2007) Hare Psychopathy Checklist Revised profiles of male patients with Asperger's syndrome detained in high security psychiatric care. *Journal of Forensic Psychiatry and Psychology*, **18**, 120–126.

National Autistic Society (2008) *Being Me*. A National Autistic Society DVD and CD-ROM. The National Autistic Society. Available at http://www.autism.org.uk/products/dvd-media-or-software/being-me.aspx (accessed January 2015).

National Centre for Social Research (2009) *Autism Spectrum Disorders in Adults Living in Households throughout England: Report from the Adult Psychiatric Morbidity Survey 2007*. NHS Information Centre for Health and Social Care.

National Institute for Health and Clinical Excellence (2012) *Autism Recognition, Referral, Diagnosis and Management of Adults on the Autism Spectrum (CG142)*. NICE.

O'Neill, M. & Jones, R. (1997) Sensory-perceptual abnormalities in autism: a case for more research? *Journal of Autism and Developmental Disorders*, **27**, 283–293.

Radley, J. & Shaherbano, Z., (2011) Asperger syndrome and arson: a case study. *Advances in Mental Health and Intellectual Disabilities*, **5**, 32–36.

Robinson, L., Spencer, M., Thomson, L., *et al* (2012) Evaluation of a screening instrument for autistic spectrum disorders in prisoners. *PLoS ONE*, **7**, e36078.

Royal College of Psychiatrists (2011) *Diagnostic Interview Guide for the Assessment of Adults with Autism Spectrum Disorder*. RCPsych.

Royal College of Psychiatrists (2014) *Good Practice in the Management of Autism (including Asperger Syndrome) in Adults (CR191)*. Royal College of Psychiatrists.

Scragg, P. & Shah, A. (1994) Prevalence of Asperger's syndrome in a secure hospital. *British Journal of Psychiatry*, **165**, 679–682.

Sherry, J.L. (2001) The effects of violent video games on aggression: a meta-analysis. *Human Communication Research*, **27**, 409–431.

Siddles, R., Mills, R. & Collins, M., *et al* (1997) SPELL – The National Autistic Society Approach to Education. *Communication*, Spring, 8–9.

Siegel, D.J. & Minshew, N.J. (1996) Wechsler IQ Profiles in Diagnosis of High-Functioning Autism. *Journal of Autism and Developmental Disorders*, **26**, 389–406.

Skuse, D., Warrington, R., Bishop D., *et al* (2004) The Developmental, Dimensional and Diagnostic Interview (3di): a novel computerized assessment for autism spectrum disorders. *Journal of the American Academy of Child & Adolescent Psychiatry*, **43**, 548–558.

Stokes, M., Newton, N. & Kaur, A. (2007) Stalking, and social and romantic functioning among adolescents and adults with autism spectrum disorder. *Journal of Autism and Developmental Disorder*, **37**, 1969–1986.

Sverd, J. (2003) Psychiatric disorders in individuals with pervasive development disorder. *Journal of Psychiatric Practice*, **9**, 111–127.

Tuchman, R. & Rapin, I. (2002) Epilepsy in autism. *Lancet Neurology*, **1**, 352–358.

Webster, C., Douglas, K., Eaves, D., *et al* (1997) *HCR-20 Assessing Risk for Violence Version 2*. Mental Health, Law and Policy Institute, Simon Fraser University.

Wechsler, D. (2010) *Wechsler Adult Intelligence Scale, Fourth UK Edition (WAIS-IV UK)*. Pearson.

Williams, K., Wheeler, D.M., Silove, D., *et al* (2011) Cochrane review: selective serotonin reuptake inhibitors (SSRIs) for autism spectrum disorders (ASD). *Evidence-based Child Health*, **6**, 1044–1078.

Wing, L. (1981) Asperger's syndrome: a clinical account. *Psychological Medicine*, **11**, 115–129.

Wing, L. & Gould, J. (1979) Severe impairments of social interaction and associated abnormalities in children: epidemiology and classification. *Journal of Autism and Developmental Disorders*, **9**, 11–29.

Wing, L. & Potter, D. (2002) The epidemiology of autistic spectrum disorders: is the prevalence rising? *Mental Retardation and Developmental Disabilities Research Reviews*, **8**, 151–161.

Wilson, B.A., Evans, J.J., Emslie, H., *et al* (1998) The development of an ecologically valid test for assessing patients with a dysexecutive syndrome. *Neuropsychological Rehabilitation*, **8**, 213–228.

Wing, L., Leekam, S.R., Libby, S.J., *et al* (2002) The Diagnostic Interview for Social and Communication Disorders: background, inter-rater reliability and clinical use. *Journal of Child Psychology and Psychiatry*, **43**, 307–325.

Woodbury-Smith, M., Robinson, J., Wheelwright, S., *et al* (2005) Screening adults for Asperger syndrome using the AQ: a preliminary study of its diagnostic validity in clinical practice. *Journal of Autism and Developmental Disorders*, **35**, 331–335.

Woodbury-Smith, M., Clare, I., Holland, A., *et al* (2006) High functioning autistic spectrum disorders, offending and other law-breaking: findings from a community sample. *Journal of Forensic Psychiatry & Psychology*, **17**, 108–120.

World Health Organization (2008) *ICD-10: International Statistical Classification of Diseases and Related Health Problems (10th revised edition)*. WHO.

CHAPTER 11

Acquired brain injury, trauma and aggression

Nick Alderman

Introduction

Outcome from acquired brain injury is characterised by a range of physical, functional, cognitive, behavioural and psychosocial problems. Behaviour disorders are enduring and create severe difficulties for patients and their families (Hall *et al*, 1994). The term 'neurobehavioural disability' is used to highlight the combination of neurological and neuropsychological origins of deficits in behaviour observed among survivors of acquired brain injury (Wood, 1990). The condition comprises elements of executive and attentional dysfunction, poor insight, problems of awareness and social judgement, labile mood, poor impulse control and a range of personality changes (Wood, 2001). These result in serious long-term social handicap and poor psychosocial outcome (Kreutzer *et al*, 1996).

Among the constellation of symptoms of neurobehavioural disability, aggression is the most overt and debilitating (Fleminger *et al*, 2006). It creates special challenges in rehabilitation units and constrains achievement of rehabilitation potential (Burke *et al*, 1988). Some individuals are excluded from rehabilitation altogether (Prigatano, 1987). When this happens, people with acquired brain injury gravitate to placements for management purposes that are ill-equipped to meet their rehabilitation needs, including forensic services (Alderman, 2001).

Prevalence and progression of aggression after acquired brain injury

Aggressive behaviour is a legacy of acquired brain injury that has particularly damaging effects, but how characteristic a consequence it is remains uncertain. Tateno *et al* (2003) established that reports in the literature of aggression among survivors of traumatic brain injury varied from 11 to 96%. In their own study, 33.7% had engaged in significant aggressive behaviour within 6 months of injury. Baguley *et al* (2006) investigated outcome among a large sample of survivors of traumatic brain injury at

6 months, 24 months and 5 years post-injury. Each time, 25% met the study's criteria for 'significant' aggressive behaviour. They concluded it was a frequent and long-term sequela of traumatic brain injury. Kelly *et al* (2008) investigated challenging behaviour profiles of people with acquired brain injury living in community settings. Aggression was very characteristic, with nearly 86% engaging in verbal aggression, 41.1% in assaults on other people and 35.3% in physical aggression towards objects. This study also highlighted longevity of aggression as mean time since injury was nearly 10 years, with the longest being 41.3 years.

Variability between studies regarding prevalence of aggressive behaviour is partly attributable to the non-homogeneous nature of acquired brain injury (Wilson, 1991). However, a more consistently reported finding is that in the absence of rehabilitation there is an alarming tendency for symptoms of neurobehavioural disability, including aggression, to increase over time. Brooks *et al* (1987) reported that 64% of individuals with traumatic brain injury had temper control problems 5 years post-injury and 20% exhibited increased violent behaviour. Fifteen percent of relatives of people with acquired brain injury reported 'threats of violence' 1 year after injury, but 54% complained of this after 5 years. Similarly, whereas Johnson & Balleny (1996) found that a small minority of acquired brain injury patients presented with verbal and physical aggression while still in hospital (6%), this increased significantly as reported by relatives 18 months or more after they had been discharged home (55.5%).

Services specifically organised to manage challenging behaviour arising from neurobehavioural disability have been in existence for some time; however, information about levels of aggression they are required to manage has only recently become available. This also suggests considerable variability. For example, in a neurobehavioural service that supports people with acquired brain injury, challenging behaviour and long-term needs, Giles *et al* (2005) reported 49 incidents of aggression shown by 40 patients over a 20-month period. In contrast, Alderman (2007) described 5548 episodes, including 729 physical assaults on other people. Although this was exhibited by a larger group of patients (108 altogether), observations were made over a much shorter time (14 days). One explanation for the discrepancy was that Alderman's sample comprised patients engaged in active rehabilitation, whereas the other consisted of patients in a slow-stream care pathway where expectations were lower.

Management and treatment of acquired brain injury aggressive behaviour: general considerations

There are a range of options available to clinicians for the management of acquired brain injury aggressive behaviour disorders. To maximise the benefits of intervention, clinical teams use a structured, procedurally driven approach to management that is clearly embedded in a conceptual framework

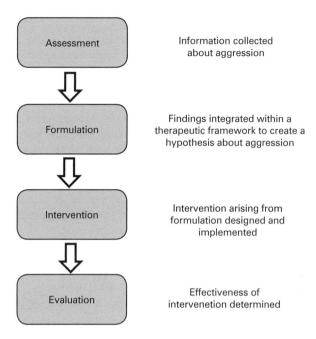

Fig. 11.1 A protocol for the management of acquired brain injury aggressive behaviour disorders.

that underpins decision-making and is supported by evidence-based practice and outcomes. An example of such a protocol is shown in Fig. 11.1, which is a simplified version of the Process Model for guiding interventions described by Alderman (2001). This will structure the remainder of this chapter.

Assessment

Deciding it is 'right' to intervene

Management of acquired brain injury aggression benefits from a multidisciplinary process that begins with comprehensive assessment (Yody *et al*, 2000). It is essential that agreement is obtained that it is acceptable to try to change a person's behaviour, and the subsequent debate brings a moral and ethical dimension to clinical decision-making. Tolerance of behaviour and perceiving it is 'right' to intervene will vary within teams and is dependent on age, culture, the context the behaviour takes place in, local norms, expectations and the belief structures and values of individual clinicians. With regard to acquired brain injury it has been suggested that behaviours that increase vulnerability, limit or delay access to community resources and decrease the likelihood of attaining full recovery potential are factors likely to warrant intervention (Alderman, 2001). In the UK, the government have encouraged a 'zero tolerance' approach regarding aggression directed against healthcare staff as it has long been recognised that such behaviour has serious consequences (Stubbs *et al*, 2009). Nevertheless, agreeing intervention is necessary must involve consideration of context, risks to self and others of allowing it to continue, appreciation of what will be lost and gained by not intervening, and determining whether the clinical team has the skills and resources required.

Patients presenting with frequent and/or severe aggression, such as those described by Alderman (2007), will require admission to in-patient neurobehavioural facilities that operationalise aspects of physical, procedural and relational security. For example, services will require an appropriate staff/patient ratio to maintain a safe and therapeutic environment, staff trained in the management of aggression and violence, and the ability to legally detain patients.

Collecting relevant information about aggression

Having made the decision to intervene, information is collected to make a formulation which identifies those factors which drive and maintain aggression for the individual. From this formulation intervention planning aimed at addressing these factors can commence. It is beyond the scope of this chapter to completely catalogue what should be considered, but it would ordinarily include obtaining a detailed history, including onset and progression of aggressive behaviour. Whenever possible, patients should contribute, although disorders of self-awareness result in unrealistic self-appraisals and a tendency to understate difficulties, casting doubt on the validity of self-report in reliably informing treatment (Hillier & Metzer, 1997; Port *et al*, 2002).

Although it is useful to collate knowledge about aggressive behaviour retrospectively, ensuring there is a system in place to collect prospective information is desirable. Asking relatives, carers and clinicians to recall details about previous events should not be entirely relied on. Events may have taken place some time ago and the level of detail recalled degraded as a consequence. Formation of new memories is not a passive process and it is subject to bias from beliefs, knowledge, expectations and emotions, which shape and potentially distort recall of events. Observing or being subject to an act of aggression is a stressful experience; consequently, high levels of cortisol released into the bloodstream have a further degrading effect on memory for events. Different neural systems process information, resulting in emotion-induced memory enhancement and amnesia, and there is evidence that recall of emotional experience is enhanced, whereas that of neutral stimuli degraded (Buchanan *et al*, 2006). Consequently, memories of behaviour are fragmented and disorganised. A further point is that beliefs and attitudes also prejudice perception of why the person with acquired brain injury is behaving as they are, having an adverse impact on the formulation and relevance of the treatment implemented.

These sources of bias can be mitigated through the use of observational recording measures. These prompt documentation of standardised variables as soon as possible after aggressive incidents which might otherwise be neglected, and provide objective information which can be used to test assumptions about behaviour. Furthermore, they have known psychometric qualities underpinned by operational definitions of what constitutes aggression. One reason for variability in prevalence of aggressive behaviour disorders, such as the 11–96% reported by Tateno and colleagues (2003), is inconsistency in definitions employed. Concepts used by clinicians, such as 'violence', 'irritability' and 'agitation', are inadequate for collecting reliable, valid measures; it is also important to distinguish between different types of aggression to achieve consistent reporting. Operational definitions of behaviours within observational recording scales enable reliable and valid measurement of aggressive behaviour that informs treatment and can also be used to measure outcome.

Measures of aggression

The Overt Aggression Scale – Modified for Neurorehabilitation (OAS-MNR; Alderman *et al*, 1997) was developed using an operant conceptual framework to create a standardised method of reporting aggression in residential neurorehabilitation programmes that is both valid and reliable. It captures information regarding type and severity of individual episodes of aggression, along with associated setting events, antecedents and interventions. It has good interrater reliability, seen widespread use, and been successfully employed in clinical work, research, outcome measurement and service evaluation (Alderman *et al*, 1999; Watson *et al*, 2001; Alderman, 2003). While there are many measures of aggression, only the OAS-MNR and its extended version (Giles & Mohr, 2007) have been specifically validated for use with acquired brain injury patients. With the OAS-MNR, a set of codes can be used as a shorthand means of capturing complex sequences of behaviour.

Whereas 'focal' measures such as the OAS-MNR yield the best-quality and most sensitive information, in some settings it is not possible to capture every incident. Use of 'global' assessment tools that provide an overview of behaviour will still make a valuable contribution to assessment. The Overt Behaviour Scale (OBS; Kelly *et al*, 2006) was developed to record challenging behaviours, including aggression, displayed by people with acquired brain injury in community settings. The St Andrew's–Swansea Neurobehavioural Outcome Scale (SASNOS; Alderman *et al*, 2011) consists of 49 items that measure five domains of neurobehavioural disability, including aggression, differentiating between provocative behaviour, irritability and overt aggression. Both the OBS and SASNOS were conceptualised for acquired brain injury, are straightforward to administer and score, provide a profile of strengths and weaknesses that aids rehabilitation planning, and have known psychometric properties, making them valuable contributions to the assessment/formulation process and determining outcome.

Formulation

This stage considers information gleaned from assessment and uses an appropriate conceptual framework to create a hypothesis about factors that cause and maintain acquired brain injury aggression. This drives treatment.

The formulation process also considers what is known from the literature concerning acquired brain injury aggression. Interpreting results from the assessment stage within this wider context further enriches understanding of behaviour and helps ensure formulations are valid, reliable and consequently likely to result in effective treatment.

Causes of acquired brain injury aggressive behaviour disorders

Neurobehavioural disability, including aggression, has complex origins. Alterations in behaviour are the product of interaction between damaged neural systems, neurocognitive impairment and premorbid personality traits, exacerbated by post-injury learning as a result of environmental influences (Alderman *et al*, 2011). The diverse, complex aetiology of behaviour change has resulted in numerous attempts in the literature to produce taxonomies of factors believed to underpin acquired brain injury aggression. These generally distinguish between explanations of behaviour change that have a predominantly neurological basis from those attributable to neurocognitive impairment (Wood, 2001).

With regard to neurological causes, damage to several brain sites has been associated with aggression, particularly the orbitofrontal cortex (OFC) and its connections with other brain structures. These include the orbito-temporal-limbic feedback loop, in which the inhibitory function of the cortex over the amygdala is disrupted, depriving the cognitive functions of any ability to suppress instinctive emotional reactions (Starkstein & Robinson, 1991). This type of aggression has clear antecedents that provoke it (Medd & Tate, 2000). Reduction in inhibitory control probably accounts for increased aggressive behaviour in people with a premorbid history of violence (Dyer *et al*, 2006).

Another category of neurologically mediated aggression is the episodic dyscontrol syndrome (EDS), one of the post-traumatic tempero-limbic disorders characterised by paroxysmal changes that reflect behavioural sequelae of electrophysiological disturbance in the brain. Episodic dyscontrol syndrome aggression tends to be brief, clear-cut and 'out of character', without obvious triggers, or preceded by minor frustration to which the magnitude of the behavioural response is grossly out of proportion (Eames, 2001).

Aggression may also be influenced by other factors, including neurocognitive impairment and especially executive function disorders. Reduced ability to initiate use of preserved abilities, monitor performance and utilise feedback effectively to regulate behaviour results in lack of 'error awareness' observed as disinhibition, impulsiveness and poor response to cues. This can result in frustration and aggression because of concurrent difficulties with response inhibition, as described above (Alderman, 2003).

The effect of the environment is also important (Medd & Tate, 2000; Demark & Gemeinhardt, 2002; Kim, 2002), including interaction with carers and clinicians (Pryor, 2004). Post-injury learning is also significant, especially when aggression serves an avoidance/escape function (Alderman, 2001).

However, while taxonomies regarding individual causes of aggressive behaviour are useful in helping to inform the formulation process, causes of post-morbid acquired brain injury aggression are likely to be multifarious (Dyer *et al*, 2006). Alderman (2007) reported data that showed how interactions between individual patient characteristics and environmental factors resulted in different types of aggression. Distinguishing these, understanding what individual and environmental factors drive them and how they interact is an important goal of assessment in creating effective treatment interventions. Utilising knowledge from the literature about acquired brain injury aggression, information about the patient themselves and data from assessment measures such as the OAS-MNR are essential in facilitating this process.

Treatment (intervention) and evaluation

As there are different combinations of reasons that drive acquired brain injury behaviour disorders, it is desirable to have a broad range of treatment options to draw from. Fortunately, many types evolved from different conceptual frameworks have been described, including pharmacological and rehabilitative interventions (Rao & Lyketsos, 2000). Non-pharmacological treatment methods include cognitive therapies, relaxation-based therapies, skills-training programmes, exposure-based treatments, cathartic treatments, behavioural interventions and multicomponent treatments (Demark & Gemeinhardt, 2002; Alderman, 2003, 2004). The importance of thorough assessment has been highlighted, and will assist in indicating the relevance of particular types of treatment: for example, a person with severe amnesia is unlikely to benefit from 'talking therapies'.

Outcome studies examining efficacy of different types of interventions are of variable quality regarding the degree of scientific rigour employed, and the evaluation stage of the protocol described here should ideally utilise scientific methods to determine them, including single-case experimental design methodologies (Alderman, 2002). Continuous monitoring of aggression using an observational recording scale such as the OAS-MNR will enable treatment effects to be closely scrutinised and fine tuned, while intermittently rating patients on global measures, including the OBS and SASNOS, will generate rehabilitation 'snapshots' that can be compared to determine progress. The principal treatment methods are now discussed.

169

Pharmacological management

Pharmacological approaches may have particular application when aggression is primarily driven by organic factors (Rao & Lyketsos, 2000; Eames, 2001; Kim, 2002). Dopamine agents are especially relevant when anterior brain structures are implicated, while anticonvulsants have a potentially important role to play in the treatment of episodic dyscontrol syndrome (Alderman, 2004). However, lack of trained, experienced neuropsychiatrists, temptation to sedate patients, and the sensitivity of people with acquired brain injury to debilitating side-effects remain potential areas of concern (Alderman, 2003). Surprisingly, a comprehensive review of pharmacological management of acquired brain injury aggressive behaviour disorders concluded there was no firm evidence this is effective and that large-scale randomised controlled trials are required to substantiate claims from small studies and anecdotal case descriptions (Fleminger *et al*, 2006).

Cognitive–behavioural therapy

Cognitive–behavioural therapy (CBT) draws on an information processing model (Hawton *et al*, 1989) which suggests that how people perceive and interpret their experience alters and shapes their behaviour. Bias or faulty processing of information may result in disorders of mood and behaviour, including aggression. CBT attempts to help patients understand links between beliefs, thinking and behaviour, identify thinking distortions, and help them generate rational interpretations of events. The 'hypothesis testing' approach to therapy ideally results in a shift in how experience is perceived and with this replacement of distorted cognitive schema used to process information and change in belief systems. CBT is successfully employed with many clinical populations, covering a broad range of disorders (Scott, 1997). It is popular, time-limited and perceived as effective. CBT has been successfully applied to the management of anger in users of mental health services (Bradbury & Clarke, 2007) and has high face validity for treatment of similar difficulties in acquired brain injury, with 'how to' manuals being available (O'Neill, 2006).

Although successful outcomes have been demonstrated regarding mood disorders (Arundine *et al*, 2012), the evidence base for acquired brain injury challenging behaviour is lacking. It may be because it remains an under-researched area and consequently robust conclusions regarding CBT cannot yet be made (Manchester & Wood, 2001). There are few case reports conducted with appropriate scientific rigour: those there are show programmes required heavy modification and implementation over much longer periods than 'standard treatments'. Challenges to implementing CBT include neurocognitive impairment, disorders of self-awareness and severity of challenging behaviour (Alderman, 2003). However, accounts of group-delivered CBT for managing aggression among people with acquired brain injury are more prolific (Whitehouse, 1994; Medd & Tate, 2000; Demark & Gemeinhardt, 2002; Walker *et al*, 2010). Group treatment has obvious benefits for resource allocation, costs and mutual support, so using this platform is an attractive proposition (Alderman, 2003; Psalia & Gracey, 2009). However, inclusion criteria for participation can be highly selective, including the need to be fully oriented, to have good communication skills, preserved ability to learn, capability of attaining goals, and ability to cooperate with requests, and have no drug/alcohol dependency and no premorbid psychiatric history. Consequently, many may be excluded from such programmes.

Behavioural interventions

Interventions derived from learning theory delivered within the context of a neurobehavioral approach to manage acquired brain injury challenging behaviour have been reported in the literature for over three decades. The neurobehavioural approach also provides a conceptual structure that facilitates understanding of the relationship between behaviour and environmental contingencies, while also accommodating constraints to new learning imposed by neurocognitive impairment. Two recent reviews have highlighted the success of this approach to managing aggression in both children and adults with acquired brain injury (Ylvisaker *et al*, 2007; Wood & Alderman, 2011).

Methods from operant theory are most frequently reported. The importance of consequences in maintaining aggression is especially highlighted. The probability of behaviour operating on the environment and reoccurring is in part dependent on whether or not it is rewarded (positive and negative reinforcement), whether an expected reward is being withheld (extinction), and whether it results in aversive consequences (positive punishment) or in loss of something of value (negative punishment). The functional analytical approach provides a methodology that highlights relationships between behaviour and the environment, and tools such as the OAS-MNR are especially useful (Alderman *et al*, 1999). Identifying the purpose behaviour serves through functional analysis directly informs the formulation. A frequent finding is that aggressive behaviour fulfils an escape or avoidance function, for example in response to therapy demands, and is therefore maintained through positive reinforcement (Alderman, 2007). Having a clear understanding of the function of the behaviour and what is maintaining it will signpost relevant operant methods that are likely to be effective.

An important contribution of the operant conceptual framework in the management of acquired brain injury aggression is the pragmatic, structured, 'step-by-step' approach it brings to rehabilitation. This expands on the assessment–formulation–treatment–evaluation schema used to structure this chapter and includes (Alderman, 2001):

171

1   Designation of a clear set of procedures followed when designing and implementing treatment interventions, to ensure a consistent and objective approach by staff.

2   Detailed assessment of social and environmental contingencies that drive aggression.

3   Individually designed interventions derived from a functional analysis of antecedents that trigger aggression or consequences that maintain it.

4   Continuous monitoring once an intervention has been implemented using objective criteria.

5   Attempts to withdraw interventions when goals have been met and to generalise benefits to other environments.

6   Further functional analysis if intervention is unsuccessful to re-evaluate the original formulation.

A wide range of operant interventions are available, including differential reinforcement, shaping, response cost and time out. Managing antecedents so that triggers of aggression are avoided are also relevant, especially in long-stay residential settings (Narevic *et al*, 2011).

A potential criticism of behavioural approaches is that for new learning to take place, especially in a clinical population in whom neurocognitive impairment is endemic, a high level of consistency is required. This need has led to the establishment of neurobehavioural rehabilitation services characterised by high levels of structure capable of delivering these treatment programmes. However, there are also examples in the literature where aggressive behaviour has successfully been remediated using operant methods in non-specialised settings (Crane & Joyce, 1991; Watson *et al*, 2001; Alderman, 2003; Woodhead & Edelstein, 2008).

Another criticism is that behavioural approaches are oversimplistic in accounting for behaviour through its relationship with the environment. While external factors may play a role in the evolution and maintenance of acquired brain injury aggression, many other factors contribute too. For example, poor 'error awareness' as a consequence of neurocognitive impairment is associated with unresponsiveness to cues and lack of knowledge regarding appropriateness of behaviour. Results of neuropsychological assessment are especially informative in such cases. Some operant methods help circumvent this problem by providing a structured and consistent method for staff to give frequent feedback about behaviour at regular intervals (for example, differential reinforcement). A cognitive–operant approach to acquired brain injury aggressive behaviour disorders can prove informative regarding both formulation and intervention, and illustrate the point made by some researchers that assessment and treatment using behavioural methods are inseparable (Wilson, 1989).

A further criticism of using methods from learning theory is that they reduce people to a mechanistic level that lacks humanity. I strongly refute such a view. Functional analysis has shown that aggressive behaviour exhibited

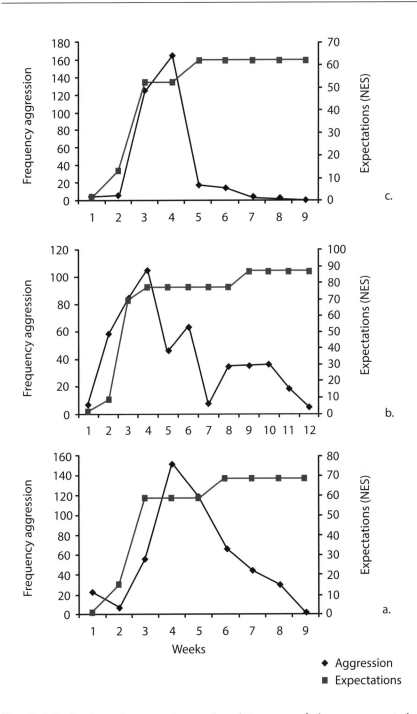

Fig 11.2 Reduction of aggression and maintenance of therapy expectations in three patients with acquired brain injury participating in neurobehavioural rehabilitation. NES, Neurobehavioural Expectations Scale.

by patients with acquired brain injury can be unwittingly maintained by those charged with their care (Rahman *et al*, 2010). One of the reasons this clinical population is unpopular with rehabilitation professionals is because of aggression (Miller & Cruzat, 1981). Consequently, this behaviour is often maintained as it leads to avoidance-escape from therapeutic activities. Staff and carers reduce expectations and may avoid 'problematic' patients altogether, resulting in their social isolation. When people are habitually ignored for long periods of time, social contact may be limited to when staff intervene to manage aggressive behaviour, thereby paradoxically further strengthening it.

However, behavioural interventions can reverse these unfortunate contingencies, first by requiring staff to interact with patients previously ignored, and second, by ensuring social reinforcement is directed at desirable, rather than challenging behaviour (Alderman, 2003). Well-managed operant methods delivered by a multidisciplinary (and preferably a transdisciplinary) team are instrumental in creating enriched environments that in the first instance change staff behaviour. This encourages the emergence of a positive social climate that promotes therapeutic relationships and good treatment outcomes (Alderman & Groucott, 2012). Provision of behavioural interventions in this way discourages aggression while actively promoting new learning, skill acquisition, independence and a collaborative approach to rehabilitation, giving patients more choice, control and freedom as they progress.

Examples of how these environments assist patients are illustrated in Fig. 11.2. This shows how exposure to a positive social climate underpinned by operant interventions typically has an impact on the frequency of aggression tracked using the OAS-MNR for three patients in a neurobehavioural rehabilitation service. Figure 11.2 also shows ratings from the Neurobehavioural Expectations Scale (NES; Swan & Alderman, 2004), a simple measure that quantifies expectations made on patients. Consistent with the avoidance-escape hypothesis, it can be seen that as expectations increased, so did frequency of aggressive behaviour. However, it is also evident the avoidance-escape function of this behaviour becomes redundant as rehabilitation demands were maintained over time. In all three cases, prolonged exposure to programmes that encouraged achievement within a positive social environment resulted in reduction of aggression.

Conclusions

The presence of neurobehavioural disability as a sequela of acquired brain injury is associated with poor prognosis; aggression is a particularly severe handicapping factor. Lack of standardised operational definitions of what 'aggression' comprises has led to uncertainty regarding prevalence, but there is good evidence that aggressive behaviour disorders get worse over time, so intervention is essential.

This chapter was pragmatically structured using a schema that can be applied to the rehabilitation of the aggressive patient. It begins with assessment: collection of good-quality information is essential for the purpose of creating a hypothesis about behaviour that drives treatment. Interpreting data using a conceptual framework will further enhance understanding and facilitate formulation. Behaviour has primarily an organic or neurocognitive basis, but is shaped further by other factors, including the environment. The multivariate origins of acquired brain injury aggression confirm there is no single 'one fix' solution and further highlights the need for detailed, individual assessment.

Treatment follows formulation, and is subject to constant evaluation and modification as required. Many treatments have been proposed and some briefly considered here. There are insufficient large-scale randomised controlled studies available to underpin effectiveness of pharmacological approaches in the management of acquired brain injury aggressive behaviour disorders. There is a similar lack of evidence for CBT, but formal evaluations published in the literature may be subject to too rigorous inclusion/exclusion criteria. Nonetheless, the multivariate origins of acquired brain injury aggression and presence of neurocognitive impairment challenge application of CBT to the extent that it has been successfully used with other clinical populations. In contrast, there is a good evidence base for the efficacy of behavioural approaches for reducing acquired brain injury aggression.

In conclusion, a wide range of interventions are available for the management of acquired brain injury aggressive behaviour disorders. More evidence regarding what works with whom and with what type of aggression using appropriate scientific methodologies is required. The need to reduce risk can mitigate against use of these, but there are workarounds to this conflict, such as multiple case descriptions that show a similar response to comparable treatments (as illustrated in Fig. 11.2). The need to conduct a proper analysis to get the best formulation and treatment is fundamental to success. Again, this process must be balanced against the need to do something to reduce risk, especially when managing physical aggression. Input from skilled, experienced practitioners will increase the likelihood of arriving at a reliable formulation in the shortest time. While such clinicians are embedded in neurobehavioural services, the need to increase such resources highlighted over a decade ago by McMillan & Oddy (2001) remains outstanding. More acquired brain injury behaviour consultants need to be trained so the challenge of aggression exhibited by people with acquired brain injury in forensic, residential and community settings can be adequately met.

References

Alderman, N. (2001) Management of challenging behaviour. In *Neurobehavioural Disability and Social Handicap Following Traumatic Brain Injury* (eds R.L. Wood & T. McMillan): pp. 175–207. Psychology Press.

Alderman, N. (2002) Individual case studies. In *Evidence in Mental Health Care* (eds S. Priebe & M. Slade): pp. 142–157. Brunner-Routledge.

Alderman, N. (2003) Contemporary approaches to the management of irritability and aggression following traumatic brain injury. *Neuropsychological Rehabilitation*, **13**, 211–240.

Alderman, N. (2004) Disorders of behaviour. In *Rehabilitation of Neurobehavioural Disorders* (ed J. Ponsford): pp. 269–298. Guilford Press.

Alderman, N. (2007) Prevalence, characteristics and causes of aggressive behaviour observed within a neurobehavioural rehabilitation service: predictors and implications for management. *Brain Injury*, **21**, 891–911.

Alderman, N. & Groucott, L. (2012) Measurement of social climate within neurobehavioural rehabilitation services using the EssenCES. *Neuropsychological Rehabilitation*, **22**, 768–793.

Alderman, N., Knight, C. & Morgan, C. (1997) Use of a modified version of the Overt Aggression Scale in the measurement and assessment of aggressive behaviours following brain injury. *Brain Injury*, **11**, 503–523.

Alderman, N., Davies, J.A., Jones, C., *et al* (1999) Reduction of severe aggressive behaviour in acquired brain injury: case studies illustrating clinical use of the OAS-MNR in the management of challenging behaviours. *Brain Injury*, **13**, 669–704.

Alderman, N., Wood, R.Ll. & Williams, C. (2011) The development of the St Andrew's–Swansea Neurobehavioural Outcome Scale: validity and reliability of a new measure of neurobehavioural disability and social handicap. *Brain Injury*, **25**, 83–100.

Arundine, A., Bradbury, C.L., Dupuis, K., *et al* (2012) Cognitive behavior therapy after acquired brain injury: maintenance of therapeutic benefits at 6 months post-treatment. *Journal of Head Trauma Rehabilitation*, **27**,104–112.

Baguley, I.J., Cooper, J. & Felmingham, K. (2006) Aggressive behaviour following traumatic brain injury: how common is common? *Journal of Head Trauma Rehabilitation*, **21**, 45–56.

Bradbury, K.E. & Clarke, I. (2007) Cognitive behavioural therapy for anger management: effectiveness in adult mental health services. *Behavioural and Cognitive Psychotherapy*, **35**, 201–208.

Brooks, D.N., McKinlay, W., Symington, C., *et al* (1987) The effects of severe head injury upon patient and relative within seven years of injury. *Journal of Head Trauma Rehabilitation*, **2**, 1–13.

Buchanan, T.W., Tranel, D. & Adolphs, R. (2006) Impaired memory retrieval correlates with individual differences in cortisol response but not autonomic response. *Learning and Memory*, **13**, 382–387.

Burke, H.H., Wesolowski, M.D. & Lane, I. (1988) A positive approach to the treatment of aggressive brain injured clients. *International Journal of Rehabilitation Research*, **11**, 235–241.

Crane, A.A. & Joyce, B.G. (1991) Brief report: cool down: a procedure for decreasing aggression in adults with traumatic head injury. *Behavioural Residential Treatment*, **6**, 65–75.

Demark, J. & Gemeinhardt, M. (2002) Anger and its management for survivors of acquired brain injury. *Brain Injury*, **16**, 91–108.

Dyer, K.F.W., Bell, R., McCann, J., *et al* (2006) Aggression after traumatic brain injury: Analysing socially desirable responses and the nature of aggressive traits. *Brain Injury*, **20**, 1163–1173.

Eames, P.G. (2001) Distinguishing the neuropsychiatric, psychiatric, and psychological consequences of acquired brain injury. In *Neurobehavioural Disability and Social Handicap Following Traumatic Brain Injury* (eds R.L. Wood & T. McMillan): pp. 29–45. Psychology Press.

Fleminger, S., Greenwood, R.J. & Oliver, D.L. (2006) Pharmacological management for agitation and aggression in people with acquired brain injury. *Cochrane Database Systematic Review*, **4**, doi: 10.1002/14651858.CD003299.pub2.

Giles, G.M. & Mohr, J.D. (2007) Overview and inter-rater reliability of an incident-based rating scale for aggressive behaviour following traumatic brain injury: the Overt Aggression Scale-Modified for Neurorehabiltation-Extended (OAS-MNR-E). *Brain Injury*, **21**, 505–511.

Giles, G.M., Wagner, J., Fong, L., *et al* (2005) Twenty-month effectiveness of a non aversive, long-term, low-cost programme for persons with persisting neurobehavioural disability. *Brain Injury*, **19**, 753–764.

Hall, K.M., Karzmark, P., Stevens, M., *et al* (1994) Family stressors in traumatic brain injury: a two-year follow-up. *Archives of Physical Medicine and Rehabilitation*, **75**, 876–884.

Hawton, K., Salkovskis, P.M., Kirk, J., *et al* (eds) (1989) *Cognitive Behaviour Therapy for Psychiatric Problems: A Practical Guide*. Oxford University Press.

Hillier, S.L. & Metzer, J. (1997) Awareness and perceptions of recovery post traumatic brain injury. *Brain Injury*, **7**, 525–536.

Johnson, R. & Balleny, H. (1996) Behavioural problems after brain injury: incidence and need for treatment. *Clinical Rehabilitation*, **10**, 173–181.

Kelly, G., Todd, J., Simpson, G., *et al* (2006) The Overt Behaviour Scale (OBS): a tool for measuring challenging behaviours following acquired brain injury in community settings. *Brain Injury*, **20**, 307–319.

Kelly, G., Brown, S., Todd, J., *et al* (2008) Challenging behaviour profiles of people with acquired brain injury living in community settings. *Brain Injury*, **22**, 457–470.

Kim, E. (2002) Agitation, aggression, and disinhibition syndromes after traumatic brain injury. *NeuroRehabilitation*, **17**, 297–310.

Kreutzer, J.S., Marwitz, J.H., Seel, R., *et al* (1996) Validation of a neurobehavioural functioning inventory for adults with traumatic brain injury. *Archives of Physical Medicine and Rehabilitation*, **77**, 116–124.

Manchester, D. & Wood, R.L. (2001) Applying cognitive therapy in neuropsychological rehabilitation. In *Neurobehavioural Disability and Social Handicap Following Traumatic Brain Injury* (eds R.L. Wood & T.M. McMillan): pp. 157–174. Psychology Press.

McMillan, T. M. & Oddy, M. (2001) Service provision for social disability and handicap after acquired brain injury. In *Neurobehavioural Disability and Social Handicap Following Traumatic Brain Injury* (eds R.L. Wood & T.M. McMillan): pp. 257–273. Psychology Press.

Medd, J. & Tate, R.L. (2000) Evaluation of an anger management therapy programme following acquired brain injury: a preliminary study. *Neuropsychological Rehabilitation*, **10**, 185–201.

Miller, E. & Cruzat, A. (1981) A note on the effects of irrelevant information on task performance after mild and severe head injury. *British Journal of Social and Clinical Psychology*, **20**, 69–70.

Narevic, E., Giles, G.M., Rajadhyax, R., *et al* (2011) The effects of enhanced program review and staff training on the management of aggression among clients in a long-term neurobehavioral rehabilitation program. *Aging and Mental Health*, **15**, 103–112.

O'Neill, H. (2006) *Managing Anger, 2nd edn*. Whurr.

Port, A., Willmott, C. & Charlton, J. (2002) Self-awareness following traumatic brain injury and implications for rehabilitation. *Brain Injury*, **16**, 277–289.

Prigatano, G.P. (1987) Psychiatric aspects of head injury: problem areas and suggested guidelines for research. *BNI Quarterly*, **3**, 2–9.

Pryor, J. (2004) What environmental factors irritate people with acquired brain injury? *Disability and Rehabilitation*, **26**, 974–980.

Psalia, K. & Gracey, F. (2009) The mood management group. In *Neuropsychological rehabilitation: theory, models, therapy and outcome* (eds B.A. Wilson, F. Gracey, J.J. Evans, *et al*): pp. 112–122. Cambridge University Press.

Rahman, B., Oliver, C. & Alderman, N. (2010) Descriptive functional analysis of challenging behaviours shown by adults with acquired brain injury. *Neuropsychological Rehabilitation*, **20**, 212–238.

177

Rao, V.R. & Lyketsos, M.D. (2000) Neuropsychiatric sequelae of traumatic brain injury. *Psychosomatics*, **41**, 95–103.

Scott, J. (1997) Advances in cognitive therapy. *Current Opinion in Psychiatry*, **10**, 256–260.

Starkstein, S.E. & Robinson, R.G. (1991) The role of the human lobes in affective disorder following stroke. In *Frontal Lobe Function and Dysfunction* (eds H.S.Levin, H.M.Eisenberg & A.L.Benton): pp. 288–303. Oxford University Press.

Stubbs, B., Winstanley, S., Alderman, N., *et al* (2009) The risk of assault to physiotherapists: beyond zero tolerance? *Physiotherapy*, **95**, 134–139.

Swan, L. & Alderman, N. (2004) Measuring the relationship between overt aggression and expectations: a methodology for determining clinical outcomes. *Brain Injury*, **18**, 143–160.

Tateno, A., Jage, R.E. & Robinson, R.G. (2003) Clinical correlates of aggressive behaviour after traumatic brain injury. *Journal of Neuropsychiatry and Clinical Neurosciences*, **15**, 155–160.

Walker, A.J., Nott, M.T., Doyle, M., *et al* (2010) Effectiveness of a group anger management programme after severe traumatic brain injury. *Brain Injury*, **24**, 517–524.

Watson, C., Rutterford, N., Shortland, D., *et al* (2001) Reduction of chronic aggressive behaviour ten years after brain injury. *Brain Injury*, **15**, 1003–1015.

Whitehouse, A.M. (1994) Applications of cognitive therapy with survivors of head injury. *Journal of Cognitive Psychotherapy: An International Quarterly*, **8**, 141–160.

Wilson, B. (1989) Injury to the central nervous system. In *The Practice of Behavioural Medicine* (eds S. Pearce & J. Wardle): pp. 51–81. Oxford University Press.

Wilson, B.A. (1991) Behavior therapy in the treatment of neurologically impaired adults. In *Handbook of Behavior Therapy and Psychological Science: An Integrative Approach* (ed P.R. Martin): pp. 227–252. Pergamon Press.

Wood, R. L. (1990) Conditioning procedures in brain injury rehabilitation. In *Neurobehavioural Sequelae of Traumatic Brain Injury* (ed R. L. Wood): pp. 153–174. Psychology Press.

Wood, R.L. (2001) Understanding neurobehavioural disability. In *Neurobehavioural Disability and Social Handicap Following Traumatic Brain Injury* (eds R.L. Wood & T. McMillan): pp. 3–27. Psychology Press.

Wood, R.L. & Alderman, N. (2011) Applications of operant learning theory to the management of challenging behaviour after traumatic brain injury. *Journal of Head Trauma Rehabilitation*, **26**, 202–211.

Woodhead, E.L. & Edelstein, B.A. (2008) Decreasing physical aggression and verbal abuse in a brain injured nursing home resident. *Clinical Case Studies*, **7**, 301–311.

Ylvisaker, M., Turkstra, L., Coehlo, C., *et al* (2007) Behavioural interventions for children and adults with behaviour disorders after traumatic brain injury: a systematic review of the evidence. *Brain Injury*, **21**, 769–805.

Yody, B.B., Schaub, C., Conway, J., *et al* (2000) Applied behavior management and acquired brain injury: approaches and assessment. *Journal of Head Trauma Rehabilitation*, **15**, 1041–1060.

CHAPTER 12

Managing aggression and violence in older people

Graeme A. Yorston

Introduction

Historical context

In the past, older people with mental health problems received the same treatment as younger adults. They were admitted to the same hospitals and the same wards. Older mentally disordered offenders who committed serious offences were admitted to hospitals for the criminally insane (East, 1944). In the UK the differentiation of generic mental health services into more specialist clinical services started slowly, but by the 1970s it had gathered enough momentum for both old age psychiatry and forensic psychiatry to split off from general psychiatry and develop along parallel service model lines. This led to the emergence of totally separate in-patient and community services often on geographically separate sites. Despite the obvious advantages of this approach in terms of developing expertise and research, the downside was that older adults were neglected as a group by developing forensic services which concentrated on young men with psychosis. The result was that only 1% of patients newly admitted to high and medium secure beds in England and Wales between 1988 and 1994 were over the age of 60 (Coid *et al*, 2002). In 1999, I highlighted the paucity of services for older adults and called for greater collaboration between old age and forensic psychiatrists (Yorston, 1999) and over the next few years a number of specialist secure services were established in the independent sector in the UK.

Much of the published research on older offenders includes a preliminary discussion of the issue of age. All figures based on chronological age, however, are arbitrary and it is better to consider age-related needs arising from life-cycle events, multiple physical comorbidities and neurodegenerative disorders, that is biological age rather than chronological age.

Though older patients have some similarities with one another owing to their age, the range of problems they present and their needs are just as varied as those of younger patients. It would be wrong therefore to confine them all together solely on grounds of chronological age. This was explored in a qualitative study at Broadmoor high secure hospital (Yorston & Taylor, 2009) which found that, despite having a ward specifically for older patients, the 16 patients over the age of 65 were spread across nine different wards in the hospital, demonstrating the heterogeneity of older mentally disordered offenders in terms of diagnosis, needs and preferences.

Violence and aggression in older adults

The rate of offending across the lifespan peaks between the ages of 18 and 22 years, thereafter going down with increasing age. This has led to youth offending being a higher priority for criminological research and criminal justice initiatives in the past, with the issues affecting older offenders being all but ignored. However, violence and aggression is extremely common in older people with mental health problems. Most of this is low severity reactive aggression, occurring in people with dementia; 78% of elderly patients in French institutional settings exhibited such behaviour (Léger et al, 2002) and similar rates have been found in many different cultures, including those with much lower base rates of violent crime, such as Japan (Ko et al, 2012). This suggests that the sociobiological mechanisms that lead to this type of aggression may be different from the mechanisms that lead to aggression in other contexts. Instrumental aggression, which is directed towards a clear goal such as revenge, intimidation, financial reward or sexual gratification, is very different in character. It is much less commonly encountered by professionals working with older people, but it does occur in Huntington's disease, frontotemporal dementia and other conditions affecting judgement and impulse control. Though typically less frequent than reactive aggression, instrumental aggression can be much more serious, and it requires very careful management, often in an environment with high staff supervision and close monitoring of potential weapons. Serious aggression may be directly linked to the psychopathology of a functional illness or the disinhibiting effects of a brain injury, cerebrovascular event or neurodegenerative process on premorbid personality traits. The effect on behaviour of lesions in the frontal lobes, especially the orbitofrontal cortex, is well known, but lesions in other brain areas that have important connections with the frontal lobes can have similar consequences, for example infarcts in the right caudate nucleus (McMurtray et al, 2008). When assessing the likely contribution of a cerebral lesion on behaviour it is important to assess premorbid personality, as a small and otherwise insignificant lesion may have a major effect on someone with a previously abnormal personality.

Crime statistics in the UK show that the homicide rate for older adults has been remarkably constant over the past 20 years, though there is a possibility that it is now starting to increase (Hunt et al, 2010). The figures have to be interpreted with caution, however, as not all cases of homicide are recorded as such. When people with severe dementia push or carry out a minor assault on a co-resident that results in injuries from which they do not recover, these are not always recorded as homicides. There have been few psychiatric studies of elderly homicide offenders, although the individual case study literature is much richer. Rollin (1973) described a case of a 71-year-old man with a history of depressive illness who battered his wife to death after becoming convinced she was beginning to fail in health and believing she was too proud to allow herself to be looked after by carers. Large homicide case series often include a small number of elderly cases: for example, in a series of 400 homicides in Scotland there were only three men aged over 65 and the oldest woman was 54. Unlike the majority of people accused of homicide who were deemed 'mentally normal' (82%), all three of the older men had psychotic illnesses (Gillies, 1976).

Reflecting on his experience as a forensic pathologist in Wales, Knight (1983) highlighted the differences between homicides occurring in older and younger intimate relationships. In contrast to typical younger couple homicides, which usually occurred against a background of long-standing interpersonal problems arising from infidelity, jealousy and money disputes often inflamed by drugs or alcohol, elderly homicides were often sudden and had no apparent warning signs. He described a case of a woman in her seventies who killed her husband with repeated brutal blows to the back of his head with the heavy iron base of an ice cream display sign while he was sitting watching television. No rational explanation for the act could be obtained.

Though the psychiatric literature emphasises the differences between elderly homicide offenders and younger homicides, criminological data from US studies show that homicide rates among the elderly mirror the non-elderly rates. The latter are strongly correlated with urbanisation and poverty, suggesting that the same factors in society are influencing the behaviour of younger and older people (Willbanks, 1984). Other US studies have shown that the elderly are more likely to kill family members, to use firearms and to carry out the offence in the home (Kratcoski & Walker, 1988).

Sexually disinhibited behaviour is relatively common in dementia, occurring in up to 17% of cases (Series & Dégano, 2005). Thankfully, most of it is mild in severity and never reaches the attention of the police or criminal justice system. However, it is important to accurately assess and monitor patients presenting such behaviour as it can escalate to more serious sexually assaultive behaviour. The routine use of a standardised rating scale such as the St Andrew's Sexual Behaviour Assessment (SASBA) is recommended to ensure systematic and consistent collection of risk data (Knight *et al*, 2008). Older people do engage in unlawful activities that end up being processed and recorded as sex crimes, however, and older adults make up around 1% of the total convictions for these offences in the UK, with broadly comparable figures from other countries, although the proportion of older adults is rather higher for those convicted of sexual offences against children. In recent years there has been a much greater willingness by prosecuting authorities to proceed with historical sexual abuse cases, including those committed many years previously in children's homes or by religious figures.

Of course, not all older adults who commit acts of aggression or sexual violence are diagnosed with a mental disorder and it is right and proper that the prison system should be able to manage older inmates. The number of older people in prison in the UK has risen sharply over the past 20 years, from a few hundred in the early 1990s to several thousand now (House of Commons Justice Committee, 2013). In the USA the number of older inmates has shown a similar dramatic rise, increasing fourteenfold between 1981 and 2012 (American Civil Liberties Union, 2012). These increases appear to be caused largely by changes in sentencing practices by the courts. In the past, the elderly were treated with a degree of leniency at all stages of the criminal justice process and they received shorter sentences. This has changed, particularly in relation to sexual offences, and in some areas there is evidence that the elderly are now dealt with more harshly than younger offenders for certain offences. The biggest reason for what has been described as the 'greying' or 'geriatrification' of prisons, however, is almost certainly the changes in mandatory sentencing practice. 'Three strikes and out' sentences were first introduced in the USA in 1993 and in the UK in 1998, with the result that recidivist violent offenders in particular remain in prison well into old age. To cope with the numbers and increasing physical frailty of older inmates, nursing home wings have been set up in prisons in most US states. In the UK, the prison service appeared oblivious to the needs of older inmates prior to the publishing of *No Problem – Old and Quiet* by Her Majesty's Inspectorate of Prisons in 2004. This report highlighted the unmet physical, mental and social care needs of older prisoners and pointed to the fact that, as a group, they tended to be quiet and pose no management problems for staff, and as a result were largely ignored.

In a recent study of sentenced male prisoners aged 50 and over (Kingston *et al*, 2011), depression was diagnosed in 41%, yet only a small proportion (18%) were prescribed medication of the appropriate class. An important finding of this study was that prisoners were able to self-report symptoms of mental illness using a simple questionnaire with high reliability, which begs the obvious question: why are such scales not in routine use?

Awareness of dementia by prison staff was extremely limited until recently, but training courses on this and other late-life issues are now available in most UK prisons. Although few cases of dementia have been detected in research studies, the applicability of the standard screening instruments in prison populations is unclear. Dementia does occur in older prisoners, and it can present major practical difficulties for prison governors trying to ensure that inmates receive adequate social care without being put at risk. A number of initiatives using fellow inmates as buddies or paid carers for prisoners with dementia have been piloted, along with projects to promote community reintegration, advocacy and safeguarding for older prisoners (Department of Health, 2007). At present most of these remain local initiatives, often funded or run by charities, or championed by enthusiasts; as such, they are subject to sudden loss of funding and personnel, and there are increasing calls for a national strategy to be developed for older prisoners encompassing their health and social care needs and offender management issues.

Assessment

Offending behaviour can occur in all of the mental disorders that affect people in late life. Generally, changes in behaviour as a result of mental disorder are recognised as such either by the individual themselves or, more commonly, by a family member or carer. Sometimes the behaviour can be so sudden and so severe, or the individual so isolated, that health services are not involved until after an offence has been committed and assessment has to take place in police cells or prison.

Trial

The Pritchard criteria used in England and Wales to determine fitness to plead and stand trial date back to 1838 and have been much criticised as there is abundant evidence that they are interpreted inconsistently by psychiatrists advising the courts (Law Commission, 2010). For older adults, mental health issues have to be considered alongside physical health and perceptual issues. For example: is the defendant able to see and hear adequately, do they need shorter court sessions because of fatigability, do they require extra toilet breaks or different seating? Although the courts are open to suggestions from psychiatrists to help ensure defendants are able to function at their best, in practice special measures are rarely recommended. The most important question to be addressed in determining fitness to plead and stand trial in older adults, however, is whether the defendant is able to follow the course of the proceedings in court. Though this may be obvious for someone with severe dementia, or someone with mild, well-managed mental health problems, in cases of mild to moderate dementia the issue is often far from clear. Standard cognitive testing in such cases can be helpful, but in serious cases fuller neuropsychological evaluation is recommended which should include tests of malingering and suggestibility.

Physical health

It is known that younger prisoners have worse physical health than age-matched controls. There is also evidence that such ill health continues into old age, with the elderly having more physical health problems than younger inmates and age-matched community-living elders (Fazel *et al*, 2001). A US study of older prisoners (Lewis *et al*, 2006) revealed high rates of cerebrovascular disease and sexually transmitted disease and the authors emphasise the importance of taking a thorough medical history and carrying out a careful physical examination, to ensure that appropriate treatment and secondary preventive measures can be taken for these and other medical conditions. Constipation, infections and metabolic imbalances, either alone or in combination with other medical problems, can all cause delirium. If this occurs in the early stages of dementia or on top of a pre-existing depressive illness it can cause marked confusion, fear and paranoia which can lead to feelings of threat and, in turn, to serious aggression in response to the perceived threat. Sudden onset and severe cases of delirium accompanied by agitation are usually obvious and most present acutely to emergency medical services. Milder, more insidious or fluctuating cases of delirium may go unrecognised, however, and clinicians working in secure psychiatric services for older people regularly encounter cases of severe violence and homicide committed by people in a subacute delirious state.

Cognitive assessment

Dementia can present with a change in behaviour: either the emergence of new behaviours that were not present at all previously or a change in the type, frequency and character of existing behaviour. Old age psychiatrists are familiar with the evaluation of such issues by taking careful histories from carers and relatives. Forensic psychiatrists, however, are generally more used to assessing individuals through detailed mental state examinations, which may reveal little in early dementia. In a study of referrals of older adults to a regional medium secure unit in England (Curtice *et al*, 2003), it was found that forensic psychiatrists did not routinely use standardised rating scales for the assessment of cognitive functioning. It is to be hoped that practice has improved since this study was conducted, but there is still value in individuals presenting with offending behaviour for the first time in old age being assessed by clinicians with experience of both old age and forensic psychiatry or, if none are available, by clinicians from each specialty working closely together. The assessment of frontal lobe functioning is important in older adults presenting with behavioural change. Most standard cognitive screening instruments contain a few questions that test this, so the use of a brief but specific frontal lobe assessment instrument such as the frontal assessment battery (FAB; Dubois *et al*, 2000) is recommended alongside a more general tool.

Psychosis

In contrast to the psychotic presentations of younger adults in which fixed paranoid delusions and command hallucinations are often warning signs of impending violence, cases of homicidal psychosis in the elderly are more often associated with depressive or nihilistic delusions. These include beliefs that the perpetrator or victim or both are seriously ill, about to lose their savings or be made homeless. The depression may be relatively mild on the surface and can be easily missed by those unfamiliar with how older men in particular can be somewhat stoical or alexithymic and deny mood symptoms even when asked about them directly. The absence of cases of depression in two studies of older adults charged with serious offences in New York (Rosner *et al*, 1985, 1991) could reflect a genuinely lower prevalence in this group or, more likely, be an indication that criminal justice professionals are not flagging up potential cases for assessment or that mental health staff may be missing the diagnosis on assessment. Careful enquiry about worries, preoccupations and changes in habit is warranted. Obtaining a detailed collateral history, focusing on any changes in day-to-day functioning, can sometimes reveal a diagnosis of depression in individuals who deny any significant affective symptoms at interview.

Personality disorder

Personality disorders do not start in old age, but a change in circumstances in late life can reveal a disordered personality that has previously been contained, usually by a long-suffering partner. This is rare in dissocial personality disorder, as the nature of the disorder is such that there is usually clear evidence of conflict with society throughout life, but it does occur with dependent, emotionally unstable and narcissistic personality disorders. Another way in which pre-exiting personality disorder can lead to offending in late life is through the disinhibiting effects of dementia or a strategic infarct. Someone with paranoid personality traits, who has been seething with resentment and discontent for their entire life, may suddenly act on their anger after years of suppression. An individual with narcissistic traits may lose all sense of proportion in pursuing the things they feel they deserve.

Drug- and alcohol-related crime

Drug use was uncommon in people who grew up in the UK in the 1940s and 50s, but this changed for the baby boom generation, who enjoyed their teenage years and early adulthood in the 1960s and 70s, and old age psychiatrists are now beginning to see older people with active drug problems. Older people can be involved in organised drug crime by rising through the ranks of seniority in crime families and, from time to time, the media report high-profile prosecutions of older drug lords. Older people can also be used to smuggle drugs, sometimes unwittingly, as drug dealers regard them as having a better chance of getting past customs officials without being searched. Alcohol misuse is also being increasingly recognised as a problem in older adults, and is common in older prisoners in the USA (Lewis *et al*, 2006). When this is linked to offending behaviour it has serious implications for risk assessment. Detailed neuropsychological assessment may detect subtle deficits in executive functioning in people who have misused alcohol over a sustained period, even those with what would have previously been considered a moderate consumption (Neafsey & Collins, 2011). This has important implications in the assessment of *mens rea* or specific intent in serious criminal cases.

Risk assessment

There has been little published research on risk assessment in the elderly. However, there is now a body of work on elderly sex offenders that has consistently demonstrated lower rates of recidivism compared with younger sex offenders (Fazel *et al*, 2006). Some of the earlier studies failed to account for the reduced time at risk of reoffending among elderly men, and that the types of offences typically committed by older men (e.g. intrafamilial abuse of girls) have lower recidivism rates in all age groups. Although the lower recidivism rate for older men appears to be a robust finding across different countries, it is of little help in assessing risk in individual cases. Assessment should be approached in a structured manner and should consider offence characteristics, history, deviant sexual arousal patterns and mental and physical health issues as in any other case. Actuarial risk assessment tools that predict the risk of sexual reoffending, such as the Sex Offender Risk Appraisal Guide (SORAG; Quinsey *et al*, 2006), are of questionable validity in older people as the base rate of offending is much lower than in younger people and the samples on which the tools are based contain few older adults. The use of a structured professional judgement tool is recommended instead as these incorporate clinical judgements of the relevance of information that is collected in a systematic way, the most well-known of these being the Risk of Sexual Violence Protocol (RSVP; Hart *et al*. 2003) for sex offenders and the HCR-20 (Webster *et al*, 1997) for assessing the risk of future violence.

Management

Environment

The most important consideration in the treatment of the mental health problems of elderly offenders is environment. For less serious offenders, normal treatment by their community mental health team in conjunction with their general practitioner (GP) is usually appropriate. For those in custody, treatment by a visiting psychiatrist and prison in-reach team may be sufficient, but for others, assessment and treatment in hospital will be required. For some of these it may be appropriate for an old age psychiatrist to manage the case within their own service, with advice from the local forensic team, but in some cases the individual may need treatment in a secure hospital.

Treatment

Pharmacological treatments are no different for elderly offenders with mental health problems than for their community peers, but the risk–benefit balance is tilted more towards drug treatment than would be the case in standard old age psychiatric practice. Antipsychotics in schizophrenia tend to be used at doses more typical of working-age adult services and may be used in dementia as well. Acetylcholinesterase inhibitors need to be used with caution as they can result in increased agitation and aggression. Anti-libidinal medication can be useful in the treatment of sexual offenders with personality disorders and organic mental health problems, but the evidence base for this is still very limited. Offence-related psychological therapies are important in older offenders, but programmes usually need to be adapted to meet the needs of older people.

Women

The number of older women in prison has shown the same dramatic increase over the past 15 years as men. Many older women are long-term prisoners who have grown old in custody, though there are a few who commit serious offences for the first time in late life. It is likely that they have at least the same prevalence of mental health problems, if not greater, than their younger peers, but as numbers are small, no formal research has been carried out. Wahidin (2004) found that there were a disproportionately high number of older women from ethnic minorities in prison, who suffered the double isolation of being different because of their age and different because of their culture. Qualitative research has revealed that many older women feel they get inadequate medical care in prison, missing out on routine screening such as mammography and cervical cytology (Wahidin, 2005).

Ethnic minorities

Little is known about the needs of Black and minority ethnic elders in prison and secure mental health services, despite the fact that they make up about 10% of the 60+ prison population. The UK prison service is becoming aware of the differing final wishes of people from different ethnic and religious backgrounds, but no formal research has been carried out to investigate the needs of this group in the UK.

Secure psychiatric services

Secure hospital services were often reluctant to admit older adults in the past, partly because of concerns about their potential vulnerability to aggression from younger patients and partly because there was a perception that their offences were less serious. However, research has consistently shown that older people do commit offences that are no less serious than those of their younger counterparts, and they account for up to 3% of referrals to forensic mental health services in Europe (McLeod *et al*, 2008). Lewis and colleagues (2006) provide further evidence for this, with most of the 99 pre-sentence evaluees in their series having been charged with serious offences.

There have been several descriptive studies of the elderly in high secure hospitals but these have mainly focused on diagnostic issues (East, 1944; Wong *et al*, 1995; Rayel, 2000). The study at Broadmoor high secure hospital in England by Yorston & Taylor (2009) highlighted the wide range of diagnoses and treatment needs of older mentally disordered offenders, as well as differences in how the patients perceived their own needs and where they wanted to be treated. This important issue emerged in some of the earlier qualitative work in prisons when it was found that not all older inmates wanted to be housed together: some liked the hustle and bustle of mixed-age units and felt they enjoyed a high status in them because of their age and life experiences (Goetting, 1983).

There is a small number of middle-aged and older women scattered throughout existing secure psychiatric services who are unable to progress through rehabilitation and who continue to require in-patient care. Little is known of their needs and whether they differ from their younger peers in this regard.

Most older adults with mental health problems are treated and cared for at home or in residential and nursing homes. Care homes for older adults often cope with high levels of minor physical aggression and sexually disinhibited behavior, yet they are not equipped to deal with more serious aggression or predatory sexual behaviour. The understanding of risk issues and how to assess and manage them is often highly sophisticated for the common behavioural problems of dementia, but for behaviour driven by antisocial personality traits it is usually lacking. This means there is a shortage of suitable facilities for older offenders who have been assessed and require ongoing nursing care in an environment that is also able to manage their risky behaviour. In the UK, medium and low secure specialist hospital units have been set up for those who require in-patient assessment and treatment, but a lack of suitable places to discharge patients to once they have been stabilised, though not necessarily to a state where the risk they pose to others has been substantially reduced, means that many remain in hospital for longer than would otherwise be necessary.

Most offenders with established dementia will be unfit to plead or stand trial, and if violence has been serious, will require further care and supervision in a hospital unit specially designed to meet their mental and physical healthcare needs, with sufficient security to ensure public protection. Good procedural and relational security are likely to be more important than physical security measures for most older mentally disordered offenders. A full range of facilities in both criminal justice and health services must be developed if older mentally disordered offenders are not to be stuck in inappropriate facilities with little chance of onward progression. Specialist care homes for older offenders are beginning to appear in the UK and it is to be hoped that these will go some way to filling the gap in this area of service provision. Commissioners of services will need to monitor these new care homes carefully, however, as there is a risk that unnecessarily coercive or restrictive practices may emerge in such facilities if they do not have the checks and balances associated with multidisciplinary input into patient care.

Future challenges

Vulnerability

Any clinical service that caters for older adults will have individuals who are in declining physical health that may make them vulnerable to intimidation and aggression. It is essential that services carefully manage the case mix of patients so that frailer patients are not put at risk from more robust patients. As specialist in-patient services for older adults in the UK are exclusively in the independent sector, there may be tensions at times between maintaining a safe environment and ensuring maximum occupancy, and it is important that commissioners of such services monitor this issue.

Forensic model

The validity of the standard forensic psychiatric treatment model of progression through tiers of security with greater testing out of risk at each level has never been assessed for older patients. For patients with dementia it is known that a change of ward or hospital can have a negative effect on mental state and physical health, and it is questionable whether a return to independent living in a community very different from the one they left is much of an incentive for good behaviour for people who have been institutionalised for many years. The model also presupposes that there is an availability of appropriate services for patients to move on to when they no longer need a specific level of security. Although community-based step-down services for older offenders are currently beginning to appear in the UK, they are not yet widespread.

Inappropriate rating scales

As alluded to previously, most of the standard rating scales and assessment tools used in forensic psychiatry have not been validated with older adults. The best ways of measuring change and progress, which is of increasing importance to commissioners who want evidence of results, have also not yet been determined for this group. In the absence of specific instruments designed for use with older adults, the standard forensic tools have a value, but the results will always need careful interpretation to be meaningful.

Paucity of research

As the number of older offenders is small, much of the research published in this area is descriptive or uses a qualitative methodology. Though this can produce important findings, testing out the effectiveness of interventions in this group remains problematic because of the heterogeneity of presentations as well as the small numbers.

Conclusions

The majority of older adults who display aggressive and violent behaviour do not need treatment in secure mental health services, but a small proportion present assessment and management challenges that are sufficiently different to those of similar age peers and younger mentally disordered offenders. For this group, specialist services, drawing equally from old age and forensic psychiatry treatment models, informed by an understanding of the life cycle changes of late life and attuned to the particular physical and neuropsychiatric needs of older adults can be beneficial. How beneficial remains unclear, however, as at present there is no published research on the outcomes of such services. Therefore, one of the priorities for future study is to find ways of exploring the effectiveness of interventions with this group to ensure treatment is safe, humane, cost-effective and evidence based.

References

American Civil Liberties Union (2012) *At America's Expense: The Mass Incarceration of the Elderly*. ACLU (https://www.aclu.org/files/assets/elderlyprisonreport_20120613_1.pdf).

Coid, J., Fazel, S. & Kahtan, N. (2002) Elderly patients admitted to secure forensic psychiatry services. *Journal of Forensic Psychiatry*, **13**, 416–427.

Curtice, M., Parker, J., Wismayer, F., *et al* (2003) The elderly offender: an 11 year survey of referrals to a regional forensic psychiatry service. *Journal of Forensic Psychiatry and Psychology*, **14**, 253–265.

Dubois, B., Slachevsky, A., Litvan, I., *et al* (2000) The FAB: a frontal assessment battery at bedside. *Neurology*, **55**, 1621–1626.

Department of Health (2007) Good Practice in Offender Health. *Department of Health*.

East, W.N. (1944) Crime, senescence and senility. *Journal of Mental Science*, **90**, 836–849.

Fazel, S., Hope, T., O'Donnell., *et al* (2001) Health of elderly male prisoners: worse than the general population, worse than younger offenders. *Age and Ageing*, **30**, 403–407.

Fazel, S., Långström, N., Sjöstedt, G., *et al* (2006) Risk factors for criminal recidivism in older sexual offenders. *Sexual Abuse*, **18**, 159–167.

Gillies, H. (1976) Homicide in the West of Scotland. *British Journal of Psychiatry*, **128**, 105–127.

Goetting, A. (1983) The elderly in prison: issues and perspectives. *Journal of Research on Crime and Delinquency*, **20**, 291–309.

Hart, S.D., Kropp, P.R., Laws, D.R., *et al* (2003) *The Risk for Sexual Violence Protocol (RSVP)*. Mental Health, Law, and Policy Institute of Simon Fraser University.

Her Majesty's Inspectorate of Prisons (2004) *'No Problems – Old and Quiet': Older Prisoners in England and Wales. A Thematic Review by HM Chief Inspector of Prisons*. Ministry of Justice.

House of Commons Justice Committee (2013) *Older Prisoners: Fifth Report of Session 2013–14*. TSO (The Stationery Office) (http://www.parliament.uk/documents/commons-committees/Justice/Older-prisoners.pdf)

Hunt, I.M., Ashim, B., Swinson, N., *et al* (2010) Homicide convictions in different age groups: a national clinical survey. *Journal of Forensic Psychiatry and Psychology*, **21**, 321–335.

Kingston, P., Le Mesurier, N., Yorston, G., *et al* (2011) Psychiatric morbidity in older prisoners – unrecognised and undertreated. *International Psychogeriatrics*, **23**, 1354–1360.

Knight, B. (1983) Geriatric homicide – or the Darby and Joan syndrome. *Geriatric Medicine*, **13**, 297–300.

Knight, C., Johnson, C., Alderman, N., *et al* (2008) The St Andrew's Sexual Behaviour Assessment (SASBA): Development of a standardised recording instrument for the measurement and assessment of challenging sexual behaviour in people with progressive and acquired neurological impairment. *Neuropsychological Rehabilitation*, **18**, 129–159.

Ko, A., Takasaki, K., Chiba, Y., *et al* (2012) Aggression exhibited by older dementia clients toward staff in Japanese long-term care. *Journal of Elder Abuse & Neglect*, **24**, 1–16.

Kratcoski, P.C. & Walker, D.B. (1988) Homicide among the elderly: analysis of the victim/assailant relationship. In *Older Offenders – Perspectives in Criminology and Criminal Justice* (eds B. McCarthy & R. Langworthy), pp. 63–75. Praeger.

Law Commission (2010) *Unfitness to Plead – a Consultation Paper*. Law Commission.

Léger, J.M., Moulias, R., Robert, P., *et al* (2002) Agitation and aggressiveness among the elderly population living in nursing or retirement homes in France. *International Psychogeriatrics*, **14**, 405–416.

Lewis, C.F., Fields, C. & Rainey, E. (2006) A study of geriatric evaluees: who are the violent elderly. *Journal of the American Academy of Psychiatry and the Law*, **34**, 324–332.

McLeod, C., Yorston, G. & Gibb, R. (2008) Referrals of older adults to forensic and psychiatric intensive care services: a retrospective case-note study in Scotland. *British Journal of Forensic Practice*, **10**, 36–40.

McMurtray, A.M., Sultzer, D.L., Monserratt, L., *et al* (2008) Content-specific delusions from right caudate lacunar stroke: association with prefrontal hypometabolism. *Journal of Neuropsychiatry and Clinical Neurosciences*, **20**, 62–67.

Neafsey, E.J. & Collins, M.A. (2011) Moderate alcohol consumption and cognitive risk. *Neuropsychiatric Disease and Treatment*, **7**, 465–484.

Quinsey, V.L., Harris, G.T., Rice, M.E., *et al* (eds) (2006) *Violent Offenders: Appraising and Managing Risk, Second Edition (The Law and Public Policy)*. American Psychological Association.

Rayel, M.G. (2000) Clinical and demographic characteristics of elderly offenders at a maximum security forensic hospital. *Journal of Forensic Science*, **45**, 1193–1196.

Rollin, H.R. (1973) Deviant behaviour in relation to mental disorder. *Proceedings of the Royal Society of Medicine*, **66**, 99–104.

Rosner, R., Wiederlight, M. & Schneider, M. (1985) Geriatric felons examined at a forensic psychiatry clinic. *Journal of Forensic Science*, **30**, 730–740.

Rosner, R., Wiederlight, M., Harmon, R.B., *et al* (1991) Geriatric offenders examined at a forensic psychiatry clinic. *Journal of Forensic Science*, **36**, 1722–1731.

Series, H. & Dégano, P. (2005) Hypersexuality in dementia. *Advances in Psychiatric Treatment*, **11**, 424–431.

Wahidin, A. (2004) *Older Women and The Criminal Justice System: Running Out of Time*. Jessica Kingsley.

Wahidin, A. (2005) *'We are a Significant Minority': Old Women in English Prisons*. British Society of Criminology (http://www.britsoccrim.org/volume6/001.pdf).

Webster, C.D., Douglas, K.S., Eaves, D., *et al* (1997) *HCR-20: Assessing Risk for Violence*. Mental Health, Law, and Policy Institute, Simon Fraser University.

Willbanks, W. (1984) The elderly offender: relative frequency and patterns of offences. *International Journal of Aging and Human Development*, **20**, 269–281.

Wong, M.T.H., Lumsden, J., Fenton, G.W., *et al* (1995) Elderly offenders in a maximum security mental hospital. *Aggressive Behaviour*, **21**, 321–324.

Yorston, G. (1999) Aged and dangerous: old age forensic psychiatry. *British Journal of Psychiatry*, **174**, 193–195.

Yorston, G. & Taylor, P.J. (2009) Older patients in an English high security hospital: a qualitative study of the experiences and attitudes of patients aged 60 and over and their care staff in Broadmoor Hospital. *Journal of Forensic Psychiatry and Psychology*, **20**, 255–267.

CHAPTER 13

Firesetting in secure settings: theory, treatment and management

Theresa Gannon, Nichola Tyler, Geoffrey Dickens

Introduction

Background and aims

Firesetting confers substantial costs on society. In 2010/2011 there were 36 000 deliberately set fires in Great Britain resulting in 72 fatalities and 1700 non-fatal casualties. Around one in five deliberate fires occur in non-dwelling buildings, including hospitals (Department for Communities and Local Government, 2011). While serious fires in psychiatric hospitals are reasonably rare, incidents in UK secure mental health units in recent years, at Stockton Hall in North Yorkshire in 2010 (BBC News, 2010) and Camlet Lodge in London in 2008 (James, 2008), have demonstrated that fire can seriously disrupt service provision and endanger life. Additionally, the total number of incidents in psychiatric hospitals attended by the fire and rescue service is disproportionately greater per bed than in general medical hospitals (Grice, 2012). Around 10% of people admitted to forensic psychiatric services have committed arson (Coid *et al*, 2001) and many more may have a history of problematic firesetting behaviour (Geller *et al*, 1992). It is important therefore that staff who work in these services hold sufficient practical and theoretical knowledge to contribute to the prevention of firesetting and to the assessment, treatment and management of firesetters in secure care.

This chapter briefly reviews the epidemiology of firesetting, its relationship with mental disorder and the prevalence of firesetting among particular patient groups who may be resident in secure care. We then describe established theories of firesetting, including motivational typologies, single-factor theories and previous attempts at multifactor theories. We then present a newly developed multi-trajectory theory of adult firesetting (M-TTAF; Gannon *et al*, 2012*a*). This theory is important because it proposes different motivational drivers and prominent risk factors for firesetting across various groups, many of whom may be characterised by particular psychopathological features common in secure settings. The implication is that different groups will hold different risk factors and require varying therapeutic approaches. Some psychological treatment interventions delivered in secure settings are then examined. Finally, we discuss aspects of practical risk assessment and management of firesetters in the secure environment.

Definitions

We use the term 'firesetting' to identify any intentional act of setting fire to property or the environment for any motive or apparent reason with the exception of socially appropriate behaviours such as campfires or bonfires. 'Arson' describes a specific property crime whose definition may vary over time and between different jurisdictions. An arsonist has received a conviction for the crime, whereas a firesetter may not because, for example, they have not been apprehended or have not been prosecuted or convicted. Therefore, the prevalence of history of firesetting behaviour among secure in-patients is almost certainly greater than that of arson. 'Pyromania' is classified as an impulse control disorder in the *Diagnostic and Statistical Manual for Mental Disorder* (DSM-5; American Psychiatric Association, 2013), characterised by repeated deliberate firesetting for pleasure or tension relief and is considered very rare (Doley, 2003). While firesetting is very common among children and adolescents, especially among those in institutional care (Del Bove *et al*, 2008; MacKay *et al*, 2009), these groups are beyond the remit of the current chapter (see Kolko, 2002 for information on children and adolescents).

Prevalence of firesetting and comorbid mental disorder

Mental disorder among firesetters

Self-reported lifetime prevalence of firesetting in the general population is 1.1% (82% male) (Blanco *et al*, 2010; Vaughn *et al*, 2010). There are very high (91%) levels of any DSM-5 mental disorder among this self-reported group, chiefly alcohol use disorder (72%) and antisocial personality disorder (52%), and high rates (46%) of lifetime mental health service use relative to that of the general population (19%) (Blanco *et al*, 2010; Vaughn *et al*, 2010). A national study of arsonists in Sweden suggests that while only a small proportion (4%) of convicted arsonists have a diagnosis of schizophrenia, men with schizophrenia are more than 20 times as likely to set a deliberate fire as population controls without such a diagnosis, whereas women with schizophrenia are nearly 40 times as likely to set a fire than similar women in the community who do not have schizophrenia. Common diagnoses of arsonists referred for forensic psychiatric assessment are personality disorder (48%), non-bipolar psychosis (24.5%) and depression or other mood disorder (12.9%) (Enayati *et al*, 2008).

Firesetting in secure mental health service user samples

Lifetime prevalence of firesetting is considerably more common among samples of mental health service users than in the general population. Geller *et al* (1992) reported that 18% of adult patients in one US psychiatric hospital had deliberately set a fire in their lifetime, while 27% had recorded evidence of more widely defined firesetting behaviour (e.g. carelessness with smoking materials). In Finland (Repo *et al*, 1997), Sweden (Fazel & Grann, 2002) and the UK (Coid *et al*, 2001) around 10% of admissions have been individuals convicted of arson. The male/female ratio of firesetters in mental health service samples is lower than that of the general population (Rix, 1994; Dickens *et al*, 2009) and in higher levels of security approaches parity (Swinton & Ahmed, 2001). One recent study found that 54% of 90 consecutive admissions to a secure mental health service for women had some recorded history of firesetting (Long *et al*, 2015). While there is little evidence to support elevated prevalence of firesetting in samples of individuals with intellectual disability relative to the general population (Holland *et al*, 2002), it is certainly true that samples of firesetters referred for forensic psychiatric assessment include individuals with low IQ (Dickens *et al*, 2007) and Asperger's syndrome and autism (Enayati *et al*, 2008). In summary, firesetting history is present across a range of groups who may be found in secure healthcare settings, including men and women, those with mental illness and those with intellectual disability.

Explanations of firesetting

The key criterion for effective assessment and treatment of firesetting in the context of mental disorder is a comprehensive understanding of the aetiological theory underpinning this behaviour. Within the firesetting literature, very few comprehensive aetiological theories have been proposed and of those available, relatively little emphasis has been placed on firesetting behaviour in the context of mental health problems.

Motivators or typologies of firesetting

A somewhat prolific – yet simplistic – explanation of firesetting has been proposed via the advancement of typologies that aim to document the apparent motives of mentally disordered firesetters (O'Sullivan & Kelleher, 1987; Prins, 1994; Rix, 1994). However, few studies have examined the apparent motives of mentally disordered firesetters within secure hospital settings since samples are often obtained via psychiatric referrals/pre-trial assessments (e.g. Rix, 1994; Jayaraman & Frazer, 2006). Commonly reported motives for mentally disordered firesetters include revenge (O'Sullivan & Kelleher, 1987; Rix, 1994), excitement (Rix, 1994; Jayaraman & Frazer, 2006), cry for help/communication (Geller,

1992), and attempted suicide or self-harm (Rix, 1994; Dickens *et al*, 2007). However, although the motives of mentally disordered and non-mentally disordered firesetters appear broadly similar (see Tyler & Gannon, 2012), 'cry for help' or communicative firesetting – that is, firesetting as an expression of dissatisfaction with current accommodation or as an expression of an inability to cope – appears to be particularly prevalent within mentally disordered firesetters (Geller 1992; Tyler & Gannon, 2012). Interestingly, poor mental health and low intellectual ability have also been identified as motivators for firesetting (Prins, 1994; Rix, 1994).

Single-factor theories

A small number of theories focus on one particular area of psychiatric or psychological functioning hypothesised to facilitate and maintain firesetting. None of these theories, however, apply exclusively to mentally disordered offenders. Psychoanalytical theories associated with Freud (1932) are perhaps the most infamous. These theories hypothesise that firesetting stems from repressed sexual urges (Vreeland & Levin, 1980), however such hypotheses have not been supported by empirical data (Gannon & Pina, 2010). A more convincing link has been established between neurobiological disorder and firesetting behaviour. Key to this link are research findings (e.g. Virkkunen, 1984; Virkkunen *et al*, 1994) showing that impulsive firesetters or repeat firesetters hold neurotransmitter defects in the form of decreased cerebrospinal fluid monoamine metabolites concentrates (i.e. 5-hydroxyindoleacetic acid and 3-methoxy-4-hydroxyphenylglycol), which lead to general increases in impulsivity and risk-taking (Moore *et al*, 2002). Finally, a popular psychological perspective – social learning theory – views firesetting as being the product of learning and reinforcement contingencies. For example, Vreeland & Levin (1980) note that firesetting may be instantly reinforcing through pure sensory excitement. Furthermore, firesetting experiences may be vicarious through exposure to prominent models of firesetting behaviour (e.g. caregivers, family members; see Rice & Harris, 1991). Numerous motives linked to firesetting may be explained by social learning theory. To illustrate, fire interest may develop as a result of positive early childhood exposure to fire (e.g. a welder father). Additionally, revenge firesetting may be explained as a product of negative childhood experiences, resulting in aggression, poor coping and low assertiveness, increasing an individual's propensity to set fires in an attempt to gain environmental control (Vreeland & Levin, 1980). Furthermore, if fire as a revenge strategy is perceived as being successful, then this is likely to reinforce such behaviour. Social learning theory highlights the relative importance of developmental factors and is generally supported empirically (see Gannon & Pina, 2010). However, this perspective is less applicable to firesetting motivated by factors other than fire interest or revenge.

Established multifactor theories

There is a surprising lack of multifactor theories currently available to explain firesetting. A widely cited explanation is Jackson's functional analysis theory (Jackson *et al*, 1987; Jackson, 1994). Within this theory, firesetting is described as stemming from a complex interplay of antecedents (i.e. prior experiences) and behavioural consequences (i.e. reinforcement contingencies associated with fire experiences). Five main antecedents are described:

- psychosocial disadvantage, such as poor relationship with caregivers
- life dissatisfaction and self-loathing associated with psychosocial disadvantage
- social ineffectiveness (e.g. poor conflict resolution)
- pre-existing fire experiences (i.e. individually or vicariously experienced)
- internal or external triggers for firesetting (i.e. strong affective states or contextual factors).

Jackson and colleagues propose that reinforcement contingencies are also key to firesetting (i.e. positive reinforcement from peer acceptance and attention from neglectful caregivers). These experiences are likely to promote temporary increases in personal effectiveness that, paired with natural sensory reinforcement, may promote escalation of fire interest and future firesetting. In terms of negative reinforcement, Jackson and colleagues argue that the frequently punitive consequences of firesetting (e.g. increased supervision or punishment) are likely to intensify existing personal inadequacies, thus increasing the likelihood that these factors will act as repetitive antecedents to firesetting.

Functional analysis theory provides a clear and intuitively appealing description of how a multitude of factors interact to facilitate and maintain firesetting behaviour; in particular, the conceptualisation of firesetting as a dysfunctional attempt at resolving problems. There are, however, some gaps within this theory (Gannon *et al*, 2012a) that threaten its ability to adequately explain the range of firesetting observed in the history of individuals in secure hospital care. First, the theory does not adequately explain why firesetting might occur in the context of more general offending and appears to assume that firesetting is accompanied by some fire interest. Second, the theory does not adequately describe the range of proximal factors likely to be associated with firesetting (e.g. cognition or affect). Finally, although the theory appears to accommodate depression (i.e. as a form of perceived ineffectiveness), it does not adequately describe how a broad range of mental disorders may fit into the proposed model.

A somewhat comparable multifactor theory of firesetting is Fineman's dynamic behaviour theory (Fineman, 1980, 1995). Similarly to Jackson *et al*, Fineman proposes that firesetting results from historical psychosocial influences that form firesetting propensities via social learning mechanisms and associated conditioning principles. However, he describes firesetting using a dynamic behavioural framework in which firesetting – as a sequence of events – is represented via a formula: firesetting = G1 (social disadvantage/ineffectiveness) + G2 (previous and existing fire reinforcers) + E (instant environmental fire reinforcement). Within this formula, detailed specifications regarding proximal factors predicted to underpin and maintain firesetting are made under E through acknowledging the role of cognition and affect pre-, during and post-firesetting. This theory is useful for guiding clinical assessment of firesetting as a sequential process and is able to explain firesetting that occurs in the context of other antisocial behaviour and in the absence of fire interest. However, most of the theory's empirical base is drawn from juvenile firesetting, which greatly limits its applicability to adult firesetting more generally.

A newly developed multifactor theory: the multi-trajectory theory of adult firesetting

The final and most recent multifactor theory of firesetting – the multi-trajectory theory of adult firesetting (M-TTAF; Gannon *et al*, 2012*a*) – was developed via 'theory knitting' (Kalmar & Sternberg, 1988). This concept refers to the amalgamation of pre-existing theoretical concepts, contemporary ideas, and research evidence to generate a powerful overarching theory that subsumes the strengths of previous theories. The theory is presented as comprising two main tiers: tier 1 provides an overview of the aetiological underpinnings of the theory, whereas tier 2 summarises prototypical patterns of factors that lead to firesetting.

Tier 1. Aetiological framework underpinning the M-TTAF

The M-TTAF's framework (Fig. 13.1) aims to amalgamate a variety of factors to explain the aetiology of firesetting behaviour. In brief, the developmental factors outlined within the M-TTAF relate to the caregiver environment (i.e. either impoverished or protective), learning experiences (i.e. the development of attitudes, self-worth, communication skills, coping scripts, scripts regarding when and where fire should be used (fire scripts) via social learning), cultural forces (i.e. societal attitudes that direct and influence early social learning experiences), and biology and temperament (i.e. brain functioning and inherited personality characteristics). The developmental context as a whole is hypothesised to create a unique pattern of fire-specific and other psychological vulnerabilities associated with firesetting. These are: inappropriate fire interest/scripts, offence-supportive cognition, self-/emotional regulation issues and communication problems.

Inappropriate fire interest/scripts represent a fire-specific vulnerability. Here, an individual may feel highly attracted towards fire (i.e. owing to sensory stimulation or other reinforcing experiences associated with fire). Alternatively, an individual may have developed an inappropriate view of when and how fire should be used (i.e. fire scripts). For example, fire may

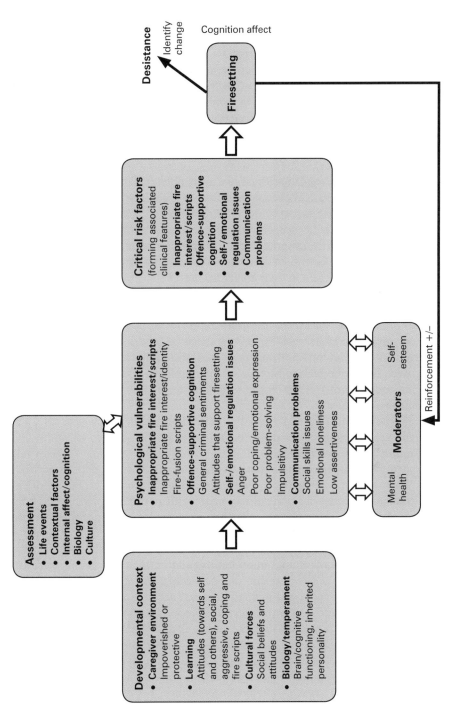

Fig. 13.1 A summary of the M-TTAF: tier 1.

Source: Gannon *et al* (2012a).

come to be viewed as representing a powerful tool for coping with various problematic situations.

Offence-supportive cognition refers to the attitudes or schemas held by individuals that function to guide social information processing in an offence-supportive manner. Ó Ciardha & Gannon (2012) have proposed that firesetters may hold any combination of five offence-supportive schemas. These schemas may function to support firesetting either directly (in the form of viewing fire as: a powerful tool, controllable and interesting/ exciting) or indirectly (through viewing violence as normal or the world as a dangerous place).

Self-/emotional regulation issues refer to an individual's ability to successfully monitor internal affect and external factors to achieve personal goals across various time periods and contexts (Baumeister & Vohs, 2004). Individuals may have problems controlling and containing strong affect (i.e. anger) or may choose inappropriate coping strategies when faced with stressful situations (e.g. drugs or alcohol). Alternatively, an individual may be extremely competent in their ability to control strong affect and so carefully plan pursuance of an inappropriate goal (e.g. to solve a dispute in the absence of verbal communication).

Finally, *communication problems* refer to an individual's ability to communicate ideas, needs and aspirations to others effectively, including generating and maintaining both platonic and intimate relationships. Individuals who lack some type of communication skills are likely to feel frustrated or distressed by their inability to obtain important needs in a prosocial manner.

A key aspect of the M-TTAF lies in its explanation of how psychological vulnerabilities become triggered to facilitate firesetting. In summary, a number of crucial proximal factors or triggers (external or internal) such as life events, contextual factors and affect are proposed to both reflect and interact with psychological vulnerabilities to produce 'critical risk factors' that facilitate firesetting. Critical risk factors are existing psychological vulnerabilities that have become greatly intensified before firesetting and present as clinical problems post-offence. For example, an individual who holds problems in the areas of inappropriate fire scripts, poor communication and emotional regulation may experience stressful life events as a direct result of poor communication and inadequate coping. These events will increase internal negative affect (e.g. anger and hopelessness) and trigger the individual's psychological vulnerabilities into critical risk factors such that use of fire is deemed to be the only viable response to the problem (Jackson, 1994). Within the M-TTAF, two main moderators – mental health and self-esteem – are hypothesised to dictate how severely proximal triggers will reflect and interact with psychological vulnerabilities to result in 'critical risk factors'. For example, good mental health and healthy self-esteem will likely reduce the interactive impact between these components. In contrast, poor mental health and low self-esteem will exacerbate the interactive impact. Nevertheless, whereas mental health is viewed as a moderator within the M-TTAF, it may present as a critical risk factor in some complex cases (e.g. command hallucinations; Gannon *et al*, 2012*a*) reflecting or disinhibiting pre-existing vulnerabilities.

The final component of the M-TTAF relates to mechanisms of firesetting maintenance and desistance. Akin to Jackson *et al*'s (1987) and Fineman's (1980, 1995) theories, the M-TTAF conceptualises positive and negative reinforcement mechanisms as playing a key role in firesetting maintenance. In line with contemporary desistence theory (Laws & Ward, 2011), it proposes that some firesetters will experience cognitive and behavioural transformations (e.g. increased social skills, prosocial attitudes and values) as a result of community interactions and opportunities (e.g. a new job) or rehabilitation (a firesetting programme) that will ultimately result in firesetting desistence.

Tier 2. Five key trajectories of the M-TTAF

Five prototypical trajectories associated with the M-TTAF are proposed by Gannon *et al* (2012*a*): antisocial, grievance, fire interest, emotionally expressive/need for recognition and multifaceted (Table 13.1). Within each trajectory, clustered patterns of characteristics are described that are hypothesised to characterise each particular firesetter subtype.

1 *Antisocial trajectory* refers to firesetters whose prominent critical risk factor revolves around antisocial cognition and values. These individuals are unlikely to hold fire interest or fire-related script issues. However, they may demonstrate other critical risk factors in the form of self-regulation issues (e.g. impulsivity). Individuals within this trajectory are likely to hold a psychiatric diagnosis of antisocial personality disorder. Proximal triggers that promote firesetting in this group are hypothesised to be largely instrumental (e.g. to evade detection for another crime). Thus, such individuals may hold lengthy criminal careers and few firesetting offences. Treatment should target general antisocial cognition and associated values rather than fire-relevant variables.

2 *Grievance* refers to firesetters whose prominent critical risk factor relates to self-regulation issues (e.g. trait aggression, passive aggressiveness). These individuals may be female or male and experience significant anger and rumination regarding perceived injustices. Thus, in the context of other critical risk factors (i.e. poor communication/assertiveness and an aggressive script linking indirect aggression with fire) individuals with a grievance use fire to send a powerful message to others who have 'wronged' them. They are likely to value fire highly as a powerful tool and may have used it in this way either repeatedly or on a single occasion. Treatment should pinpoint self-regulation and inappropriate fire scripts while increasing appropriate communication skills.

Table 13.1 A summary of the M-TTAF trajectories: tier 2

Trajectory	Prominent risk factor	Other likely risk factors	Potential clinical features	Potential motivators
Antisocial	Offence-supportive cognition (supporting general criminality)	Self-regulation issues (e.g. poor emotional modulation)	Antisocial values/attitudes Impulsivity Conduct disorder or antisocial personality disorder	Vandalism/boredom Crime concealment Profit Revenge/retribution
Grievance	Self-regulation issues	Communication problems Inappropriate fire script	Low assertiveness Poor communication Fire-aggression fusion script Anger (rumination) Hostility	Revenge/retribution
Fire interest	Inappropriate fire interest/scripts	Offence-supportive cognition (supporting firesetting)	Fire fascination/interest Impulsivity Attitudes supporting fire	Fire interest/thrill Stress/boredom
Emotionally expressive/need for recognition	Communication problems	Self-regulation issues* (e.g. poor emotional modulation)	Poor communication Impulsivity Depression Fire-coping fusion script Personality traits/disorder	Cry for help* Self-harm* Suicide* Need for recognition
Multifaceted	Offence-supportive cognition (supporting general criminality and firesetting) Inappropriate fire interest/scripts	Self-regulation issues Communication problems	Pervasive firesetting/general criminal behaviour Fire fascination/interest Antisocial values/attitudes Conduct disorder or antisocial personality disorder	Various

*Emotionally expressive subtype only. Source: Gannon et al (2012a).

3   *Fire interest* refers to firesetters whose prominent critical risk factor relates to inappropriate fire interest (note, however, that a diagnosis of pyromania (see DSM-5) is not required) or scripts. These individuals are likely to show some inappropriately focused interest in fire or fire paraphernalia and/or may have formed a deeply ingrained coping script so that, in times of stress, fire is used as a coping mechanism for tension reduction. Furthermore, these individuals may hold a further key critical risk factor in the form of fire-specific, offence-supportive cognition (e.g. 'I can control the fires that I start'). Gannon *et al* (2012a) hypothesise that inappropriate fire interest and scripts develop from interactive social learning, conditioning and cultural forces during childhood. Individuals within this trajectory may be of either gender and hold a lengthy history of firesetting yet little general offending. Thus, treatment should focus on the person's lifelong identity with fire and fire-supportive cognition to reduce firesetting recidivism.

4   *Emotionally expressive/need for recognition* refers to two variants of firesetter who hold the prominent critical risk factor of communication problems. Emotionally expressive individuals are hypothesised to hold the additional critical risk factor of self-regulation issues (e.g. poor problem-solving). When faced with proximal triggers that strain coping mechanisms, the individual feels 'unheard' and hopeless and believes that the only option available to alleviate their situation is to send a dramatic message to others – using fire – about their current emotional needs (i.e. cry for help) or to release intense negative affect. Some individuals may also hold a fire-coping script. It is this trajectory that can account for firesetting as a form of self-harm or suicide and is often observed in mental health settings. This trajectory is likely to be associated with female firesetting and borderline personality disorder. Treatment should focus on increasing effective communication of distress. Need-for-recognition firesetters tend to be male firesetters who pre-plan their firesetting to gain social attention and recognition for tackling or detecting the fire (i.e. 'hero' firesetters). Gannon *et al* (2012a) hypothesise that these firesetters – like the emotionally expressive subtype – are unable to achieve recognition via conventional outlets. This intense need for recognition may indicate the presence of personality problems (e.g. narcissism) and treatment should aim to explore these while increasing the individual's skills and opportunities to gain social recognition via prosocial outlets.

5   The final, *multifaceted trajectory* refers to firesetters who hold two coexisting prominent critical risk factors in the form of offence-supportive cognition (supporting general criminality and firesetting) and inappropriate fire interest/scripts. Other possible critical risk factors relate to self-regulation issues and communication problems. The main difference between this trajectory and the fire interest

trajectory is the combination of general criminality and inappropriate fire interest, which is likely to result in high levels of both fire- and non-fire related offending. This trajectory is likely to be more pervasive in male firesetters; particularly those diagnosed with antisocial personality disorder. It will be the antisocial attitudes and values alongside this entrenched relationship with fire that will require extensive focus in treatment.

Strengths and limitations of the M-TTAF relative to other firesetting theories

There are limitations associated with the M-TTAF that are commensurate with the lack of research literature currently available in this field (e.g. there is room for more explanatory mechanistic detail). However, the M-TTAF holds key strengths. In short, it is able to account for:

- the wide array of firesetting behaviour often documented in secure care and other settings (e.g. firesetting as self-harm, firesetting as part of a broad array of antisocial behaviour)
- the explicit and varying role that mental health plays in firesetting behaviour (i.e. as either a moderator variable or a causal critical risk factor)
- the role of intellectual disability as either a distal or proximal factor associated with firesetting, and
- the likely coexistence of personality traits and disorders as identifying clinical features associated with particular firesetting trajectories.

Furthermore, a key strength is the focus and organisation of hypothesised critical risk factors. The identification of such potentially criminogenic firesetting risk factors is critical for developing and guiding effective treatments for firesetters, both generally and in secure care settings.

Psychological treatment interventions in secure care

For many decades, adult firesetting as an offending behaviour has generally received relatively little intervention focus (Palmer *et al*, 2007). It is unclear exactly why this has been the case but presumably practitioners have been hindered by the distinct lack of research regarding the dynamic risk factors associated with firesetting (Palmer *et al*, 2010). Nevertheless, the adult firesetting interventions that have been documented appear to adopt cognitive–behavioural approaches to treatment and have been implemented in secure psychiatric settings (e.g. Hall, 1995; Swaffer *et al*, 2001; Taylor *et al*, 2002, 2004, 2006; Gannon *et al*, 2012b). The majority of programmes have been developed 'in house' and as a result vary greatly in terms of population, intervention focus and treatment length.

Swaffer *et al* (2001) describe a group firesetting treatment programme for mixed-gender patients underpinned by Jackson and colleagues' theory (1987). This programme was implemented at a high security hospital in the UK over 62 group sessions and examined: (1) education on fire danger, (2) coping skills (i.e. social skills, assertiveness, conflict resolution and problem-solving), (3) reflective insight (e.g. self-esteem and self-concept), and (4) and relapse prevention. Unfortunately, although the authors describe a case study outlining the positive effects of the programme and the range of assessments used to assess treatment progress, no treatment effectiveness data are provided. A somewhat similar programme, also implemented at a UK high security hospital, is described by Hall (1995), but again, no treatment effectiveness data are provided.

Taylor *et al* (2002) describe a group firesetting treatment programme – again underpinned by Jackson and colleagues' 1987 theory – for patients with intellectual disability implemented separately for male and female patients (8 and 6 respectively) in a low secure UK hospital. The group ran over 40 group sessions covering fire education, analysis of offending, coping skills, family problems and relapse management. Statistically significant improvements were reported on measures examining fire interest and attitudes, understanding of victim issues, risk and emotional expression, anger and self-esteem. Nevertheless, the authors note themselves that this study lacks an adequate control group comparison. In a later study describing a similar programme, Taylor and colleagues (2004) outline four case studies of male patients with intellectual disability who completed a similar programme. Positive outcomes are reported for each patient. However, the sample size was too small to draw any meaningful conclusions (see Taylor *et al* (2006) for similar findings with female patients with intellectual disability).

More recently, Gannon *et al* (2012b) have published some preliminary descriptions of a newly developed group treatment programme for use with male and female patients in secure care settings, the Firesetting Intervention Programme for Mentally Disordered Offenders (FIP-MO; Gannon & Lockerbie, 2011). The group is underpinned by the M-TTAF and runs over 28 sessions with weekly individual work. It examines: fire interest, identification and safety; self- and emotional regulation; communication and relationships; cognition that supports offending; risk management and a future 'good life' (i.e. traditional relapse prevention guided by a 'good lives model' approach; Ward & Gannon, 2006). The programme is currently being implemented across 12 UK secure care settings and the results of the evaluation, which includes pre-/post-testing and a comparison group who do not receive FIP-MO treatment, are expected to be released sometime later in 2015.

Risk assessment and management of firesetters in the secure setting

High rates of repeated firesetting (13–49%) have been reported in samples of mentally disordered and non-mentally disordered firesetters (Dickens *et al*, 2009). When the definitional threshold is set at reconviction for arson, then 8% can be classified as recidivists (Soothill *et al*, 2004). Further, risk of recidivism is not restricted to firesetting: firesetters are generally versatile offenders and high rates of violent (31%) and non-violent (57%) recidivism have been reported among those discharged from a maximum security psychiatric hospital over an 8-year period (Rice & Harris, 1996). Other potential risk factors reported in the literature include early age at onset, overall number of incidents of firesetting and severity of previous incidents, developmental history of violence, substance misuse, early onset of criminal convictions, relationship problems, fire interest, severity of psychopathology, evidence of planning in previous firesetting and personality characteristics including inwardly directed hostility, lack of assertiveness and low self-esteem (Dickens *et al*, 2009; Gannon & Pina, 2010; Doley & Watt, 2012).

Currently, there is no validated risk assessment tool for use with adult firesetters. However, many of the individual risk factors listed above are similar to those included in structured professional judgement (SPJ) tools for predicting violent recidivism in general, for example the HCR-20 (Webster *et al*, 1997). SPJ approaches to risk assessment consider much firesetting to constitute violence and recommend its exclusion from the risk assessment only in instances where there is no potential for harm to persons. The HCR-20 may therefore be used for cases of firesetting that appear to relate to violent intentionality or where it is one of many presenting violent behaviours. Like the HCR-20, the M-TTAF suggests a range of historical and dynamic risk factors for firesetting but does so within the context of an explanatory theoretical framework. This is likely to assist the formulation of risk for firesetting recidivism for an individual in terms of their motivation, disinhibitors and destabilisers. In turn, this will inform risk management strategies, including the focus of therapeutic intervention. For example, firesetters who hold clinical features associated with the grievance trajectory are likely to be at increased risk when exposed to situations requiring communication skills, particularly assertiveness, beyond their current personal resources. Therapeutic intervention is likely to focus on strategies to improve and extend those resources. An individual holding clinical features associated with the antisocial trajectory is likely to hold offence-supportive cognition and may be more likely to benefit from interventions more focused on criminogenic need. Further, the M-TTAF highlights the importance of critical fire-related risk factors (inappropriate fire interest, inappropriate fire scripts), the presence of which should influence overall judgement both of risk and of management strategies.

Within the context of secure care, risk for firesetting should be managed through the physical (e.g. secure perimeter) and procedural (e.g. searching) security mechanisms which are designed to minimise the opportunity for firesetting materials, including ignition sources, accelerants and fuel, to enter the premises. Such items will largely be prohibited or their surreptitious use detected through smoke alarms. In those secure units where smoking is permitted in designated areas access to lighters/matches will be controlled and smoking supervised by staff. Secure care staff should be aware that lighters can be fashioned from batteries, wire and foil, and thus access to these items should also be controlled as appropriate to the level of security. Unprevented firesetting should be managed by following all required professional guidance on fire risk assessment to ensure impact is minimised. This includes ensuring potential escape routes are accessible, that fire doors, alarms and detection systems are in good working order and that firefighting equipment is available and regularly replenished. Of utmost importance is the presence of a comprehensive emergency plan that is known to all staff and that allows for the safe removal, if required, of patients from an affected area while maintaining necessary security. A full account of fire safety in secure care has been provided by Grice (2012) and is recommended reading for providers of secure care.

Conclusions

This chapter has highlighted the relevance of deliberate firesetting to practitioners in secure care settings. The behaviour itself is rare in these settings precisely because the appropriate use of security precludes access to ignition sources and flammable fuel. Nevertheless, a significant minority of patients in secure services have some history of deliberate firesetting. The chapter has reviewed existing theories of firesetting and identified their limitations. A powerful new multi-trajectory theory of adult firesetting (M-TTAF; Gannon *et al*, 2012*a*) has been proposed and its strengths and possible limitations reviewed. The M-TTAF is able to account for a wide array of firesetting behaviour demonstrated by individuals in secure care and has much relevance to risk assessment and management. In particular, the model suggests how resources can be targeted effectively to address the risk factors held by individuals.

References

American Psychiatric Association (2013) *Diagnostic and Statistical Manual of Mental Disorders, Fifth Edition* (DSM-5). APA.

Baumeister, R.F. & Vohs, K.D. (2004) *Handbook of Self-Regulation: Research, Theory and Applications*. Guilford Press.

BBC News (2010) Psychiatric hospital damaged by 'suspicious' fire. *BBC News*, 15 May.

Blanco, C., Alegria, A.A., Petry, N.M., *et al* (2010) Prevalence and correlates of fire-setting in the United States: results from the National Epidemiologic Survey on Alcohol and Related Conditions (NESARC). *Journal of Clinical Psychiatry*, **71**, 1218–1225.

Coid, J., Kahtan, N., Gault, S., *et al* (2001) Medium secure forensic psychiatry services: comparison of seven English health regions. *British Journal of Psychiatry*, **178**, 55–61.

Del Bove, G.D., Caprara, G.V., Pastorelli, C., *et al* (2008) Juvenile firesetting in Italy: relationship to aggression, psychopathology, personality, self-efficacy, and school functioning. *European Journal of Child and Adolescent Psychiatry*, **17**, 235–244.

Department for Communities and Local Government (2011) *Fire Statistics Great Britain, 2010–2011*. Department for Communities and Local Government (http://www.communities.gov.uk/documents/statistics/pdf/568234.pdf).

Dickens, G., Sugarman, P., Ahmad, F., *et al* (2007) Gender differences amongst adult arsonists at psychiatric assessment. *Medicine, Science and the Law*, **47**, 233-238.

Dickens, G., Sugarman, P., Ahmad, F., *et al* (2009) Recidivism and dangerousness in arsonists. *Journal of Forensic Psychiatry and Psychology*, **20**, 621–639.

Doley, R. (2003) Pyromania: fact or fiction? *British Journal of Criminology*, **43**, 797–807.

Doley, R.M. & Watt, B.D. (2012) Assessment of firesetters. In *Firesetting and Mental Health: Theory, Research and Practice* (eds G.L. Dickens, P.A. Sugarman & T.A. Gannon): pp. 184–205. RCPsych Publications.

Enayati, J., Grann, M., Lubbs, S., *et al* (2008) Psychiatric morbidity in arsonists referred for forensic psychiatric assessment in Sweden. *Journal of Forensic Psychiatry and Psychology*, **19**, 139–147.

Fazel, S. & Grann, M. (2002) Older criminals: a descriptive study of psychiatrically examined offenders in Sweden. *International Journal of Geriatric Psychiatry*, **17**, 907–913.

Fineman, K.R. (1980) Firesetting in childhood and adolescence. Child psychiatry: contributions to diagnosis, treatment and research. *Psychiatric Clinics of North America*, **3**, 483–500.

Fineman, K.R. (1995) A model for the qualitative analysis of child and fire deviant behavior. *American Journal of Forensic Psychology*, **13**, 31–60.

Freud, S. (1932) The acquisition of power over fire. *International Journal of Psychoanalysis*, **13**, 405–410.

Gannon, T. A. & Lockerbie, L. (2011) *Firesetting Intervention Programme for Mentally Disordered Offenders (FIP-MO)*. CORE-FP, University of Kent and Kent Forensic Psychiatry Services: NHS.

Gannon, T.A. & Pina, A. (2010) Firesetting: psychopathology, theory and treatment. *Aggression and Violent Behavior*, **15**, 224–238.

Gannon, T.A., Ó Ciardha. C., Doley, R.M., *et al* (2012*a*) The multi-trajectory theory of adult firesetting. *Aggression and Violent Behavior*, **17**, 107–121.

Gannon, T.A., Lockerbie, L. & Tyler, N. (2012*b*) A long time coming? The Firesetting Intervention Programme for Mentally Disordered Offenders (FIP-MO). *Forensic Update*, **106**, 1–10.

Geller, J.L. (1992) Communicative arson. *Hospital and Community Psychiatry*, **43**, 76–77.

Geller, J.L., Fisher, W.H. & Moynihan, K. (1992) Adult lifetime prevalence of firesetting behaviours in a state hospital population. *Psychiatric Quarterly*, **63**, 129–142.

Grice, A. (2012) Fire risk and fire safety in psychiatric care. In *Firesetting and Mental Health: Theory, Research and Practice* (eds G.L. Dickens, P.A. Sugarman & T.A. Gannon): pp. 254–269. RCPsych Publications.

Hall, G. (1995) Using group work to understand arsonists. *Nursing Standard*, **9**, 24–28.

Holland, T., Clare, I.C.H. & Mukhopadhyay, T. (2002) Prevalence of 'criminal offending' by men and women with intellectual disability and the characteristics of 'offenders': implications for research and service development. *Journal of Intellectual Disability Research*, **44**, 6–20.

Jackson, H.F. (1994) Assessment of fire-setters. In *The Assessment of Criminal Behaviours in Secure Settings* (eds M. McMurran, & J. Hodge), pp. 94–126. Jessica Kingsley.

Jackson, H.F., Glass, C. & Hope, S. (1987) A functional analysis of recidivistic arson. *British Journal of Clinical Psychology*, **26**, 175–185.

James, A. (2008) Patients evacuated after psychiatric unit fire. PsychMinded, 23 October. Available at http://psychminded.co.uk/news/news2008/October08/psychiatric_unit_fire_London005.htm (accessed January 2015).

Jayaraman, A. & Frazer, J. (2006) Arson: a growing inferno. *Medicine, Science and the Law*, **46**, 295–300.

Kalmar, D.A. & Sternberg, R.J. (1988) Theory knitting: an integrative approach to theory development. *Philosophical Psychology*, **1**, 153–170.

Kolko, D. J. (2002) *Handbook on Firesetting in Children and Youth*. Academic Press.

Laws, D.R. & Ward, T. (2011) *Desistance from Sex Offending: Alternatives to Throwing Away the Keys*. Guilford Press.

Long, C.G., Fitzgerald, K.-A. & Hollin, C.R. (2015) Women firesetters admitted to secure psychiatric services: characteristics and treatment needs. *Victims and Offenders*, 1–13, published online 6 January.

MacKay, S., Paglia-Boak, A., Henderson, J., *et al* (2009) Epidemiology of firesetting in adolescents: mental health and substance use correlates. *Journal of Child Psychology and Psychiatry*, **50**, 1282–1290.

Moore, T.M., Scarpa, A. & Raine, A. (2002) A meta-analysis of serotonin metabolite 5-HIAA and antisocial behaviour. *Aggressive Behaviour*, **28**, 229–316.

Ó Ciardha, C. & Gannon, T.A. (2012) The implicit theories of firesetters: a preliminary conceptualization. *Aggression and Violent Behaviour*, **17**, 122–128.

O'Sullivan, G.H. & Kelleher, M.J. (1987) A study of firesetters in South-West Ireland. *British Journal of Psychiatry*, **151**, 818–823.

Palmer, E.J., Caulfield, L.S. & Hollin, C.R. (2007) Interventions with arsonists and young fire setters: a survey of the national picture in England and Wales. *Legal and Criminological Psychology*, **12**, 101–116.

Palmer, E.J., Hollin, C.R., Hatcher, R.M., *et al* (2010) Arson. In *Handbook of Crime* (eds F. Brookman, T. Bennett, M. Maguire, *et al*): pp. 380–392. Willan.

Prins, H. (1994) *Fire-Raising: Its Motivation and Management*. Routledge.

Repo, E., Virkkunen, M., Rawlings, M., *et al* (1997) Criminal and psychiatric histories of Finnish arsonists. *Acta Psychiatrica Scandinavica*, **95**, 318–323.

Rice, M.E. & Harris, G.T. (1991) Firesetters admitted to a maximum security psychiatric institution. *Journal of Interpersonal Violence*, **6**, 461–475.

Rice, M. & Harris, G. (1996) Predicting the recidivism of mentally disordered firesetters. *Journal of Interpersonal Violence*, **11**, 364–375.

Rix, K.J.B. (1994) A psychiatric study of adult arsonists. *Medicine, Science and the Law*, **34**, 21–24.

Soothill, K., Ackerley, E. & Francis, B. (2004) The criminal careers of arsonists. *Medicine, Science, and the Law*, **44**, 27–40.

Swaffer, T., Haggett, M. & Oxley, T. (2001) Mentally disordered firesetters: a structured intervention programme. *Clinical Psychology and Psychotherapy*, **8**, 468–475.

Swinton, M. & Ahmed, A. (2001) Arsonists in maximum security: mental state at time of fire-setting and relationship between mental disorder and pattern of behaviour. *Medicine, Science and the Law*, **41**, 51–57.

Taylor, J.L., Thorne, I., Robertson, A., *et al* (2002) Evaluation of a group intervention for convicted arsonists with mild and borderline intellectual disabilities. *Criminal Behaviour and Mental Health*, **12**, 282–293.

Taylor, J.L., Thorne, I. & Slavkin, M.L. (2004) Treatment of firesetting behaviour. In *Offenders with Developmental Disabilities* (eds W. Lindsay, J. Taylor & P. Sturmey), pp. 221–241. Wiley.

Taylor, J.L., Robertson, A., Thorne, I., *et al* (2006) Responses of female fire-setters with mild and borderline intellectual disabilities to a group intervention. *Journal of Applied Research in Intellectual Disabilities*, **19**, 179–190.

Tyler, N. & Gannon, T.A. (2012) Explanations of firesetting in mentally disordered offenders: a review of the literature. *Psychiatry: Interpersonal and Biological Processes*, **75**, 150–166.

Vaughn, M.G., Fu, Q., DeLisi, M., *et al* (2010) Prevalence and correlates of fire-setting in the United States: results from the National Epidemiological Survey on Alcohol and Related Conditions. *Comprehensive Psychiatry*, **51**, 217–223.

Virkkunen, M. (1984) Reactive hypoglycemic tendency among arsonists. *Acta Psychiatrica Scandinavica*, **69**, 445–452.

Virkkunen, M., Kallio, E., Rawlings, R., *et al* (1994) Personality profiles and state aggressiveness in Finnish alcoholic, violent offenders, fire setters, and healthy volunteers. *Archives of General Psychiatry*, **51**, 28–33.

Vreeland, R. & Levin, B. (1980) Psychological aspects of firesetting. In *Fires and Human Behaviour* (ed. D. Canter), pp. 31–46. Wiley.

Ward, T., & Gannon, T.A. (2006) Rehabilitation, etiology and self-regulation: the comprehensive good lives model of treatment for sexual offenders. *Aggressive and Violent Behaviour*, **11**, 77–94.

Webster, C., Douglas, K., Eaves, D., *et al* (1997) *HCR-20 Assessing Risk for Violence Version 2*. Mental Health, Law and Policy Institute, Simon Fraser University.

CHAPTER 14

Specialist psychological treatment programmes in secure mental healthcare

Clive Long and John Shine

Introduction

Psychological treatments in secure mental health settings comprise a wide range of interventions that are delivered at the individual, group and ward milieu level. Different forms of structured psychological treatments have evolved in these settings to offer remediation of mental health problems and symptoms and to reduce risk. The past 20 years have witnessed a significant expansion of psychological therapies facilitated by government-driven initiatives to improve access to talking therapies. Over the same time period there has been an expansion in the provision of psychological, educational and behavioural intervention programmes for offenders, including those detained in secure psychiatric settings, based on the 'what works' in reducing reoffending literature (Lipsey & Wilson, 1993; Lösel, 1996; Hollin, 1999). In the UK, much progress in secure services has been driven by the National Health Service's (NHS's) Improving Access to Psychological Therapies (IAPT) programme (www.iapt.nhs.uk). The National Institute for Health and Care Excellence (NICE) guidelines for specific disorders have highlighted the evidence base for psychological therapies and the development of minimum standards for patients in secure services has been paralleled by an increased focus on high-quality in-patient care (Doyle *et al*, 2012). This has had an impact on the model of service delivery for psychological treatments. Accordingly, psychologists have been less involved in directly providing interventions and more involved in treatment development, training and consultative capacities, for example in the development of manualised treatments that aim to improve treatment integrity and facilitate treatment delivery by (trained) non-psychology staff (Hollin, 2006). Psychological therapies are therefore currently provided by clinical and forensic psychologists, and also by psychiatrists, specially trained mental health nurses, occupational therapists, psychotherapists and art and drama therapists.

This chapter is intended as a general guide to evidence-based psychological interventions for patients in secure psychiatric settings. It draws on evidence from a growing international literature on the effectiveness of interventions in criminal justice settings, with specific examples of programmes that operate in the UK, such as Controlling Anger and Learning how to Manage it (CALM; Ministry of Justice, 2010a). These programmes, whose primary goal is reduction of recidivism, are not routinely transferable into forensic mental health settings, where the emphasis is on reducing the risk posed by factors such as mental illness and substance misuse in addition to index offence-based work (Long *et al*, 2008).

The chapter starts with an overview of specialist psychological treatment approaches including cognitive–behavioural therapy (CBT), dialectical behaviour therapy (DBT) and behavioural interventions. It then moves on to a review of illness-focused and offence-focused psychological treatments and programmes. Following this, the trans-diagnostic issue of substance misuse is considered. Finally, we summarise the current state of knowledge and offer some thoughts for future directions.

Specialist psychological treatment approaches

Three of the most widely practised forms of psychotherapy in forensic mental health services are CBT, DBT and behavioural interventions. It is important to note, however, that treatment trials that provide the evidence base for these therapies have not been conducted with forensic mental health in-patients and there is a relative lack of evidence about 'what works' with this group (Davies & Oldfield, 2009). To date, the evidence for the effectiveness of the treatments in secure hospitals comes from service evaluations (e.g. Hughes *et al*, 1997; Long *et al*, 2014).

CBT

CBT grew in the 1970s from the integration of behaviour therapy with research on cognitive psychology (Ellis, 1962; Meichenbaum, 1977; Beck *et al*, 1979). CBT requires strict adherence to an empirical approach and emphasises working therapeutically in the present moment and planning for the future. It is time limited and usually carried out over 5–20 sessions, depending on the nature and severity of the presenting problem. However, in more complex conditions such as personality disorder, CBT can continue for 1–2 years.

The main elements of most CBT-based interventions in secure mental health settings include: assessment, clinical formulation, goal-setting, psychoeducation linked to diagnosis; and identification of core beliefs, rules for living and unhealthy cycles of behaviour, feelings and behaviours that may lead to relapse. Other elements include experiments to drop familiar but unhelpful safety behaviours; learning how to challenge 'cognitive distortions', such as catastrophic interpretations of events, with more balanced appraisals; and development of a relapse prevention plan. CBT is offered as an individual therapy or in a group format such as the Systems Training for Emotional Predictability and Problem Solving programme (STEPPS; Black et al, 2004) and in conjunction with pharmacological treatments (Smedley, 2010).

CBT has gained increasing acceptance as the psychological 'treatment of choice' for mental health problems, particularly for anxiety and depression. It owes its current status and popularity to a strong evidence base. A seminal paper by Butler et al (2006) reviewed 16 rigorous meta-analyses of CBT for a range of disorders to assess whether the positive outcomes reported in previous research were robust. The authors reported large treatment effect sizes for unipolar depression, generalised anxiety disorder, panic disorder with or without agoraphobia, social phobia, post-traumatic stress disorder and childhood depressive and anxiety disorders. Moderate effect sizes were reported for CBT for marital distress, anger, childhood somatic disorders and chronic pain. The authors found that that CBT was 'somewhat superior to antidepressants in the treatment of adult depression' (Butler et al, 2006: p. 17) and was 'equally effective as behaviour therapy in the treatment of adult depression and obsessive–compulsive disorder' (ibid.: p. 17). CBT was also reported to be effective for bulimia nervosa and schizophrenia. The authors concluded that their review supported the effectiveness of CBT for many common psychological disorders.

In the UK, CBT in some form is commonly recommended as the psychosocial treatment of choice by NICE for many disorders, including anxiety (NICE, 2004a; 2005a,b), depression (NICE 2004b; 2012a) and schizophrenia (NICE, 2014). However, in key areas specific to secure hospital settings, such as antisocial personality disorder, the value of CBT does not justify its use above other interventions (Gibbon et al, 2010). The current evidence for CBT is mainly derived from non-forensic populations, yet its efficacy is widely considered to be relevant to secure mental health settings. It is common practice to adapt CBT to meet the learning needs of different diagnostic groups. For example, Gaus (2007) describes the use of adapted CBT for people with autism spectrum disorder. Service evaluations within secure forensic settings point to the value of gender-specific manualised CBT group treatments for women diagnosed with personality disorder (Long et al, 2014).

DBT

Despite its success, CBT has not proved equally effective for all diagnostic groups. When applied to patients diagnosed with borderline personality disorder, standard CBT has often met with considerable difficulties. Borderline personality disorder is characterised by frequent and unrelenting personal crises and high levels of emotional dysregulation. Swales & Heard (2008) have described how a person diagnosed with borderline personality disorder might bring multiple problems to weekly therapy sessions, including panic attacks, social avoidance, binging and vomiting, and acute suicidal crisis. Further, the emphasis on change inherent in the CBT approach could be experienced as invalidating by such a patient, while teaching new coping skills can prove problematic in the context of treating their frequent suicidal behaviours. These issues create problems for standard CBT, which emphasises the importance of adherence to therapy agendas and session structure.

In response to the challenges of delivering CBT to this group, Marsha Linehan and colleagues developed a dialectical behaviour therapy which, while involving major adaptations to CBT, retained its underlying principles (Linehan, 1993). The changes incorporated by Linehan (1993) are best conceptualised as principles for therapy rather than protocols as in standard CBT. Central was the inclusion of the principles of validation and acceptance of the patient's current capabilities and functioning. The addition of these principles to a CBT model that emphasised change led to the use of the term 'dialectical' to describe the synthesis of opposites: a blend of both validation and acceptance strategies within the context of change. This helps counter the tendency for individuals with borderline personality disorder to become stuck in polemical positions, including preoccupation with past grievances or prior experiences of hurt or rejection.

In DBT, skills are learnt through a combination of weekly skills groups and individual therapy. The skills groups comprise four modules: mindfulness, distress tolerance, emotional regulation and interpersonal effectiveness. The skills group modules typically run over a 6-month period and there is an expectation that patients repeat the cycle two or three times. Additionally, therapy may take place via telephone coaching in times of crisis. Homework assignments may be set and meetings with key significant others held to help the client generalise new skills to the wider environment. The therapy is organised into three sequential stages. Stage one targets life-threatening behaviours such as self-harm, suicide attempts or, in forensic units, violence towards others. Stage two focuses on therapy-interfering behaviours. In DBT it is recognised that patients with borderline personality disorder often terminate therapy prematurely and so the specific factors that may affect a patient's continuation in therapy, such as the need to work on trauma arising from childhood events, are targeted. When the patient has developed skills to control life-threatening urges, and has learnt to tolerate and manage distressing emotions, work on stage three targets aimed at improving the quality of life for clients is undertaken.

DBT is an empirically supported treatment. Swales & Heard's (2008) review reported that nine randomised controlled trials of the effectiveness of DBT for borderline personality disorder have been conducted. Results showed that DBT reduced suicide attempts, non-suicidal self-injury, depression, hopelessness, anger, substance dependence and impulsiveness. It was found to increase social and general adjustment, and positive self-esteem. DBT has also been successfully extended to patients with other psychiatric diagnoses, including substance misuse, eating disorder, anxiety and depression. A multi-site clinical trial on the use of a new form of DBT for treatment-resistant depression named 'radically open DBT' (RO-DBT) is currently underway, although the results will not be known for some time (www.reframed.org.uk/about). Although most research on DBT has involved out-patient settings, a recent summary of research on DBT for in-patients in non-forensic settings noted that most studies reported improvements in relation to suicidal ideation, self-injurious behaviours and symptoms of depression and anxiety, whereas the results for reducing anger and violent behaviours were mixed (Bloom *et al*, 2012). Most recently, a service evaluation of a 1-year low secure DBT programme for women reported formal improvement on staff- and patient-rated outcome measures in addition to a reduction in risk behaviours (Fox *et al*, 2014).

Behavioural interventions

Behavioural interventions aim to modify a measurable and unwanted aspect of challenging behaviour such as aggression or self-harm. Interventions are generally predicated on theories of operant or classical conditioning. A detailed account of behavioural methods, particularly with reference to acquired brain injury, is presented in Chapter 11, 'Acquired brain injury, trauma and aggression'. Many different techniques have been devised to address specific problems but they share a number of common characteristics:

- clear identification and definition of measurable target behaviours for modification
- conduct of a full functional analysis of the target behaviour for the individual through assessment of the relationships between the antecedents and consequences of the behaviour
- collection of data about the frequency, severity and topography of challenging behaviours to establish the baseline rate
- testing of hypotheses about which functions are driving the target behaviour
- monitoring the progress of interventions to test their effectiveness through production of data, often presented in a graphical format.

Finally, all interventions are rigorously evaluated to test their efficacy in modifying the target behaviour before alternative approaches are trialled. In this way an informed and unique understanding of what works for whom can be acquired.

Behaviour therapy continues to be practised in secure in-patient units, notably for patients diagnosed with acquired brain injury, intellectual disability and autism spectrum disorder. Recent guidelines for autism spectrum disorder have recommended that behavioural approaches should be utilised to manage challenging behaviour (NICE, 2012*b*). Interestingly, radical behavioural approaches are returning in new forms in 'third wave' CBT approaches such as acceptance and commitment therapy (ACT; Hayes *et al*, 2006) and functional analytical psychotherapy (FAP; Kohlenberg & Tsai, 1991). Behaviour therapies frequently form part of the philosophy of care for in-patient units and are used to support patient recovery. Commonly used approaches include exposure-based treatments for anxiety, relaxation training and skills training such as developing assertiveness skills. RAID (reinforce appropriate/implode destructive behaviours; Davies, 2011) constitutes a behavioural philosophy which was established to help manage extreme behaviours. RAID is predicated on helping staff to work effectively with extreme, challenging behaviour through the relentless and creative reinforcement of positive behaviour to extinguish destructive behaviours as the patient's appropriate behaviours increase.

Other approaches

Mentalisation-based treatment (MBT) is a psychodynamic approach with roots in attachment theory and cognitive psychology. Mentalisation refers to the ability to focus and reflect on one's own mental state, an ability that is compromised in borderline personality disorder. Its benefit has been demonstrated in an 8-year follow up of MBT *v.* treatment as usual (Bateman & Fonagy, 2008). Other treatments that may be employed in forensic settings include mindfulness (Howells *et al* 2010), cognitive analytic therapy (CAT; Kellet *et al*, 2013) and eye movement desensitisation and reprocessing (EMDR; Bisson *et al*, 2007).

Treatment models and programmes

Secure mental health services have a dual responsibility for treating mental illness/disorder and for simultaneously managing and minimising risk. If risky behaviour is directly associated with the current episode of mental illness, then the treatment of that illness is the first priority. First, so that with improved insight and understanding patients can take on a greater role in maintaining their mental health in the future, and second, so that treatment interventions that target offending can be implemented. The psychological contribution to each aspect of treatment is outlined below.

Interventions to address mental health issues

Forensic mental health services work with patients who have a range of mental disorders, including schizophrenia, antisocial and borderline personality disorder, major affective disorder and mild intellectual disability. In addition, there are high rates of comorbidity, with many patients fulfilling diagnostic criteria for more than one disorder (dual diagnosis). In services for men the most common diagnosis is schizophrenia, whereas in women's services borderline personality disorder is most common. NICE guidelines for schizophrenia (NICE, 2014), antisocial personality disorder (NICE, 2009*a*), depression (NICE, 2012*a*) and borderline personality disorder (NICE, 2009*b*) provide a guideline for treatment development in the secure setting but are evidenced, in the main, on studies conducted with different populations. Within secure hospital settings treatment outcome is a function of acculturation to a treatment milieu which is generally more effective for those transferred from hospital rather than prison settings (Long *et al*, 2012). Interventions such as RAID (Davies, 2011) are provided at a ward milieu level to aid stabilisation of psychiatric state, and at an individual level through the development of a therapeutic alliance (for issues in delivering effective psychological treatment see Long, 2013). Best practice dictates that treatment programmes be based on a thorough needs analysis of patients admitted. Surveys of interventions in medium secure psychiatric setting show a wide range of philosophy and treatment (Davies & Oldfield, 2009).

Individual and group CBT for schizophrenia as an adjunct to medication has largely focused on interventions for delusions and hallucinations (Roberts *et al*, 2006). These interventions target insight, relapse prevention, symptomatology and medication adherence. The evidence base for their use is evolving and, with few exceptions (Pinkham *et al*, 2004), studies have been concerned with out-patient groups. The treatment protocol for a typical 12-session CBT group for voices would cover the establishment of a therapeutic alliance; education about voices and sharing voice experiences; content and behavioural analysis of voices; and coping skills (Roberts *et al*, 2006).

Within a secure service for women, manualised psychosocial interventions have been deemed as core (i.e. relevant to all) or non-core (relevant to a subgroup) (Long *et al*, 2011). Core CBT groups include: getting the most from your treatment, emotional regulation, social problem solving, interpersonal effectiveness, developing social confidence, and living skills. Non-core groups include overcoming substance misuse, firesetting, understanding personality disorder, living with mental illness, body image, and self-care and physical healthcare. These treatments have been found to be effective in real-world, uncontrolled evaluations (e.g. Long *et al*, 2014).

Interventions to address offending behaviours

The risk–need–responsivity model and the Good Lives Model

In the 1970s, reviews of psychological and educational interventions for offending behaviours offered pessimistic conclusions about their effectiveness (Martinson, 1974). In later years more sophisticated meta-analyses of 'what works' for the reduction of reoffending combined the results of individual studies to gauge overall treatment effect. These results were more supportive of psychological, educational and behavioural interventions. A number of influential researchers (Lipsey, 2009; Andrews & Bonta, 2010) proposed that the most effective interventions adhered to three key principles and incorporated these into a risk–need–responsivity (RNR) model for offender assessment and rehabilitation (Bonta & Andrews, 2007). In the RNR model, the 'risk' principle proposes that interventions should be targeted at high-risk offenders because they produce the greatest reductions in recidivism. The 'need' principle indicates that interventions should target the specific risk areas known to be associated with reoffending, including membership of antisocial peer groups, antisocial behaviours, personality characteristics and thinking styles. Finally, the 'responsivity' principle involves therapists delivering interventions using a structured cognitive–behavioural or skills-based approach and in an active, motivational style that takes account of the learning styles and needs of the individual offender. The responsivity principle is of crucial importance and considerable attention has focused on identifying the specific factors in the therapeutic style of facilitators that are associated with the successful delivery of interventions (Kozar, 2010). Increased optimism about offending interventions was associated with widespread adoption of RNR principles in the 1990s and a large-scale increase in programmes aimed at reducing recidivism. Although these methods are used in secure mental health settings, most evaluative work has been undertaken with males in correctional facilities. The suite of programmes described below are under continuous development, with newer approaches added where they are able to meet strict accreditation criteria.

While the RNR model was the dominant paradigm of intervention for offenders throughout the 1990s, the strengths-based Good Lives Model (GLM; Ward et al, 2007) has more recently gained credence as an alternative approach in forensic mental health settings. GLM concentrates on strengthening the positive aspects of patients' interests in pursuit of their goals in life. It is built on the notion that individuals who offend have similar aims and needs as non-offenders but have developed maladaptive ways of meeting these needs. GLM approaches seek to build on the individual's strengths and help them to find pro-social ways of meeting their needs. The model has been influential in a number of areas but particularly in the treatment of sex offenders (Whitehead et al, 2007; Marshall et al, 2011). As McMurran (2011) points out, offenders report that they want to avoid criminal behaviour and lead satisfying lives. Mental health practitioners accordingly need to identify and focus on risk factors but in ways which motivate patients and build on their strengths as well as addressing their deficits. In this way both the RNR and GLM approaches have a role to play in offender and secure hospital interventions (see Mann & Carter (2012) for a further elaboration of this integrative approach). Although the GLM is attractive to practitioners, it lacks the empirical support of the RNR model.

Thinking/cognitive skills programmes

The underlying premise of thinking or cognitive skills programmes is that many offenders have high levels of impulsivity and hold deficits in their ability to reason and solve life's problems in a healthy and pro-social manner. Offenders may fail to sufficiently consider the outcomes or risks associated with a particular course of action and may show insufficient consideration of the perspectives of others. They may persist with flawed problem-solving approaches, including aggression and violence, because they have used them successfully in the past. Cognitive skills programmes typically focus on helping participants learn thinking skills to help them solve problems more effectively. Programmes can be delivered in group or individual mode. Methods used to keep participants engaged and stimulated include frequent use of role-play, modelling by facilitators of key skills, and the use of workbooks. Thought-storming, where an idea is presented and participants are encouraged to generate associations, and games linked to session objectives may also be used. Participants may engage in creativity exercises and the use of 'step-by-step' guides to thinking and problem-solving. Homework assignments are linked to reviews of learning and applications of skills to real-life situations.

Recently, the Thinking Skills programme run by the National Offender Management Service (NOMS) has had some success in enhancing engagement and the quality of working alliance between facilitators and participants. Participants are also assigned individual sessions to support learning from the programme (see Clarke (2010) for a summary of these changes). 'Cognitive skills' programmes are effective in improving pro-social thinking styles and reducing recidivism rates (Hollin, 2006; Tong & Farrington, 2006) and impulsivity (McDougall *et al*, 2009), which is a well-established risk factor for offending. Other studies, using large databases and controlling for demographic and risk factors, have shown significant reductions in reoffending rates (Hollis, 2007; Ministry of Justice, 2010*a*; Sadlier, 2010). The cognitive deficits targeted by Thinking Skills programmes are common among patients in mental health settings, indicating that there is scope to increase their provision. Accordingly, they have been increasingly adopted in forensic mental health settings with positive results (Tapp *et al*, 2010).

Violence and anger management programmes

Research evidence shows that factors that are empirically linked to violent offending, include associations with criminal peers, antisocial attitudes, deficits in social-cognitive skills such as problem-solving, poor social perspective-taking skills, impulsivity, low IQ, psychopathy, lack of insight into violence, rehearsal of violent thoughts, substance misuse and poor emotional management (Ministry of Justice, 2010*b*). The NOMS currently runs programmes for violent offenders based on this research and programmes based on similar principles have been run in high secure psychiatric settings (Jones & Hollin, 2004). The CALM programme runs for 24 weekly 2-hour sessions and is designed for medium- to high-risk participants whose offending is linked to anger. The goals of the programme are to assist participants in understanding the factors that trigger their anger and aggression and in developing skills to manage emotional arousal. Participants learn about the main thinking processes that create and sustain anger and about ways of challenging these with pro-social alternatives. Relaxation techniques to reduce anger arousal are also taught, along with methods of reducing conflict without using anger inappropriately. Emotional states which are linked to anger, such as jealousy and depression, are also addressed. An evaluation of the Canadian equivalent of the CALM programme showed that the 3-year reoffending rate for programme completers was less than 10%, compared with 30% for the comparison group (Ministry of Justice, 2010b). The Cognitive Self-Change Programme (CSCP) is aimed at high-risk offenders and runs for much longer than CALM (8–15 months), depending on the level of need (Ministry of Justice, 2010b).

An anger treatment programme designed for people with developmental disability (Taylor & Novaco, 2005) uses similar methods to the CALM programme, including self-monitoring, relaxation and recognition of anger triggers. In addition, the programme includes a pre-treatment preparatory phase to identify the costs of anger and aggression to self and others. Participants identify and rank order the types of situations that they find most stressful and anger-provoking, and repeatedly work through each situation in a structured manner using techniques to lower arousal and to imagine themselves dealing with the situation effectively.

There is considerable evidence that interventions for violent offenders based on cognitive–behavioural principles lead to reductions in reconviction for both general and violent recidivism, and that participation in these interventions leads to changes in self-reported measures of anger and aggression. A recent controlled trial of a cognitive–behavioural anger management programme for patients with developmental disability and severe problems of aggression detained in a secure mental health facility found that those who received treatment had lower scores on assessments of anger and aggression, and improved behaviour as reported by institutional staff (Taylor *et al*, 2010).

Sex offender treatment programmes

About 7% of individuals admitted to medium and high secure forensic mental health services have been convicted of a sexual offence (Rutherford & Duggan, 2007). Reconvictions for sexual offending from secure forensic services were much lower than comparable rates from prison. The Ministry of Justice (2010c: p. 1) has identified that the sex offender treatment programmes (SOTPs) that have the best prospects of reducing the risk of recidivism should focus on:

'sexual preoccupation; sexual preference for children; preference for sex involving violence or humiliation; rare sexual interests; offence-supportive attitudes; seeking emotional intimacy with children rather than adults; lack of emotional intimacy with adults; impulsive lifestyle; poor problem solving; resistance to rules; generalised grievance against others; having criminal friends.'

Interestingly, research indicates that other treatment targets commonly included in SOTPs, such as reducing denial and increasing personal responsibility for offending, victim empathy and social skills, have not been found to be empirically related to sexual offending recidivism rates (Mann & Carter, 2012).

CBT approaches are the best supported interventions for sex offenders, particularly when paired with pharmacological treatment, whereas approaches based on counselling and psychodynamic methods are not effective (Ministry of Justice, 2010c). Group CBT has been found to be most effective with medium-risk sex offenders, whereas reported treatment effect sizes are smaller with high-risk offenders. Further, because reoffending rates are very low, specialised sex offender treatment is not justified for most low-risk offenders. In a meta-analysis, Hanson *et al* (2009) reported that offenders that received treatment had lower reconviction rates than untreated comparison groups. The strongest treatment effects were found for programmes that followed RNR principles. Schmucker & Lösel (2008) conducted a review including only high-quality studies to evaluate the efficacy of sex offender treatment and reported an average reduction in reoffending rates of 27% for those receiving treatment compared with untreated samples. Although the current balance of evidence is generally favourable, it is generally agreed that there is a need for better-quality sex offender treatment research. Mann & Carter (2012) outline a set of organising principles to inform the next generation of programmes, including targeting neurocognitive functioning through greater use of problem-solving, medication and mindfulness, and strengthening social resources and social networks. An important development in this respect is the use of social networks such as Circles of Support and Accountability (Wilson *et al*, 2008), whose evaluation has provided encouraging evidence about reducing recidivism rates. These developments are likely to be very influential in shaping sex offender treatment programmes in the future, both in mental health and in criminal justice settings.

Psychological approaches to substance misuse

Individuals with severe mental health problems are at increased risk for the development of substance misuse and dependence disorders. Such disorders are common in secure psychiatric hospital settings, with prevalence estimates ranging from 50 to 90% (Scott *et al*, 2004; Steel *et al*, 2004). Substance misuse by individuals with mental disorder (i.e. dual diagnosis) doubles the likelihood of poor prognosis (Lehman, 1995). The high prevalence of early-onset alcohol misuse by mentally disordered offenders (Lumsden *et al*, 2005) and the association between substance misuse, violent recidivism and psychiatric relapse make treatment a priority in secure settings (Springer *et al*, 2003).

Treatment goals and components

The principal treatment goals in dual disorder programmes include control of the patient's symptoms; the acquisition of skills; preservation of the patient's safety and that of others; and the cultivation of motivation and determination to develop self-control for recovery. Engagement strategies are of primary importance for patients in secure settings and include individual motivational interviewing (MI; Miller & Rollnick, 1991) to enhance motivation to reduce drug use outside of hospital. Motivational interviewing is a counselling approach designed to help patients become aware of their substance misuse problems through articulation and pursual of their own personal goals. A more directive form of motivational interviewing has been developed for patients with serious and persistent mental illness (Bellack *et al*, 2007). Many patients know little about their psychiatric illness, the principles of its treatment and its interaction with stress or with alcohol and drugs. Education about the reasons for substance use, and about the particular risks of substance use for people with schizophrenia or personality disorder, is used to shift the decisional balance towards decreased use. In group settings, discussion of the negative effects of substance use can be balanced by an understanding of individual motivating factors. Other key treatment components include structured goal-setting to identify realistic, short-term goals for abstinence or decreased use; social skills and drug refusal training to deal with social pressure and provide success experiences that can increase self-efficacy for change; dealing with drug-related thinking; and relapse prevention training that focuses on behavioural skills for coping with urges and dealing with high-risk situations and lapses. Psychosocial rehabilitation also addresses substance misuse indirectly by building compensatory skills and activities (lifestyle changes) that undermine the patient's need and desire to use substances. This emphasis is consistent with the use of social learning approaches to teaching social and independent living skills to long-term psychiatric in-patients (Paul & Lentz, 1977). A number of good-practice examples of dual diagnosis treatment programmes can be found in the literature (e.g. Graham *et al*, 2003; Mueser *et al*, 2003; Bellack *et al*, 2007). Such programmes take into account the cognitive deficits of patients through the use of highly structured sessions that emphasise behavioural rehearsal and the 'over learning' of specific skills for key high-risk situations. Training is typically done in a small-group format.

In prison settings CBT approaches have been found to be effective in reducing alcohol consumption and alcohol-related aggression (McCullough & McMurran, 2008) as well as recidivism in drug users (Pearson *et al*, 2002). There is also some evidence for the success of integrated approaches in reducing rates of hospitalisation, symptoms of mental illness and substance use. There remains, however, a need for controlled trials to establish the effectiveness of psychological interventions for substance misuse with psychiatric comorbidity (Cleary *et al*, 2008).

Treatment for substance misuse in secure hospital settings

Many patients in secure psychiatric settings have a dual diagnosis. Although such settings offer the opportunity for integrated treatment approaches (i.e. concurrent treatment of both psychiatric and substance misuse problems by the same team), there are a number of issues that need to be considered in treatment design and delivery. These include inadequate identification of substance misuse problems, poor motivation to engage, current mental health status, cognitive impairment and polydrug use. Motivation to work on substance misuse problems in hospital may be situation specific. However, the assessment of treatment outcome is complicated by the need for the 'success' of an intervention to be known before patients are placed in situations where they have free access to alcohol and other drugs (Long & Hollin, 2009). On a positive note, hospitalisation presents a valuable opportunity to engage in treatment patients who might otherwise be inaccessible to clinicians. Involuntary exposure to intervention can sometimes 'break the ice' of treatment refusal and resistance and engage patients with their treatment teams; indeed, the majority of those who have been involuntarily hospitalised hold positive views of their treatment on discharge (Hiday, 1996).

Evaluation of substance misuse treatment in secure settings

Despite the fact that patients with substance misuse problems discharged from medium secure settings were more likely than other patients to re-offend, a survey of units found that formal substance misuse treatment programmes were rare (Scott *et al*, 2004). Thus research describing treatment programmes and outcomes for patients in secure settings is limited and concerns small, largely male samples (Derry & Batson, 2008; Morris & Moore, 2009; Oddie & Davis, 2009). For example, Miles *et al* (2007) report on the evaluation of a three-stage model of integrated treatment for substance misuse problems in a medium secure unit for men. Stages 1 and 2 consist of 12 weekly group sessions and target individuals in the pre-contemplation, contemplation, action, maintenance and relapse stages of the stage of change model of addictive behaviours (Prochaska *et al*, 1992). Stage 3, entitled 'Just Say No', is a maintenance phase aimed at maintaining motivation to sustain therapeutic gains and abstinence. The authors report that of 19 patients admitted in 2005 who received treatment for substance misuse, approximately three-quarters were abstinent by the end of June 2006. Participants' self-reported insight and confidence to make changes to their substance use had also increased. In an evaluation of a gender-sensitive group programme for women in medium security, Long *et al* (2010) found that treatment was successful in engaging two-thirds of patients to completion. Positive outcomes were identified for treatment completers in terms of improved substance-related self-efficacy, lower perceived costs and greater benefits of change. A further series of group sessions develops themes for application in conditions of low security where patients have, by virtue of community leave arrangements, access to alcohol and other substances.

Conclusions

Within the criminal justice system, the best validated and most widely disseminated psychological approaches are 'manualised' cognitive–behavioural programmes that have a structured content, concrete goals and are focused on the acquisition of skills and on risk factors for criminal recidivism (Tong & Farrington, 2006; Lipsey *et al*, 2007). Such approaches, many of which derive from the Canadian criminal justice system, have been widely adopted in the prison and probation service in England and Wales (Hollin & Palmer, 2006). The results of meta-analytic research indicate that such programmes can reduce the recidivistic behaviour of offenders who complete them (Hatcher, 2012).

Research in secure psychiatric settings to date has focused on the admission characteristics of patients, with a dearth of studies on outcomes (Edwards *et al*, 2002; Bartlett, 2007). A study of discharges from secure services shows a mortality rate of 10%, a readmission rate of 38% and a reconviction rate of 49% (Davies *et al*, 2007). Despite problems of methodology, it is clear that a large proportion of individuals continue to present a risk to themselves and others following treatment, and that a sizeable group are readmitted to secure care. Whether findings from the correctional literature can be extrapolated to mentally ill offenders in secure psychiatric settings is a moot point. Mentally ill offenders frequently have a dual diagnosis and many pose a risk to themselves as well as others.

Despite the treatment challenge posed by patients in secure care, there is a scarcity of literature describing the treatment of offending behaviour in secure settings and very little on treatment effectiveness. To date, most evaluations have used quasi-experimental or pre-post designs to evaluate psychological treatment programmes. Published works have focused on service evaluations for secure populations with a predominant diagnosis of personality disorder or mental illness and on specific programmes for skills development. Despite rapid expansion in evidence-based psychological therapies over the past two decades, these approaches are not always adopted widely and may struggle to be accepted (Shafran *et al*, 2009). The secure psychiatric sector has adopted a predominantly CBT-oriented (and variants) approach to patient care on the basis of research in related fields. It has also responded to incorporate the so-called third wave of CBT that has been strongly influenced by spiritual and contemplative traditions such as Buddhism and which uses mindfulness to facilitate coping and alleviate distress (Howells *et al*, 2010). There is a concurrent re-emphasis on behavioural approaches in different forms, including DBT and ACT. It is, of course, important not to view psychological therapies in isolation from other effective approaches, particularly pharmacology. It is of interest, for example, that while medication is identified as a key target in 70% of individuals admitted to secure care, psychological treatment is identified in fewer than 50% (Melzer *et al*, 2004). The complementary natures of psychological and pharmacological approaches are evident in the treatment approach to sexual offending and depression (Beech & Mitchell, 2005; Mann & Carter, 2012; NICE, 2012*a*).

This chapter has reviewed the dominant themes and psychological approaches at the time of writing. It has been of necessity selective and it is of its time. In a rapidly changing field it is anticipated that subsequent overviews of this field may reach substantially different conclusions. Currently, questions exist about whether transmission of empirically supported treatments from prison and probation to mental health settings is possible. Further, there is little guidance about how to adapt treatments for appropriate use in forensic mental health settings while maintaining fidelity to essential treatment principles. McHugh *et al* (2009) offered transdiagnostic interventions (principle-based treatments) which add flexibility of delivery while maximising fidelity to treatment principles. This affords a way of synthesising effective principles of forensic treatment drawn from the criminal justice system with findings from the general clinical treatment outcome literature.

Overall, psychological treatments for addressing problem behaviours in secure settings are emergent. Issues including engagement, non-completion of treatment, small sample size and lack of adequate control groups have limited the conclusions to be drawn from evaluations. There remains an urgent need to develop an evidence base for risk- or offence-focused treatments in secure settings. Studies undertaken to date in forensic mental health settings are best viewed as pilot evaluations that have nevertheless provided promising indications that psychological treatment can be effective.

Acknowledgements

We thank Adam Carter, Head of SOTP and Research, National Offender Management Service for providing the latest research on programme evaluation.

References

Andrews, D. A. & Bonta, J. (2010) *The Psychology of Criminal Conduct*, 5th edn. Anderson.

Bartlett, A. (2007) *Second Expert Paper: Social Division and Difference – Women*. NHS National Programme on Forensic Mental Health Research and Development.

Bateman, A.W. & Fonagy, P. (2008) Eight year follow-up of patients treated for borderline personality disorder: mentalization-based treatment versus treatment as usual. *American Journal of Psychiatry*, **166**, 1355–1364.

Beck, A.T., Rush, A.J., Shaw, B.F., *et al* (1979) *Cognitive Therapy of Depression*. Guilford Press.

Beech, A. R. & Mitchell, I.J. (2005) A neurobiological perspective on attachment problems in sexual offenders and the role of selective serotonin re-uptake inhibitors in the treatment of such problems. *Clinical Psychology Review*, **25**, 153–182.

Bellack, A.S., Bennett, N.E. & Gearon, J.S. (2007) *Behavioural Treatment for Substance Abuse in People with Serious and Persistent Mental Illness*. Routledge.

Bisson, J.I., Ehlers, A., Matthews, R., *et al* (2007) Psychological treatments for chronic post-traumatic stress disorder: systematic review and meta-analysis. *British Journal of Psychiatry*, **190**, 97–104.

Black, D.W., Blum, N., Pfohl, B., *et al* (2004) The STEPPS group treatment program for outpatients with borderline personality disorder. *Journal of Contemporary Psychotherapy*, **34**, 193–210.

Bloom, J.N., Woodward, E.N., Susmaras, T., *et al* (2012) Use of dialectical behaviour therapy in in-patient treatment for borderline personality disorder: a systematic review. *Psychiatric Services*, **63**, 881–888.

Bonta, J. & Andrews, D.A. (2007) *Risk–Need–Responsivity Model for Offender Assessment and Rehabilitation (User Report 2007 06)*. Public Safety Canada.

Butler, A.C., Chapman, J.E., Formen, E.M., *et al* (2006) The empirical status of cognitive behaviour therapy: a review of meta-analyses. *Clinical Psychology Review*, **26**, 17–31.

Clarke, D. (2010) Therapy and offending behaviour programmes. In *Psychological Therapy in Prison and Other Secure Settings* (eds J. Harvey & K. Smedley), pp. 234–256. Willan Publishing.

Cleary, M., Hunt, G.E., Matteson, G.L., *et al* (2008) Psychosocial interventions for people with both serve mental illness and substance misuse. *Cochrane Database of Systematic Reviews*, **1**, CD001088.

Davies, J. & Oldfield, K. (2009) Treatment need and provision in medium secure care. *British Journal of Forensic Practice*, **11**, 24–30.

Davies, S., Clarke, M., Hollin, C., *et al* (2007) Long term outcomes after discharge from medium secure care: a cause for concern. *British Journal of Psychiatry*, **191**, 70–74.

Davies, W. (2011) *The RAID Course*, 9th edn. APT Press.

Derry, A. & Batson, A. (2008) Getting out and staying out: does substance use treatment have an effect on the outcome of mentally disordered offenders after discharge from a medium secure service? *British Journal of Forensic Practice*, **10**, 13–17.

Doyle, M., Logan, C., Ludlow, A., *et al* (2012) Milestones to recovery: preliminary validation of a framework to promote recovery and map progress through the medium secure inpatient pathway. *Criminal Behaviour and Mental Health*, **22**, 53–64.

Edwards, J., Steed, P. & May, K. (2002) Clinical and forensic outcome 2 years and 5 years after admission to medium secure unit. *Journal of Forensic Psychiatry*, **13**, 68–87.

Ellis, A. (1962) *Reason and Emotion in Psychotherapy*. Lyle Stuart.

Fox, E., Krawczyk, K., Staniford, J., *et al* (2014) A service evaluation of a 1-year dialectical behaviour therapy programme for women with borderline personality disorder in a low secure unit. *Behavioural and Cognitive Psychotherapy*, 13 February, doi:10.1017/S1352465813001124.

Gaus, L. (2007) *Cognitive-Behavioral Therapy for adult Asperger Syndrome*. Guilford Press.

Gibbon, S., Duggan, C., Stoffers, J., *et al* (2010) Psychological intervention for antisocial personality disorder (review). *Cochrane Database of Systematic Reviews*, **6**, CD007668.

Graham, H.L., Copello, A., Birchwood, M.J., *et al* (2003) Cognitive behavioural integrated treatment approach for psychosis and problem substance use. In *Substance Misuse and Psychosis* (eds H.L. Graham, A. Copello, M. Birchwood, *et al*), pp. 181–207. Wiley.

Hanson, R.K., Bourgon, G., Helmus, L., *et al* (2009) The principles of effective correctional treatment also apply to sexual offenders: a meta-analysis. *Criminal Justice and Behavior*, **36**, 865–891.

Hatcher, R. (2012) Risk assessment and offender programmes. In *Forensic Psychology: Crime, Justice, Law, Interventions*, 2nd edn (eds G. Davies & A. Beech): pp. 327–348. BPS Blackwell.

Hayes, S.C., Luoma, J.B., Bond, F.W., *et al* (2006) Acceptance and commitment therapy: model, processes and outcomes. *Behaviour Research and Therapy*, **44**, 1–25.

Hiday, V.A. (1996) Involuntary commitment to psychiatric technology. *International Journal of Technology Assessment in Healthcare*, **12**, 585–603.

Hollin, C.R. (1999) Treatment programmes for offenders: meta-analysis, 'what works' and beyond. *International Journal of Law and Psychiatry*, **22**, 361–372.

Hollin, C.R. (2006) Offending behaviour programmes and contention: evidence based practice manuals, and programme evaluation. In *Offending Behaviour Programmes: Development, Application and Controversies* (eds C.R. Hollin & E.J. Palmer): pp. 33–68. John Wiley & Sons.

Hollin, C.R. & Palmer, E.J. (eds) *(2006) Offending Behaviour Programmes: Development, Application and Controversies*. John Wiley & Sons.

Hollis, V. (2007) *Reconviction Analysis of Programme Data using Interim Accredited Programmes Software (IAPS)*. National Offender Management Service.

Howells, K., Tennant, A., Day, A., *et al* (2010) Mindfulness in forensic mental health: does it have a role? Mindfulness, 1, 4–9.

Hughes, G., Hugue, T., Hollin, C., *et al* (1997) First stage evaluation of a treatment programme for personality disordered offenders. *Journal of Forensic Psychiatry*, **8**, 515–527.

Jones, D. & Hollin, C.R. (2004) Managing problematic anger: the development of a treatment programme for personality disordered patients in high security. *International Journal of Forensic Mental Health*, **3**, 197–210.

Kellett, S., Bennett, D., Ryle, T., *et al* (2013) Cognitive analytic therapy for borderline personality disorder: therapist competence and therapeutic effectiveness in routine practice. *Clinical Psychology and Psychotherapy*, **20**, 216–225.

Kohlenberg, R.J. & Tsai, M. (1991) *Functional Analytic Psychotherapy: A Guide for Creating Intense and Curative Therapeutic Relationships*. Plenum.

Kozar, C. (2010) Treatment readiness and the therapeutic alliance. In *Transitions to Better Lives: Offender Readiness and Rehabilitation* (eds A. Day, S. Casey, T. Ward, *et al*), pp. 195–213. Willan Publishing.

Lehman, A.F. (1995) Editorial. In: *Double Jeopardy. Chronic Mental Illness and Substance Use Disorders* (eds A.F. Lehman & L.B. Dixon): pp. 3–7. Harwood Academic Publishers.

Linehan, M. (1993) *Cognitive Behavioural Treatment of Borderline Personality Disorder*. Guilford Press.

Lipsey, M.W. (2009) The primary factors that characterise effective interventions with juvenile offenders: a meta analysis overview. *Victims and Offenders*, **4**, 124–147.

Lipsey, M. & Wilson, D.B. (1993) The efficacy of psychological, educational and behavioural treatment: confirmation from meta-analysis. *American Psychologist*, **48**, 1181–1209.

Lipsey, M.W., Landenberger, N.A. & Wilson, S.J. (2007) Effects of cognitive-behavioral programs for criminal offenders. *Campbell Systematic Reviews*, **6**, doi: 10.4073/csr.2007.6.

Long, C.G. (2013) Delivering affective cognitive behavioural group treatment for women in secure psychiatric settings. *Journal of Forensic Practice*, **15**, 55–67.

Long, C.G. & Hollin, C.R. (2009) Assessing co-morbid substance use in detained psychiatric patients: issues and instruments for evaluating treatment outcome. *Substance Use and Misuse*, **44**, 1602–1641.

Long, C.G., Fulton, B. & Hollin, C.R. (2008) The development of a 'best practice' service for women in a medium secure psychiatric setting: treatment component and evaluation. *Clinical Psychology and Psychotherapy*, **15**, 304–319.

Long, C.G., Fulton, B., Fitzgerald, K., *et al* (2010) Group substance abuse treatment for women in secure services. *Mental Health and Substance Use: Dual Diagnosis*, **3**, 227–237.

Long, C.G., Collins, L., Mason, F., *et al* (2011) Effective therapeutic practice in a secure women's service: from vision to reality. *International Journal of Clinical Leadership*, **17**, 79–82.

Long, C.G., Dolley, O., Barron, R., *et al* (2012) Women transferred from prison to medium secure psychiatric care: the therapeutic challenge. *Journal of Forensic Psychiatry and Psychology*, **23**, 261–273.

Long, C.G., Dolley, O. & Hollin, C.R. (2014) Personality disordered women in secure care: a treatment evaluation. *Journal of Criminal Psychology*, **4**, 44–58.

Lösel, F. (1996) Effective correctional programming: what empirical research tells us and what it doesn't. *Forum on Corrections Research*, **6**, 33–37.

Lumsden, J., Headfield, J., Littler, S., *et al* (2005) The prevalence of early onset alcohol abuse in mentally disordered offenders. *Journal of Forensic Psychiatry and Psychology*, **16**, 651–659.

Mann, R.E. & Carter, A.J. (2012) Organising principles for the treatment of sexual offending. In *Behandlung von Straftätern: Sozialtherapie, Maßregelvollzug, Sicherungsverwahrung [Offender treatment: Social Therapy, Special Forensic Hospitals, and Indeterminate Imprisonment]* (eds B. Wischka, W. Pecher & H. van der Boogaart). Centaurus.

Marshall, W.L., Marshall, L.E., Serran, G.A., *et al* (2011) *Rehabilitating Sex Offenders: A Strength-Based Approach*. American Psychological Association.

Martinson, R. (1974) What works? Questions and answers about prison reform. *Public Interest*, **10**, 22–54.

McCulloch, A. & McMurran, M. (2008) An evaluation of a treatment programme for alcohol related aggression. *Criminal Behaviour and Mental Health*, **18**, 224–231.

McDougall, C., Perry, A.E., Clarbour, J., *et al* (2009) *Evaluation of HM Prison Service Enhanced Thinking Skills Programme: Report on the Outcome from a Randomised Controlled Trial*. Ministry of Justice.

McHugh, R.K., Murray, H.W. & Barlow, D.H. (2009) Balancing fidelity and adaption in the dissemination of the empirically-supported treatments: the promise of trans diagnostic interventions. *Behaviour, Research and Therapy*, **49**, 946–953.

McMurran, M. (2011) Motivational interviewing with offenders: a systematic review. *Legal and Criminological Psychology*, **14**, 83–100.

Meichenbaum, D. (1977) *Cognitive Behaviour Modification: An Integrative Approach*. Plenum Press.

Melzer, D., Tom, B.D.M., Brugha, T., *et al* (2004) Access to medium secure psychiatric care in England and Wales: the clinical needs of assessed patients. *Journal of Forensic Psychiatry and Psychology*, **15**, 50–65.

Miles, H., Dutheil, L., Welsby, I., *et al* (2007) 'Just Say No': a preliminary evaluation of a three-stage model of integrated treatment for substance use problems in conditions of medium security. *Journal of Forensic Psychiatry and Psychology*, **18**, 141–159.

Miller, W.R. & Rollnick, S. (1991) *Motivational Interviewing: Preparing People to Change Addictive Behaviours*. Guilford.

Ministry of Justice (2010*a*) *Do Cognitive Skills Programmes Work with Offenders?* (Factsheet). National Offender Management Service (https://www.swmcrc.co.uk/wp-content/uploads/2010/06/What-works-Cognitive-skills.pdf).

Ministry of Justice (2010*b*) *What Works with Violent Offenders?* (Factsheet). National Offender Management Service (https://www.swmcrc.co.uk/wp-content/uploads/2010/06/What-works-violence.pdf).

Ministry of Justice (2010*c*) *What Works with Sex Offenders?* (Factsheet). National Offender Management Service (http://www.justice.gov.uk/downloads/information-access-rights/foi-disclosure-log/prison-probation/foi-75519-annex-a.pdf).

Morris, C.E. & Moore, E. (2009) An evaluation of group work as an intervention to reduce the impact of substance misuse for offender patients in a high secure hospital. *Journal of Forensic Psychiatry and Psychology*, **20**, 559–576.

Mueser, K.T., Noordsy, D.L., Drake, R.E., *et al* (2003) *Integrated Treatment for Dual Disorders: A Guide to Effective Practice*. Guilford Press.

National Institute for Health and Clinical Excellence (2004*a*) *Anxiety: Management of Anxiety (Panic Disorder, With and Without Agoraphobia, and Generalised Anxiety Disorder) in Adults in Primary, Secondary and Community Care* (CG22). NICE.

National Institute for Health and Clinical Excellence (2004b) *Depression: Management of Depression in Primary and Secondary Care* (CG23). NICE.

National Institute for Health and Clinical Excellence (2005a) *Post-Traumatic Stress Disorder: The Management of PTSD in Adults and Children in Primary and Secondary Care (CG26)*. NICE.

National Institute for Health and Clinical Excellence (2005b) *Obsessive-Compulsive Disorder: Core Interventions in the Treatment of Obsessive-compulsive Disorder and Body Dysmorphic Disorder (CG31)*. NICE.

National Institute for Health and Clinical Excellence (2009a) *Antisocial Personality Disorder (CG77)*. NICE.

National Institute for Health and Clinical Excellence (2009b) *Borderline Personality Disorder (CG78)*. NICE.

National Institute for Health and Clinical Excellence (2012a) *Depression in Adults (update) (CG90)*. NICE.

National Institute for Health and Clinical Excellence (2012b) *Autism: Recognition, Referral, Diagnosis and Management of Adults on the Autistic Spectrum (CG142)*. NICE.

National Institute for Health and Care Excellence (2014) *Psychosis and Schizophrenia in Adults (CG178)*. NICE.

Oddie, S. & Davies, J. (2009) A multi-method evaluation of a substance misuse programme in a medium secure forensic mental health unit. *Journal of Addiction Nursing*, **20**, 132–141.

Paul, G.L. & Lentz, R.J. (1977) *Psychosocial Treatment of Chronic Mental Patients: Milieu versus Social Learning Programmes*. Harvard University Press.

Pearson, F.S., Lipton, D.S., Cleland, C.M., *et al* (2002) The effects of behavioural/cognitive-behavioural programs on recidivism. *Crime and Delinquency*, **48**, 476–496.

Pinkham A.E., Gloege A.T., Flanagan, S., *et al* (2004) Group cognitive behavioural therapy for auditory hallucinations: a pilot study. *Cognitive and Behavioural Practice*, **11**, 93–98.

Prochaska, J.O., DiClemente, C.C. & Norcross, J.C. (1992) In search of how people change: applications to addictive behaviours. *American Psychologist*, **47**, 1102–1114.

Roberts D.L., Pinkham A.E. & Penn D.L. (2006) Schizophrenia. In *Cognitive Behavioural Therapy in Groups* (eds P.J. Bieling, R.E. McCabe & M.M. Antony), pp. 350–376. Guilford Press.

Rutherford, M. & Duggan, S. (2007) *Forensic Mental Health Services – Facts and Figures on Current Provision*. Sainsbury Centre for Mental Health (http://www.centreformentalhealth.org.uk/pdfs/scmh_forensic_factfile_2007.pdf).

Sadlier, G. (2010) *Evaluation of the Impact of the HM Prison Service Enhanced Thinking Skills Programme on Reoffending: Outcomes of the Surveying Prisoner Crime Reduction (SPCR) Sample*. Ministry of Justice (http://www.justice.gov.uk/downloads/publications/research-and-analysis/moj-research/eval-enhanced-thinking-skills-prog.pdf).

Scott, F., Whyte, S., Bernette, R., *et al* (2004) A national survey of substance misuse and treatment outcome of psychiatric patients in medium security. *Journal of Forensic Psychiatry & Psychology*, **15**, 595–605.

Schmucker, M. & Lösel, F. (2008) Does sexual offender treatment work? A systematic review of outcome evaluations. *Psicothema*, **20**, 10–19.

Shafran, R., Clark, D.M., Fairburn, C.G., *et al* (2009) Mind the gap: improving the dissemination of CBT. *Behaviour Research and Therapy*, **47**, 902–909.

Springer, D.W., McNeece, C.A. & Arnold, E.N. (2003) *Substance Abuse Treatment for Criminal Offenders: An Evidence-Based Guide for Practitioners*. American Psychological Association.

Smedley, K. (2010) Cognitive behaviour therapy with adolescents in secure settings. In *Psychological Therapy in Prisons and Other Secure Settings* (eds J. Harvey & K. Smedley), pp. 71–101. Willan Publishing.

Steel, J., Darjee, R. & Thomson, L.D. (2004) Substance dependence in schizophrenia in patients with dangerous, violent and criminal propensities: a comparison of comorbid and non-comorbid patients in a high secure setting. *Journal of Forensic Psychiatry & Psychology*, **14**, 596–584.

Swales, M.A. & Heard, H.L. (2008) *Dialectical Behaviour Therapy: Distinctive Features*. Taylor & Francis.

Tapp, J., Fellowes, E., Wallis, N., *et al* (2010) An evaluation of the enhanced thinking skills (ETS) programme with mentally disordered offenders in a high security hospital. *Legal and Criminological Psychology*, **14**, 201–212.

Taylor, J.L., Lindsay, W.R., Hastings, R., *et al* (eds) (2010) *Psychological Therapies for Adults with Intellectual Disabilities*. John Wiley & Sons.

Taylor, J.L. & Novaco, R.W. (2005) *Anger Treatment for People with Developmental Disabilities: A Theory, Evidence, and Manual Based Approach*. John Wiley & Sons.

Tong, S.J. & Farrington, D.P. (2006) How effective is the reasoning and rehabilitation (programme) in reducing re-offending? A meta analysis of evaluations of three countries. *Psychology, Crime and Law*, **12**, 3–34.

Ward, T., Mann, R.E. & Gannon, T.A. (2007) The good lives model of offender rehabilitation: clinical implications. *Aggression and Violent Behaviour*, **12**, 87–107.

Whitehead, P.R., Ward, T. & Collie, R.M. (2007) Time for a change: applying the 'good lives' model of rehabilitation to a high-risk violent offender. *International Journal of Offender Therapy and Comparative Criminology*, **51**, 578–598.

Wilson, R.J., McWhinnie, A.J., & Wilson, C. (2008) Circles of support and accountability: an international partnership in reducing recidivism. *Prison Service Journal*, **138**, 26–36.

CHAPTER 15

Nursing in secure mental healthcare settings

Geoffrey Dickens

Introduction

This chapter appraises the evidence for nursing in secure mental health environments as a specialty branch of mental health nursing. It opens with a brief history of nursing in secure and forensic mental health settings in England, describes the claims made for specialist status and identifies the main definitions and theories of mental health nursing in secure care. The worldwide empirical research evidence about the distinguishing features of the role is reviewed. It is concluded that nursing in secure care requires specialist skills and knowledge related to security, risk, therapeutic activity and clinical specialism. However, nurses working in secure services share many key mental health nursing attributes with those working in mainstream mental health services. Shared characteristics include teamwork, communication and professional development. Core values of both include a recovery and equality focus and commitment to evidence-based practice. Nurses should utilise the best evidence from all settings to support their practice, adapting where necessary to meet the clinical and security needs of the diverse groups for whom they provide care.

A brief history of nursing in secure mental healthcare

In England, nursing in conditions of security is rooted in the development of asylums for the criminally insane (Dale *et al*, 2001), the first at Broadmoor (opened 1863) and the second at Rampton (1914). Also in 1914, a state institution for people with intellectual disability (then known as mental retardation) of 'dangerous or violent propensities' (Mental Deficiency Act 1913) was opened at Moss Side on Merseyside (McGrath, 1966). However, there were no nurses, only 'attendants', at Broadmoor until the introduction in 1938 of a nursing examination (Hamilton, 1980). A nursing school was opened at Rampton hospital in 1950 (Nottinghamshire Healthcare NHS Trust, 2007). Until the Mental Health Act 1959 designated all three institutions as 'special hospitals' responsible to the Ministry for Health they had been an arm of the criminal justice system responsible to the Home Office. Despite the new healthcare alignment of the hospitals, nurses were solely represented in employment negotiations by the Prison Officers Association until the mid-1990s (Murphy, 1997). Nurses were also considered to be civil servants, until 1979 subject to the Official Secrets Act, resulting in a climate of secrecy about nursing activity in the special hospitals during this period (Kirby, 2000).

A note by the medical superintendent of Broadmoor offers the best available description of how nurses and patients experienced life in the special hospitals:

> 'Life inside the hospital differs... from that in conventional psychiatric units. High security demands rules; these rules... demand people to enforce them, and sanctions to uphold them; an authoritarian orientation is thus imposed on nursing staff. Warm and productive relationships do grow up between patients and nursing staff, but this reflects the skill of the nurses, not the virtues of the situation' (McGrath, 1966: p. 700).

The 'rules' comprised a complex system of social and monetary incentives and disincentives, which were viewed by patients as 'rewards and punishments' (McGrath, 1966: p. 700). One former Rampton patient described how rule transgression resulted in enforced repeated scrubbing of the same small area of stone floor over extended periods (*Hansard*, 1957). The recurrent suspicion that maltreatment of patients was widespread culminated in a 1979 television documentary *The Secret Hospital*, an exposé of nursing practice at Rampton hospital which alleged routine cruelty and brutality. The ensuing major police investigation resulted in only a small number of convictions (*Hansard*, 1982) and a government inquiry (Boynton, 1980) praised the vast majority of nurses' dedication and care and made numerous recommendations for systemic change across the special hospitals. Overcrowding was identified as particularly anti-therapeutic and a clear cause of inappropriately custodial care by nurses. Further recommendations led to reduced emphasis on the provisions of the Official Secrets Act and an opening up of the hospital for scrutiny.

As a result of separate major mental health inquiries in the mid-1970s (the 'Butler report' (Home Office & Department of Health, 1975), the 'Glancy report' (Department of Health and Social Security, 1974); see Chapter 1, 'The evolution of secure and forensic mental healthcare'), the early 1980s witnessed the development of a network of regional secure units (RSUs, now called medium secure units). They were intended to accommodate patients stepping down from the high secure special hospitals and those stepping up from inappropriate placements in unlocked acute wards. This expansion of provision, comprising smaller units based closer to local communities and staffed by mental health nurses who were members of nursing and healthcare trade unions, provided the context for the emergence of the first descriptive accounts of nursing activity within UK secure environments (Benson, 1992; Burnard, 1992). From this time onwards the term forensic mental health (FMH) nurse became commonly accepted to describe nurses working in secure hospital settings (Mason, 2002). Recent years have seen the development and further specialisation of secure services to include a tier of 'low secure services' (see Chapter 1). As a result, mental health and intellectual disability nurses work across the full range of secure services, caring for a diverse group of patients, some of whom are convicted offenders and some who display seriously challenging behaviours that place them at risk to others and/or to themselves. Although the United Kingdom Central Council for Nursing and Midwifery's report *Nursing in Secure Environments* (UKCC, 1999) attempted to recognise the limitations of the term 'forensic' to describe nursing work with people who had not been diverted from the criminal justice system, the term 'FMH nurse' has become largely synonymous with nurses working at all levels of security. Some authors have expanded the FMH nurse definition to include nurses working in community settings, for example nurses in community forensic mental health teams (Coffey & Jones, 2008). However, by far the greatest proportion of literature and research about FMH nurses in the UK addresses the role of mental health nurses working in secure mental health hospitals. In this chapter, therefore, the terms 'FMH nurse' and 'nursing in secure environments' are used interchangeably.

The nursing role in secure mental healthcare

In the 20 years since the emergence of the first descriptive accounts of FMH nursing there has been an accumulation of literature, much of which has aimed to identify the specialist nature of the role (e.g. Chaloner & Coffey, 2000; Dale *et al*, 2001; Aiyegbusi & Clarke-Moore, 2008; National Forensic Nurses Research and Development Group, 2008, 2010). There are a variety of voices and opinions. This chapter deals separately with expert commentary and opinion and evidence from empirical research.

Expert opinion on FMH nursing

Early expert accounts emphasised a dichotomy in secure settings that required nurses to negotiate a pathway comprising competing elements of care and containment (Peternelj-Taylor, 2009). The distinguishing element of the nursing role was, in effect, believed to be the therapeutic use of security (Burrow, 1991; Kitchiner *et al*, 1992; Caplan, 1993; Mason & Mercer, 1996). Other proposed distinguishing attributes were risk management (Benson, 1992; Kitchiner *et al*, 1992; Burrow, 1993; Tarbuck, 1994), multidisciplinary working (Mason & Carton, 2002; Mason *et al*, 2002) and the therapeutic use of self (Burnard, 1992; Burrow, 1993). Further, it was claimed that FMH nurses used distinct interventions comprising the application of mainstream mental health nursing techniques in a forensic context, for example cognitive behavioural work specifically for sex offending behaviours (McCourt, 1999). Similarly, Kettles & Robinson (1999) argued that the FMH nurse performs similarly to the mainstream mental health nurse but 'more so… in backup; in awareness of the patient's potential; in dealing with violence and greater complexity and therefore had to cope with more; in being more team based' (p. 32).

A recurring theme suggests an added role complexity for nurses in secure settings because they are required to work with patients who may invoke abjection or fear in them (Mason, 2002; Jacob *et al*, 2009). Collins & Davies (2005) have more recently argued that security management is a specific key FMH nursing skill that involves assessment of each patient's precise physical, procedural and relational security needs. Differentiation from other professional disciplines has also been proffered as a distinguishing attribute of the FMH nurse: Lynch & Standing Bear (1999) claimed that an FMH nurse provides a more comprehensive, holistic evaluation than a psychiatrist and has the physiological knowledge necessary to identify critical issues in diagnosis that are outside the remit of the psychologist. In contrast, Rogers & Soothill (2008) claimed that without a separate specialist training and stronger evidence base of its own, FMH nursing should not be considered a specialty in its own right.

FMH nursing literature reviews

Previous reviews of the literature on FMH nursing have drawn somewhat different conclusions. Mason's (2002) extensive review of the forensic and related literature concluded that the FMH nurse's role was underpinned by six domains of practice or 'binary constructs'. Each domain is characterised by binary oppositions, broadly described as positive and negative features (success *v.* failure; win *v.* lose; transference *v.* countertransference; use *v.* abuse; confidence *v.* fear; medical knowledge *v.* lay knowledge; Table 15.1). The clear strength of the model is that the proposed theoretical domains lend themselves to testable predictions. While Mason articulated clear hypotheses that nurses in high secure environments would be characterised by higher 'negative' and lower 'positive' scores, it is unclear what the implications of this are for nursing practice. Further, it is unclear how some of the domain descriptors, for example 'use *v.* abuse' and 'win *v.* lose', apply specifically to FMH and not to mainstream mental health nursing. Nevertheless, Mason *et al* (2009*a,b*) later developed the domains into a questionnaire instrument, and binary construct theory is the only theory of FMH nursing that has been subject to empirical investigation. Results are discussed later in the chapter.

Bowring-Lossock's (2006) review concluded that the specialist attributes of FMH nurses lay in four domains: task-oriented competence (e.g. escorting, observation, searching), knowledge (e.g. legal, symptom-related, theoretical), skills (e.g. advocacy, emotional self-management, therapeutic skills) and personal qualities (e.g. honesty, maturity, assertiveness). Hers is a clear exposition, but, like other reviews, it draws extensively on the

Table 15.1 The six binary constructs model of forensic psychiatric nursing

Positive pole	Terms of reference	Negative pole	Terms of reference
Success	Nurse viewed as effective, accomplished, capable, skilled	Fail	Discrepancy between knowledge and ability, frustrated with failures
Win	Focus on maintaining control, need for managerial support, act in the patient's best interest	Lose	Others govern, loss of power, not listened to, no support, small 'cog' syndrome
Transference	Withdrawal from treatment, refusal of therapy, denial of responsibility, therapist as controller	Counter-transference	Early prediction of failure for the patient, emphasises compliance, desires non-release, told-you-so
Use	Proactive, interaction is welcomed, avoidance of task orientation, low absenteeism, low sick rates, feelings of being appreciated and effective	Abuse	Reactive, low self-esteem, unappreciated, feelings of retribution (to organisation), subversive elements, low morale, burnout, high stress
Confidence	Management of dangerousness, management of aggression, skill in violence prevention, awareness of injury, underreporting of incidents	Fear	Overemphasis on dangerousness, violence and aggression, failure of effectiveness, humiliation, shame, embarrassment, loss of face, reputation, cultural credence
Medical knowledge	Psychiatric explanations, discourse of diagnosis, care plan constructions, reliance on medication, prognosis	Lay knowledge	Belief in forensic psychiatry as a 'paper exercise', going through the motions, incurable, badness, evil, 'no hope for them'

Source: Mason *et al* (2009*a*).

non-empirical literature. Drawing on broadly the same literature, both Whyte (1997) and Martin (2001) have concluded that almost all of the skills and competencies described by studies of FMH nursing would be equally applicable in most mainstream in-patient mental health settings. This suggests that, at least in part, those espousing FMH nursing as a specialism hold a prior commitment to the concept irrespective of the empirical evidence.

A different perspective is offered by Kettles & Woods (2006), whose review resulted in a definition of FMH nursing as an advanced practice role that:

'applies and integrates evidence from general mental health, psychiatric nursing and psychological principles and evidence, along with specific forensic knowledge such as that which relates to the criminal justice system, risk, safety, security and forensic theory applied to practice, role, interventions and skills within a secure environment and in the community' (p. 25).

The model forensic nurse was proposed to be a registered nurse with 8 years' experience in a high-security environment; they would have worked with personality-disordered, substance misusing patients and hold a post-registration qualification in substance misuse and a masters degree in interventions with this group. The important contribution made by Kettles and Woods was therefore to distinguish theoretically the advanced and non-advanced FMH nurse practitioner in three domains: risk assessment, professional, legal and ethical aspects of care, and interpersonal competencies. Similarly, reviews by Kent-Wilkinson (2010) and Lyons (2009) have emphasised that FMH nursing is an advanced practice role.

Nursing models in FMH nursing practice

There have been very few accounts of the use of nursing models in FMH nursing practice. In a survey of nurses from high secure hospitals, Mason & Chandley (1990) found that a variety of models were reportedly used, including Henderson's (1966) need model, Orem's (1991) model of self-care and Roper et al's (2000) activities of living model. More recently, reports in the nursing literature (Cook et al, 2005; Doyle & Jones, 2013) have noted the adaptation of Phil Barker's Tidal Model (Stevenson et al, 2002) and Brian Hodges' Health Career Model (Hodges, 1997) for use in forensic settings. Barker's model is strongly influenced by the interpersonal theory of Hildegard Peplau (1988) and is intended to assist nurses in achieving a high level of engagement with patients. Hodges' model proposes a biological–psychological–sociological–legal framework which does not dictate practice but rather suggests domains in which to provide nursing assessment and care. Neither model has been subject to rigorous evaluation.

Empirical literature

Descriptive studies

A range of studies from the UK and Ireland, Scandinavia and North America have generated a plethora of information about FMH nurses' own narratives about their work and their particular competencies. Commonly occurring themes include risk assessment (Rask & Aberg, 2002; Timmons, 2010) and working therapeutically while maintaining security (Niskala, 1986; Scales et al, 1993; UK Central Council for Nursing and Midwifery (UKCC), 1999).

Therapeutic activity

Therapeutic activity is also commonly identified as an FMH nursing role without the security qualifier (Burnard & Morrison, 1995; Gillespie &

Flowers, 2009), although it has been noted that it is sometimes unclear what the therapeutic content of FMH nursing comprises (Burnard *et al*, 1999). Specific activities suggested or endorsed by FMH nurses as part of their therapeutic repertoire include: meeting patient needs (Burnard & Morrison, 1995); protection of patients from themselves and others, and protection of patients from abuse (Shelton, 2009; Timmons, 2010; UKCC, 1999); enabling individuals to develop meaningful relationships with others and maintain contact in isolating situations, and supporting individuals when they are distressed (Shelton, 2009); assisting with activities of daily living, including practical work on the ward, regular verbal interactions with patients, planning activities with patients, and social skills training (Rask & Hallberg, 2000; Rask & Brunt, 2007); maintaining the ward atmosphere or therapeutic milieu (Burnard & Morrison, 1995; Rask & Hallberg, 2000).

Developing relationships with patients has been identified as a key role element of FMH nurses (Burnard & Morrison, 1995; Timmons, 2010). More specific elements have included the importance of effective communication with patients (Niskala, 1986). Further, Rask & Aberg's (2002) grounded theory analysis of qualitative data led them to the conclusion that 'an interpersonal patient–nurse relationship based on trust, empathy, respect and responsibility for the patient's personal resources' (p. 531) is the essence of nursing care. Similarly, FMH nurses in the UKCC's (1999) nationwide study of nurses working in low-, medium- and high-security units reported strong endorsement of the item 'demonstration of humanity for the patient regardless of offence or behaviour'. The skill of developing relationships with patients who have sometimes committed heinous offences is highlighted by Rose *et al* (2011), who reported that nurses navigated a practical compromise to their emotive-cognitive reactions through a non-judgemental approach and an appreciation of the context of offences. Potentially less constructive approaches by FMH nurses have also been described. For example, Jacob's (2012) qualitative study reported that nurses in a Canadian correctional setting reconceptualised inmates/ patients as deviants and by so doing were more able to distance themselves from problematic patients.

Finally, a range of professional activities have been put forward by nurses in descriptive studies as central to the FMH nursing role. These were maintenance and development of the professional role (Niskala, 1986; Shelton, 2009), the potential for autonomous professional practice (Scales *et al*, 1993), clinical supervision (UKCC, 1999), managing one's case-load (Shelton, 2009), and providing an effective communication link between other disciplines (Robinson & Kettles, 1998; Baxter, 2002). Attributes rated in the descriptive empirical literature as of lesser importance to the FMH nursing role have been research and instruction of offenders (Niskala, 1986).

In summary, descriptive studies of FMH nurses' self-reported activities and role resemble earlier expert, narrative accounts. Commonly endorsed or reported role strengths relate to risk and security, to therapy and the therapeutic relationship, and to professional issues. These studies vary in sample size and methodological quality, and have been conducted with nurses working in different levels of security and across a range of countries with quite varied secure provision. They have used a range of research approaches with non-standardised data collection instruments. Results are difficult to interpret because studies lack comparison groups of nurses and other professionals against which to put the reported specialist competences of FMH nurses. Nevertheless, they have been widely cited in previous literature reviews as evidence of FMH nursing specialism.

Comparative studies: nurses working in secure environments and nurses or other professionals in other settings

Studies that compare FMH nurses with other nurses or other professionals have the potential to more accurately identify their defining characteristics, skills and knowledge. Hurst *et al* (1998) observed and documented the activities of nurses in one English high secure hospital and compared their data with equivalent information from mainstream mental health nurses. High secure nurses spent marginally less time in face-to-face patient contact and in indirect care with no patient contact (e.g. recording therapeutic activity, report-writing). They spent more time on administrative and personal tasks and in therapeutic activity. Elsewhere, no significant difference has been found between FMH and non-FMH nurses on attitudinal measures of treatment conservatism (adherence to a medical model) *v.* liberalism (more socially oriented approaches) (Kinsella & Chaloner, 1995). FMH and mainstream nurses did not differ on an overall measure of stress (Chalder & Nolan, 2001), but stress for secure care nurses emanated from intra-team relationships, while for acute care nurses it resulted from lack of resources. The authors claimed this reflected the FMH nurses' relatively strong personalities and preparedness to be assertive.

In the largest and most representative study to date, Mason *et al* (2008*a,b*) surveyed 1172 qualified and unqualified nurses working in low, medium and high secure UK psychiatric hospitals, plus mainstream mental health nurses and non-nursing professionals. Respondents were asked about the role dimensions and clinical aspects of nursing in forensic secure units. Both FMH and mainstream mental health nurses reported experience, empathy, listening and patience to be key role strengths; both reported that key skills include listening and communication. In contrast, there were clear differences between non-nursing professionals and all nurses in their views about nursing roles. Non-nursing professionals viewed clear boundaries, monitoring medication and ability to work with low staff-to-patient ratios as being among key nursing strengths. These issues were rarely mentioned by either FMH or mainstream nurses, who concentrated on personal qualities, including patience and tolerance. Nurses working in secure settings were, however, significantly more likely to name nursing people diagnosed with a personality disorder and aggression management as specific skill requirements relative to both other groups.

Subsequent research (Bowen & Mason, 2012) throws some light on the reported difference between FMH and mainstream nurses in terms of their role in working with patients with personality disorder. The researchers compared FMH nurses (defined in this study as those working in high, medium and low secure services, prison and community settings) and other nurses on their reports of the importance of various attributes and weaknesses when nursing this group. FMH nurses reported key strengths and skills as firmness, limit-setting and professional boundaries. In contrast, other nurses emphasised being non-judgemental, listening skills and risk management. While informative, it is not clear whether these differences reflect disparities in attitude between the groups, differences in the severity of symptomatology and psychopathology displayed by the patients with whom each group works, or some combination of the two.

Mason & Phipps (2010) asked 348 FMH nurses (mental health and intellectual disability nurses working in low, medium and high secure UK services) and 295 other practising mental health and intellectual disability nurses ('non-FMH nurses') about the top ten problems, skills and areas for development for nurses working with individuals with intellectual disability in secure settings. Both groups rated violence and aggression as the main problems. The main skills needed to overcome problems were risk assessment, early interventions and control of medication for FMH nurses but forming relationships and knowledge of the patient for non-FMH nurses. FMH nurses reported the most important areas for development as assessments and general interventions, whereas non-FMH nurses ranked relationship formation with patients significantly more highly. This research suggests clear differences between the two groups, with FMH nurses focused on a more active, interventional approach to management than their counterparts. However, it is somewhat limited by the data simply being ranked in importance rather than being more precisely measured, which limits further examination of the magnitude and import of this difference.

In Finland, Tenkanen et al (2011) compared 'registered mental nurses' (RNs) and 'practical mental nurses' (PMNs; nurses with practical experience but not graduates of a nursing programme) working in a secure forensic setting. The researchers employed questionnaires that provided 360-degree self-, peer and managerial appraisal ratings of variables measuring core interventions and core competencies for the nursing care of schizophrenia, including pharmacotherapy, forensic psychiatric knowledge, treatment of violent patients, emotional regulation and need-adapted treatment of the patient. Analysis of responses suggested that RNs exceeded PMNs on mastery of core interventions. The researchers therefore concluded that RNs educated to degree level were more suited to work in forensic psychiatric settings. However, other findings indicated that they still required considerable further education and that the FMH nursing role was largely viewed as custodial rather than therapeutic. Even though it was probably predictable that nurses prepared to a higher academic level should be found to have greater abilities, this is the only study of FMH nurses that demonstrates their superiority on a measure of competence in comparison with another group. The findings, however, may not be automatically generalisable to the UK and other international settings.

In summary, research that compares FMH with other nurses reveals a limited number of differences. The strongest research from a large sample of nurses (Mason *et al*, 2008*a,b*) reveals commonalities in relation to the required personal attributes and skills of FMH and non-FMH nurses alike. Reported differences are that FMH nurses say that they require particular skills or competences in relation to aggression management, work with people with intellectual disability, and work with patients with personality disorder. Even then, however, these findings are largely from self-report data that cannot be guaranteed to reflect actual skills, characteristics or effectiveness.

Comparative studies: nurses working at different levels of security

Comparing mental health nurses who work at different levels of security can inform us whether there is homogeneity in the characteristics of the proposed specialist group.

Dale & Storey (2004) examined differences between registered nurses working in low-, medium and high-security settings in terms of agreement or disagreement with the 45 competency statements devised for the UKCC (1999) study. High secure nurses were less likely to report working with the patient's family and preparation for discharge as key competencies. They were more likely to report a security–therapy dichotomy. This is interesting given the prominence of this concept in the literature as a proposed differentiator of FMH nursing as a specialist area of practice. A similar study from the USA (Shelton, 2009) found that nurses working in medium and high security differed significantly from one another in terms of their agreement with two items: 'promoting and implementing principles that underpin effective quality and practice' and 'providing and improving resources and services that facilitate organisational functioning'. Low and medium secure nurses differed from one another on their ratings of assessing, developing, implementing and improving programmes of care for individuals.

Lammie *et al* (2010) recruited nurses and nursing assistants from low and medium secure wards in two Scottish hospitals into their study of discriminatory and stigmatising practitioner attitudes towards forensic patients. Participants were asked to complete Corrigan's Attribution Questionnaire 27 (CAQ; Corrigan *et al*, 2003) in relation to a fictitious vignette about a patient with schizophrenia. The CAQ is intended to identify attitudes about issues including dangerousness, avoidance and segregation.

Participants working in the low secure wards made significantly more negative evaluations of the patient than staff in medium secure wards. This result ran counter to the prediction that nurses working in medium secure settings, presumably with more disturbed patients, would display the most stigmatising attitudes. The significance of this finding from a small study of 43 nurses is unclear.

In the most interesting comparative study to date, Mason's (2002) six binary constructs model (Table 15.1) informed the development of a questionnaire comprising statements for each positive and negative pole, each rated on a 7-point Likert scale representing strong agreement v. strong disagreement (Mason et al, 2009a,b). The questionnaire was completed by 416 nurses working in UK low, medium and high secure services. High-security nurses responded to statements on win and lose items in a manner suggesting the greatest need for control. Nurses working in all levels of security, but especially high secure nurses, endorsed lay explanations of patients' behaviour and rejected medical reasoning. The researchers suggested that this indicated a heightened perception that patients are not amenable to treatment. High secure nurses reported the most fear and least confidence, which may be unsurprising given the likely reasons for the need for high security in the patient population. Nurses working in low and high secure services differed significantly from one another on most other items, including transference and countertransference, success and failure, and use and abuse. Low secure nurses consistently scored more positively/less negatively than high secure nurses. Ratings of medium secure nurses were not consistently different from either high or low secure nurses.

The differences between nursing groups identified by Mason et al's (2009a,b) studies are difficult to interpret. To an extent, they reflect the model's predictions. However, those very differences tend to undermine the proposition that FMH nurses can be understood as a coherent specialist group with homogeneous characteristics. Further, the implications that results hold for practice are somewhat ambiguous and the link between expressed attitudes and nursing practice is unclear. There is also a lack of evidence for the psychometric properties of the scale. External validity is not established in terms of the relationship of items to established valid constructs and the factor validity of the various poles remains untested. Nevertheless, establishing the likelihood of demonstrable differences between nurses operating at different security levels has value in highlighting the importance of questioning the applicability of conclusions drawn about nursing in secure settings as a whole from studies in any one security level.

FMH nursing as an advanced practice role

Notably, the empirical evidence summarised so far is reliant on samples of nurses whose location of practice is in secure environments irrespective of their level of qualifications or experience. It is therefore unlikely that such studies are informative about FMH nursing as an advanced practice role as described by Kettles & Woods (2006), Kent-Wilkinson (2010) and Lyons (2009). Studies of well-defined advanced practice FMH nurses are almost entirely absent from the literature. In one study, the key role dimensions of forensic consultant nurses were identified as service development, workforce planning, expert practice, research and education, conducting investigations and incident command (Langton, 2008). Descriptions of advanced practice roles in non-FMH nursing share many of these elements but, interestingly, place less emphasis on strategic management and service planning and more on advanced clinical skills (Allen, 1998; Jinks & Chalder, 2007).

Key elements of nursing in secure mental healthcare

The review presented in this chapter suggests that the claims for a specialist FMH nurse role made in the UK from the early 1990s onwards have exceeded the supporting empirical evidence. This may partly result from a preponderance of uncontrolled studies that examine FMH nurses defined by their location of practice rather than their advanced practice status. Further, the premature declaration of FMH nursing as a specialty in its own right may be best viewed as an aspiration, or even as an attempt by FMH nurse leaders to increase their own influence (Sekula *et al*, 2001). There is as much variation between the attributes required by nurses working at different levels of security, and with different groups of patients, as there is between nurses working in secure settings and those in mainstream mental health services. In the final section a number of key attributes of nursing are highlighted. Each element is important in secure care but it is also probably important in mainstream services. Nurses, nurse leaders and nurse researchers should aim to interpret and determine the best evidence and carefully apply it to their own setting.

Risk assessment and management

Risk assessment and risk management play a central role in all mental health nursing practice (Department of Health, 2006; Cordall, 2009). Owing to the nature of secure services, much of the focus is on risk of aggression and violence and risk of self-harm. Evidence from meta-analysis of aggressive incidents in psychiatric in-patient settings (Bowers *et al*, 2011) suggests that, after factoring in length of stay, patient aggression is equally likely in forensic and acute psychiatric units. This suggests that nurses in both environments require skills and knowledge in the prevention and management of aggression and violence. Developments in risk assessment for in-patient settings, such as the Short Term Assessment of Risk and Treatability (START) guide (Webster *et al*, 2004), have emphasised the need both to consider the other significant risks faced by users of secure services (self-neglect, victimisation) and to bear in mind their strengths or protective factors as well as risk factors. Mental health nurses working in secure care, like other nurses, will be involved in such risk assessment and in formulating management plans. They should therefore be adequately prepared in structured professional judgement approaches to risk assessment and management. Recognition of early warning signs is particularly important (Fluttert *et al*, 2008).

Security management

Nurses are largely responsible for the day-to-day management of security. Security management is of course interconnected at every level with, and provides one of the main vehicles of, risk management (see Chapter 4, 'Risk management in secure care'). By definition, at higher levels of security nurses will be involved in more frequent and intensive security management procedures requiring different knowledge. Progress has been made in recent years to identify the core components of physical, procedural and relational security (Collins & Davies, 2005; Department of Health, 2010; Chapter 4, this volume). Nurses in secure care should participate in multidisciplinary individual assessment of the security requirements of patients to ensure that unnecessary restriction does not occur.

Therapeutic activity

The intended therapeutic activity of nurses in secure mental healthcare is multi-faceted and interconnected with risk and security issues. First, only with the appropriate management of risk and security can potentially therapeutic interventions be delivered. Second, some argue that the careful management of risk, including planned and graduated exposure to risk, may be therapeutic in itself (Doyle & Dolan, 2008). Therapeutic activities for which mental health nurses should be prepared include the five discussed in this section.

1. Developing therapeutic relationships

Clearly this is central to the mental health nursing role in any setting (O'Brien, 2001). As identified in this chapter, nurses in secure settings recognise the need to build relationships, maintain appropriate boundaries, demonstrate humanity and unconditional positive regard, to support patients in time of distress, and to display trust and empathy. Among the challenges in secure care is maintaining positive regard in the face of patients who display aggressive behaviour and when confronted with knowledge of the index offence perpetrated by some patients.

2. Managing the ward environment

Ward climate or atmosphere has long been viewed as central to the therapeutic endeavour in mental health settings (Rossberg & Friis, 2004; Schalast *et al*, 2008). Work by Schalast *et al* (2008) has identified three

243

factors that contribute to ward atmosphere in forensic psychiatric units: experienced safety (general sense of safety and freedom from aggression), patient cohesion (sense of belonging and support among patients) and therapeutic hold (feeling valued and treated as an individual). These factors are clearly related to other key elements of the mental health nursing role in secure care. Further research is required on how best to intervene to improve ward climate, but it is clear that mental health nurses would be central to the success of any such interventions.

3. Psychological interventions

Mental health nurses in secure settings are frequently involved in the delivery of psychological interventions that are based on formal psychological theory. This may involve participation in behaviour modification programmes based on incentives and rewards (e.g. Holmes & Murray, 2012) or those based on social learning theory (e.g. reinforce appropriate/implode disruptive behaviours (RAID), Davies 2001). These may sometimes be devised by psychologists, but nurses should ensure they understand the underlying theoretical principles. Nurses may also, with adequate training and education, deliver evidence-based group and individual therapies, for example cognitive–behavioural interventions for social problem-solving, life skills and body image (Long, 2013). Nurses should also recognise and meet the spiritual needs of patients (Department of Health, 2006).

4. Practical/occupational activity

The Roper–Logan–Tierney model (Roper *et al*, 2000) has been used widely by mental health nurses to support individualised care planning in relation to activities of living (ALs). While it has roots in general medical nursing, nurses working in secure settings are among those best placed to assess need and provide assistance that promotes maximum independence across ALs. In forensic settings issues related to the expression of sexuality are likely to provoke ethical concerns for nurses across all areas of secure care (Peternelj-Taylor, 1998; Mercer, 2012).

5. Physical healthcare

It is surprising and somewhat worrying that physical healthcare has so rarely been recognised as key to the role of the nurse in the secure care setting. It is a key role of the mental health nurse to improve physical well-being (Department of Health, 2006). The relatively lengthy stay of patients in secure settings (Sainsbury Centre for Mental Health, 2007), and the high rates of morbidity and mortality in this group (Cormac *et al*, 2005) suggest that this should be a particular concern for nurses working in secure settings. Recent research, including the development of the Physical Health Attitude Scale for mental health nurses (PHASe) (Robson & Haddad, 2012; Robson *et al*, 2013), should be further examined to more accurately identify how nurses in secure settings can make impactful, health-improving interventions with patients.

Advanced clinical specialism

Considerable attention has been paid within the literature to the distinct role of the nurse in secure care with regard to nursing patients with personality disorder (Mason *et al*, 2008*a,b*), and some evidence has suggested that nurses working in secure settings value particular approaches with this group (Bowen & Mason, 2012). Some nurses (e.g. McVey, 2012) advocate nursing models based on the interpersonal theory of Hildegard Peplau (1988) or its modern descendant, the Tidal Model (Barker, 2003). However, there is little evidence that such specific nursing interventions are effective with these service users; rather, psychological interventions hold the strength of evidence (Woods & Richards, 2003). Mental health nurses should be knowledgeable about aetiology, epidemiology, and diagnosis of and treatment approaches to specific patient groups. The increasing specialism evident in secure services (see Chapter 1, 'The evolution of secure and forensic mental healthcare') means that this includes not just personality disordered patients but those with intellectual disability, autism spectrum disorders, acquired brain injury and major mental disorder. In addition, nurses need to be aware of how issues of gender, age, race and physical disability affect care needs. Further, the role of comorbid substance misuse in mental disorder has a significant impact in patients who require secure care.

Interpersonal style and communication

As outlined in this chapter, interpersonal style and communication has been identified in many empirical studies as a specialist component of FMH nursing, but it is immediately clear that this cannot be the sole province of the specialist. All nurses require good listening and communication skills, and will have regular, meaningful verbal interaction, awareness of their non-verbal signals and cues, and will offer support and encouragement to patients.

Professional development

As with communication, professional development has been cited by researchers as evidence of specialism. It is of course incumbent on all nurses to keep their skills and knowledge up to date (Nursing and Midwifery Council, 2008) and mental health nurses should strive to develop new roles and skills (Department of Health, 2006).

Values

The Chief Nursing Officer's review of mental health nursing (Department of Health, 2006) recommended three value domains: recovery-oriented practice; promoting equality in care and providing evidence-based care. As discussed elsewhere in this volume (Chapter 5, 'Recovery in secure environments'), personal recovery has been described as a way of living a satisfying, hopeful and contributing life, even with limitations caused by illness (Anthony, 1993). To date, relatively little has been written about the recovery approach and nursing in secure mental health settings, and further research is needed. However, accounts are emerging in the wider forensic literature (Gill *et al*, 2010; Doyle *et al*, 2011; Drennan & Alred, 2012) and Doyle & Jones (2013) have proposed that the recovery approach is compatible with a specific nursing model in forensic mental healthcare. Considerable strides have been made in recent years to increase equality in secure service provision, for example through acknowledgement of the different needs of patient groups, including women (Bartlett, 2004) and Black and minority ethnic patients (Hackett, 2008). Finally, in relation to a commitment to evidence-based practice, the current chapter has assisted in identifying the limited scale of nursing research that specifically addresses nursing in secure environments. This echoes the general finding of the Chief Nursing Officer that the evidence for mental health nursing is, beyond pockets of excellence related to in-patient aggression and medication management, sorely limited (Department of Health, 2006).

Conclusions

Nurses comprise the largest single professional group within secure mental health services and are clearly central to the effective day-to-day management of units and wards. They are the most visible professional presence for patients, and are usually the first point of contact for them on a daily basis. Nurses are in a strong position to influence the ward environment for good and are primarily responsible for the prevention and management of risk behaviours. Nurses provide practical and emotional support, consolation and empathy 24 hours a day, 7 days per week, sometimes in the face of significant resistance and challenging behaviour. Although the research evidence for FMH nursing has grown (Kettles & Walker, 2007), the majority of evidence emanates from mainstream in-patient services rather than from secure forensic services. While this remains the case, it is sensible to utilise the best mental health nursing evidence rather than asserting a forensic specialism and applying weaker forensic evidence over stronger non-forensic evidence. A large-scale programme of research to generate an evidence base for nursing in secure settings is a priority.

References

Aiyegbusi, A. & Clarke-Moore, J. (eds) (2008) *Therapeutic Relationships with Offenders: An Introduction to the Psychodynamics of Mental Health Nursing*. Jessica Kingsley Publishers.

Allen, J. (1998) A survey of psychiatric nurses' opinions of advanced practice roles in psychiatric nursing. *Journal of Psychiatric and Mental Health Nursing*, **5**, 451–462.

Anthony, W.A. (1993) Recovery from mental illness: the guiding vision of the mental health service system in the 1990's. *Psychosocial Rehabilitation Journal*, **16**, 11–23.

Barker, P. (2003) The Tidal Model: psychiatric colonization, recovery and the paradigm shift in mental health care. *International Journal of Mental Health Nursing*, **12**, 96–102.

Bartlett, A. (2004) The care of women in forensic services. *Psychiatry*, **3**, 25–28.

Baxter, V. (2002) Nurses' perceptions of their roles and skills in a medium secure unit. *British Journal of Nursing*, **11**, 1312–1319.

Benson, R. (1992) The clinical nurse specialist in forensic settings. In *Aspects of Forensic Psychiatric Nursing* (eds P. Morrison & P. Burnard), pp. 45–60. Aldershot.

Bowen, M. & Mason, T. (2012) Forensic and non-forensic psychiatric nursing skills and competencies for psychopathic and personality disordered patients. *Journal of Clinical Nursing*, **21**, 3556–3564.

Bowers, L., Stewart, D., Papadopoulos, C., *et al* (2011) *Inpatient Violence and Aggression*. Report from the Conflict and Containment Reduction Research Programme. King's College London (http://www.kcl.ac.uk/iop/depts/hspr/research/ciemh/mhn/projects/litreview/LitRevAgg.pdf).

Bowring-Lossock, E. (2006) The forensic mental health nurse – a literature review. *Journal of Psychiatric and Mental Health Nursing*, **13**, 780–785.

Boynton, J. (1980) *Report of the Review of Rampton Hospital* (Cmnd 8073). HMSO.

Burnard, P. (1992) The expanded role of the forensic psychiatric nurse. In *Aspects of Forensic Psychiatric Nursing* (eds P. Morrison & P. Burnard), pp. 139–154. Aldershot.

Burnard, P. & Morrison, P. (1995) Evaluating forensic psychiatric nursing care. *Journal of Forensic Psychiatry*, **6**, 139–159.

Burnard, P., Morrison, P. & Philips, C. (1999) Job satisfaction amongst nurses in an interim secure forensic unit in Wales. *Australian and New Zealand Journal of Mental Health Nursing*, **8**, 9–18.

Burrow, S. (1991) The special hospital nurse and the dilemma of therapeutic custody. *Journal of Advances in Health and Nursing Care*, **1**, 21–38.

Burrow, S. (1993) The role conflict of the forensic nurse. *Senior Nurse*, **13**, 20–25.

Caplan, C.A. (1993) Nursing staff and patient perceptions of the ward atmosphere in a maximum security forensic hospital. *Archives of Psychiatric Nursing*, **7**, 23–29.

Chalder, G. & Nolan, P. (2001) The role of the forensic nurse consultant observed. *British Journal of Forensic Practice*, **3**, 23–30.

Chaloner, C. & Coffey, M. (eds) (2000) *Forensic Mental Health Nursing: Current Approaches*. Wiley-Blackwell.

Coffey, M. & Jones, R. (2008) Forensic community mental health nursing. In *Forensic Mental Health Nursing Capabilities, Roles and Responsibilities* (eds National Forensic Nurses Research and Development Group): pp. 259–272. Quay Books.

Collins, M. & Davies, S. (2005) The security needs assessment profile: a multidimensional approach to measuring security needs. *International Journal of Forensic Mental Health*, **4**, 39–52.

Cook, N.R., Phillips, B.N., & Sadler, D. (2005) The tidal model as experienced by patients and nurses in a regional forensic unit. *Journal of Psychiatric and Mental Health Nursing*, **12**, 536–540.

Cordall, J. (2009) Risk assessment and management. In *Risk Assessment and Management in Mental Health Nursing* (eds P. Woods & A.M. Kettles): pp. 9–48. Wiley-Blackwell.

Cormac, I., Ferriter, M., Benning, R., *et al* (2005) Physical health and health risk factors in a population of long-stay psychiatric patients. *Psychiatrist*, **29**, 18–20.

Corrigan, P., Markowitz, F.E., Watson, A., *et al* (2003) An attribution model of public discrimination towards persons with mental illness. *Journal of Health and Social Behavior*, **44**, 162–179.

Dale, C. & Storey, L. (2004) High, medium, and low security care: does the type of care make any difference to the role of the forensic mental health nurse? *Nursing Times Research*, **9**, 168–184.

Dale, C., Woods, P. & Thompson, T. (2001) Nursing. In *Forensic Mental Health: Issues in Practice* (eds C. Dale, T. Thompson, & P. Woods): pp. 107–121. Harcourt Publishers.

Davies, W. (2001) *The RAID Manual*. APT Press.

Department of Health (2006) *From Values to Action: The Chief Nursing Officer's Review of Mental Health Nursing*. Department of Health.

Department of Health (2010) *See, Think, Act: Your Guide to Relational Security*. Department of Health.

Department of Health and Social Security (1974) *Security in NHS Hospitals for the Mentally Ill and the Mentally Handicapped (Glancy report)*. DHSS.

Doyle, M. & Dolan, M. (2008) Understanding and managing risk. In *Handbook of Forensic Mental Health* (eds K. Soothill, P. Rogers & M. Dolan): pp. 244–266. Willan Publishing.

Doyle, M. & Jones, P. (2013) Hodges' Health Career Model and its role and potential application in forensic mental health nursing. *Journal of Psychiatric and Mental Health Nursing*, **20**, 631–640.

Doyle, M., Logan, C., Ludlow, A., *et al* (2011) Milestones to recovery: preliminary validation of a framework to promote recovery and map progress through the medium secure inpatient pathway. *Criminal Behaviour and Mental Health*, **22**, 53–64.

Drennan, G. & Alred, D. (2012) *Secure Recovery – Approaches to Recovery in Forensic Mental Health Settings*. Routledge.

Fluttert, F.A., Van Meijel, B., Webster, C., *et al* (2008) Risk management by early recognition of warning signs in patients in forensic psychiatric care. *Archives of Psychiatric Nursing*, **22**, 208–216.

Gill, P., McKenna, P., O'Neill, H., *et al* (2010) Pillars and pathways: foundations of recovery in Irish forensic mental health care. *British Journal of Forensic Practice*, **12**, 29–36.

Gillespie, M. & Flowers, P. (2009) From the old to the new: is forensic mental health nursing in transition? *Journal of Forensic Nursing*, **5**, 212–219.

Hackett, R. (2008) Improving quality of mental health care for BME clients. *Nursing Times*, **104**, 35–36.

Hamilton, J.R. (1980) The development of Broadmoor 1863–1980. *Psychiatrist*, **4**, 130–133.

Hansard (1957) HC Deb 19 December 1957 vol 580 cc. 719–738.

Hansard (1982) HL Deb 25 October 1982 vol 435 cc. 365–384.

Henderson, V. (1966) *The Nature of Nursing: A Definition and its Implications for Practice, Research, and Education*. Macmillan.

Hodges, B. (1997) *Hodges' Health Career Model*. At http://www.p-jones.demon.co.uk/hcm.htm (accessed 6 March 2015).

Holmes, D. & Murray, S.J. (2012) A critical reflection on the use of behaviour modification programmes in forensic psychiatry settings. In *(Re)Thinking Violence in Health Care Settings: A Critical Approach* (eds D. Holmes, T. Rudge & A. Perron): pp. 21–30. Ashgate Publishing.

Home Office & Department of Health (1975) *Report of the Committee on Mentally Abnormal Offenders (CMND 6244) (Butler report)*. HMSO.

Hurst, K., Whyte, L. & Robinson, D. (1998) *Analysis of Nursing Activity within a High Secure Hospital*. Nuffield Institute for Health, University of Leeds.

Jacob, J.D. (2012) The rhetoric of therapy in forensic psychiatric nursing. *Journal of Forensic Nursing*, **8**, 178–187.

Jacob, J.D., Gagnon, M. & Holmes, D. (2009) Nursing so-called monsters: on the importance of abjection and fear in forensic psychiatric nursing. *Journal of Forensic Nursing*, **5**, 153–161.

Jinks, A.M. & Chalder, G. (2007) Consensus and diversity: an action research study designed to analyse the roles of a group of mental health consultant nurses. *Journal of Clinical Nursing*, **16**, 1323–1332.

Kent-Wilkinson, A. (2010) Psychiatric mental health forensic nursing: responding to social need. *Issues in Mental Health Nursing*, **31**, 425–431.

Kettles, A.M. & Robinson, D.K. (1999) Overview of contemporary issues in the role of the forensic nurse in the UK. In *Nursing and Multidisciplinary Care of the Mentally Disordered Offender* (eds D. Robinson & A. Kettles): pp. 26–38. Jessica Kingsley Publishers.

Kettles A. & Woods P. (2006) A concept analysis of forensic nursing. *British Journal of Forensic Practice*, **8**, 16–27.

Kettles, A. & Walker, H. (2007) Forensic nursing research: how far we've come. *British Journal of Forensic Practice*, **9**, 35–44.

Kinsella, C. & Chaloner, C. (1995) Attitude to treatment and direction of interest of forensic mental health nurses: a comparison with nurses working in other specialties. *Journal of Psychiatric and Mental Health Nursing*, **2**, 351–357.

Kirby, S. (2000) History and development. In *Forensic Mental Health Nursing: Current Approaches* (eds C. Chaloner & M. Coffey): pp. 288–305. Wiley-Blackwell.

Kitchiner N., Wright I., Topping-Morris B., *et al* (1992) The role of the forensic psychiatric nurse. *Nursing Times*, **88**, 5.

Lammie, C., Harrison, T., Macmahon, K., *et al* (2010) Practitioner attitudes towards patients in forensic mental health settings. *Journal of Psychiatric and Mental Health Nursing*, **17**, 706–714.

Langton, D. (2008) Supporting role. *Nursing Standard*, **22** (31), 24–25.

Long, C. (2013) Delivery of effective cognitive behavioural group treatment for women in secure settings. *British Journal of Forensic Practice*, **15**, 55–67.

Lynch, V.A. & Standing Bear, Z.G. (1999) A global perspective in forensic nursing. Challenges *for the 21st century. In Forensic Nursing and Multidisciplinary Care of the Mentally Disordered Offender* (eds D. Robinson & A. Kettles): pp. 249–266. Jessica Kingsley Publishers.

Lyons, T. (2009) Role of the forensic psychiatric nurse. *Journal of Forensic Nursing*, **5**, 53–57.

Martin, T. (2001) Something special: forensic psychiatric nursing. *Journal of Psychiatric and Mental Health Nursing*, **8**, 25–32.

Mason T. (2002) Forensic psychiatric nursing: a literature review and thematic analysis of role tensions. *Journal of Psychiatric and Mental Health Nursing*, **9**, 511–524.

Mason, T. & Carton, G. (2002) Towards a a 'forensic lens' model of multidisciplinary training. *Journal of Psychiatric and Mental Health Nursing*, **9**, 541–551.

Mason, T. & Chandley, M. (1990) Nursing models in a special hospital: a critical analysis of efficacity. *Journal of Advanced Nursing*, **15**, 667–673.

Mason, T. & Mercer, D. (1996) Forensic psychiatric nursing: visions of social control. *Australian and New Zealand Mental Health Nursing*, **5**, 153–162.

Mason, T. & Phipps, D. (2010) Forensic learning disability nursing skills and competencies: a study of forensic and non-forensic nurses. *Issues in Mental Health Nursing*, **31**, 708–715.

Mason, T., Williams, R. & Vivian-Byrne, S. (2002) Multi-disciplinary working in a forensic mental health setting: ethical codes of reference. *Journal of Psychiatric and Mental Health Nursing*, **9**, 563–572.

Mason T., Lovell A. & Coyle D. (2008*a*) Forensic psychiatric nursing; skills and competencies. I. Role dimensions. *Journal of Psychiatric and Mental Health Nursing*, **15**, 118–130.

Mason T., Coyle D. & Lovell A. (2008*b*) Forensic psychiatric nursing; skills and competencies. II. Clinical aspects. *Journal of Psychiatric and Mental Health Nursing*, **15**, 131–159.

Mason, T., Dulson, J. & King, L. (2009*a*) Binary constructs of forensic psychiatric nursing: a pilot study. *Journal of Psychiatric and Mental Health Nursing*, **16**, 158–166.

Mason, T., King, L. & Dulson, J. (2009*b*) Binary construct analysis of forensic psychiatric nursing in the UK: high, medium and low security services. *International Journal of Mental Health Nursing*, **18**, 216–224.

McCourt, M. (1999) Five concepts for the expanded role of the forensic mental health nurse. In *Forensic Mental Health Nursing: Policy, Strategy and Implementation* (eds P. Tarbuck, B. Topping-Morris & P. Burnard): pp. 188–204. Whurr Publishers.

McGrath, P.G. (1966) The special hospitals – as they are. *Proceedings of the Royal Society of Medicine*, **59**, 699–700.

McVey, D. (2012) The role of the nurse in treating people with personality disorder. In *Treating Personality Disorder. Creating Robust Services for People with Complex Mental Health Needs* (eds N. Murphy & D. McVey): pp. 154–171. Routledge.

Mercer, D. (2012) Girly mags and girly jobs: Pornography and gendered inequality in forensic practice. *International Journal of Mental Health Nursing*, **22**, 15–23.

Murphy, E. (1997) The future of Britain's high security hospitals. *BMJ*, **314**, 1292–1293.

National Forensic Nurses Research and Development Group (eds) (2008) *Forensic Mental Health Nursing: Capabilities, Roles and Responsibilities*. Quay Books.

National Forensic Nurses Research and Development Group (eds) (2010) *Forensic Mental Health Nursing Ethics, Debates Dilemmas*. Quay Books.

Niskala, H. (1986) Competencies and skills required by nurses working in forensic areas. *Western Journal of Nursing Research*, **8**, 400–413.

Nottinghamshire Healthcare NHS Trust (2007) *History Information – Rampton Hospital, Forensic Services*. Nottinghamshire Healthcare NHS Trust.

Nursing and Midwifery Council (2008) *The Code: Standards of Conduct, Performance and Ethics for Nurses and Midwives*. NMC (http://www.nmc-uk.org/Documents/Standards/The-code-A4-20100406.pdf).

O'Brien, A.J. (2001) The therapeutic relationship: historical development and contemporary significance. *Journal of Psychiatric and Mental Health Nursing*, **8**, 129–137.

Orem, D.E. (1991) *Nursing: Concepts of Practice*, 4th edn. McGraw-Hill.

Peplau, H.E. (1988) *Interpersonal Relations in Nursing*, 2nd edn. Macmillan.

Peternelj-Taylor, C. (1998) Forbidden love: sexual exploitation in the forensic milieu. *Journal of Psychosocial Nursing and Mental Health Services*, **36**, 17–23.

Peternelj-Taylor, C. (2009) Forensic psychiatric nursing: the paradox of custody and caring. *Journal of Psychosocial Nursing and Mental Health Services*, **37**, 9–11.

Rask, M. & Aberg, J. (2002) Swedish forensic nursing care: nurses' professional contributions and educational needs. *Journal of Psychiatric and Mental Health Nursing*, **9**, 531–539.

Rask, M. & Brunt, D. (2007) Verbal and social interactions in the nurse–patient relationship in forensic psychiatric nursing care: a model and its philosophical and theoretical foundation. *Nursing Inquiry*, **14**, 169–176.

Rask, M. & Hallberg, I.R. (2000) Forensic psychiatric nursing care – nurses' apprehension of their responsibility and work content: a Swedish survey. *Journal of Psychiatric and Mental Health Nursing*, **7**, 163–177.

Robinson, D. & Kettles, A. (1998) The emerging profession of forensic nursing: myth or reality? *Psychiatric Care*, **5**, 214–218.

Robson, D. & Haddad, M. (2012) Mental health nurses' attitudes towards the physical health care of people with severe and enduring mental illness: the development of a measurement tool. *International Journal of Nursing Studies*, **49**, 72–83.

Robson, D., Haddad, M., Gray, R., *et al* (2013) Mental health nursing and physical health care: A cross-sectional study of nurses' attitudes, practice, and perceived training needs for the physical health care of people with severe mental illness. *International Journal of Mental Health Nursing*, **22**, 409–417.

Rogers, P. & Soothill, K. (2008) Understanding forensic mental health and the variety of professional voices. In *Handbook of Forensic Mental Health* (eds K. Soothill, P. Rogers & M. Dolan): pp. 3–18. Willan Publishing.

Roper, N., Logan, W. & Tierney, A.J. (2000) *The Roper-Logan-Tierney Model of Nursing Based on Activities of Living*. Elsevier Health Sciences.

Rose, D.N., Peter, E., Gallop, R., *et al* (2011) Respect in forensic psychiatric nurse–patient relationships: A practical compromise. *Journal of Forensic Nursing*, **7**, 3–16.

Rossberg, J.I. & Friis, S. (2004) Patient's and staff perceptions of the psychiatric ward environment. *Psychiatric Services*, **55**, 798–803.

Sainsbury Centre for Mental Health (2007) *Forensic Mental Health Services: Facts and Figures on Current Provision*. Sainsbury Centre for Mental Health.

Scales, C.J., Mitchell, J.L. & Smith, R.D. (1993) Survey report on forensic nursing. *Journal of Psychosocial Nursing and Mental Health Services*, **31**, 39–44.

Schalast, N., Redies, M., Collins, M., *et al* (2008) EssenCES, a short questionnaire for assessing the social climate of forensic psychiatric wards. *Criminal Behaviour and Mental Health*, **18**, 49–58.

Sekula, K., Holmes, D., Zoucha, R., *et al* (2001) Forensic psychiatric nursing: discursive practices and the emergence of a specialty. *Journal of Psychosocial Nursing and Mental Health Services*, **39**, 51–57.

Shelton, D. (2009) Forensic nursing in secure environments. *Journal of Forensic Nursing*, **5**, 131–142.

Stevenson, C., Barker, P. & Fletcher, E. (2002) Judgement days: developing an evaluation for an innovative nursing model. *Journal of Psychiatric and Mental Health Nursing*, **9**, 271–276.

Tarbuck, P. (1994) The therapeutic use of security: a model for forensic nursing. In *Lyttle's Mental Health and Disorder*, 2nd edn (eds T. Thompson & P. Mathias): pp. 613–637. Bailliere Tindall.

Tenkanen, H., Tiihonen, J., Repo-Tiihonen., *et al* (2011) Interrelationship between core interventions and core competencies of forensic psychiatric nursing in Finland. *Journal of Forensic Nursing*, **7**, 32–39.

Timmons, D. (2010) Forensic psychiatric nursing: a description of the role of the psychiatric nurse in a high secure psychiatric facility in Ireland. *Journal of Psychiatric and Mental Health Nursing*, **17**, 636–646.

United Kingdom Central Council for Nursing and Midwifery (1999) *Nursing in Secure Environments*. UKCC.

Webster, C.D., Martin, M., Brink, J., *et al* (2004) *Short-Term Assessment of Risk and Treatability (START)*. St. Joseph's Healthcare Hamilton, Ontario, and Forensic Psychiatric Services Commission.

Whyte, L.A. (1997) Forensic nursing: a review of concepts and definitions. *Nursing Standard*, **11**, 46–47.

Woods, P. & Richards, D. (2003) Effectiveness of nursing interventions in people with personality disorders. *Journal of Advanced Nursing*, **44**, 154–172.

CHAPTER 16

Prescribing for specialist populations

Camilla Haw

Introduction

This chapter examines good prescribing practice for patient groups in secure psychiatric care settings. Guidance on and principles of good prescribing practice are first considered, followed by a discussion of off-label prescribing with particular reference to antipsychotics for behavioural and psychiatric symptoms of dementia, clozapine for borderline personality disorder, the pharmacological management of aggression in acquired brain injury, rapid tranquillisation, antipsychotics for challenging behaviour in people with intellectual disabilities and prescribing for children and young people. The pharmacological management of treatment-resistant schizophrenia is also described, including the use of clozapine and clozapine augmentation strategies. A final section discusses high-dose antipsychotic prescribing and antipsychotic polypharmacy for patients with treatment-resistant schizophrenia.

Good prescribing practice

General guidance on good prescribing

There are some general principles of good prescribing practice that are relevant to prescribing for specialist patient populations. These are outlined in three documents that UK psychiatrists should be familiar with. First, the General Medical Council (GMC) in *Good Medical Practice* (2013*a*) states that as a doctor you should 'recognise and work within the limits of your competence' (paragraph 14), 'prescribe drugs … only when you have adequate knowledge of the patient's health and are satisfied that the drugs … serve the patient's needs' (paragraph 16a) and 'consult colleagues when appropriate' (paragraph 16d). Second, in *Good Practice in Prescribing and Managing Medicines and Devices*, the GMC (2013*b*) says that to ensure their prescribing is appropriate and responsible, doctors must keep up to date and be aware of current guidance given by the *British National*

Formulary (BNF), the National Institute for Health and Care Excellence (NICE) (in England), the Department of Health and medical Royal Colleges. Other important elements of good practice include giving patients appropriate information about side-effects, prescribing dosages appropriate for the patient and their condition, and arranging monitoring where this is necessary. Guidance is also provided about off-label prescribing, for example ensuring there is a sufficient evidence base and/or experience of using the medicine to demonstrate its safety and efficacy. Third, the Royal College of Psychiatrists, in *Good Psychiatric Practice* (2009) reiterates the GMC guidance but also adds to it. This document states that psychiatrists must be aware of clinical guidance from national bodies and be able to justify clinical decisions that lie outside of accepted guidance, as well as being mindful of the limits of their own competence. Thus, it may in some situations be appropriate to seek specialist advice when prescribing psychotropic medication.

Principles of good prescribing practice for specialist populations

Prescribing for specialist secure populations can generate therapeutic challenges. Patients often have multiple comorbid psychiatric disorders and some of these disorders may have proved resistant to mainstream evidence-based therapies (e.g. treatment-resistant schizophrenia). In addition, some patients are so mentally unwell that they lack capacity to give informed consent to treatment. Clearly, it is good practice to supply patients with appropriate information about psychotropic medication, including the likely benefits, risks and side-effects and, by explaining the treatment options, providing patients with choice. However, features of the patient's mental state, such as severe psychotic symptoms, challenging behaviour and severe intellectual disability, may prevent a full and open discussion about the best drug(s) to alleviate the patient's symptoms. In any event, the choice of drugs may be quite limited when a detailed medication history reveals that there have been multiple past treatment failures. Medicines with the best risk–benefit analysis should be tried first, but for patients with treatment-resistant illnesses, where there has been a poor response to previous pharmacotherapy, it may be necessary to carry out a therapeutic trial of a medicine with a lesser, though still favourable, risk–benefit profile. Indeed, the side-effect profile is usually an important determinant of the choice of drug.

Other principles of good prescribing are to use the lowest effective dose of a drug, to prescribe as simple a medication regime as possible, and to minimise the use of multiple antipsychotics. It is essential to take into account the patient's medical history. For example, the use of olanzapine and clozapine would not be contraindicated by the presence of diabetes mellitus but both these antipsychotics can cause and exacerbate diabetes (Haupt & Newcomer, 2001). Therefore, their use should be accompanied by careful monitoring of blood glucose and/or glycated haemoglobin (HbAIc) and may necessitate further measures to improve glucose intolerance, such as the addition of oral hypoglycaemics or insulin. Patients should be regularly screened for side-effects using recognised rating scales, for example the Liverpool University Neuroleptic Side Effect Rating Scale (Day *et al*, 1995). Sexual dysfunction, a side-effect of many antidepressants and antipsychotics, is common and should be enquired about. Patients' physical health should be monitored. Those receiving antipsychotics should have their pulse, blood pressure, body mass index (BMI), electrocardiogram (ECG), blood lipids and glucose monitored. Second-generation antipsychotics have a wide variety of metabolic side-effects which have potential long-term implications for patients' physical health and life expectancy. Finally, there needs to be regular review of the effectiveness of the medication regime. This particularly applies to high-dose antipsychotic prescribing, polypharmacy and off-label use of medication. Should the medication tried prove ineffective, it should be gradually withdrawn and alternative treatment strategies discussed and implemented.

Off-label prescribing

The term off-label prescribing refers to the use of a medicine outside the terms of its licence, known in the UK as its 'marketing authorisation' and previously called the 'product licence'. In the UK the national body that licenses drugs for medicinal use is the Medicines and Healthcare Products Regulatory Agency (MHRA). A medicine may be prescribed off-label in a number of different ways, for example when the dosage is in excess of that specified by the marketing authorisation, when it is prescribed for an unlicensed indication or for a patient group outside that given in the marketing authorisation, or by altering the dosage form, for example by crushing tablets. Pharmaceutical companies are not allowed to promote the off-label use of their products and risk being fined if they do. However, off-label prescribing is very common in psychiatry, and indeed has been described by a consensus of expert clinicians as being a necessary part of the art of medicine (Healy & Nutt, 1998). Much useful information and guidance about off-label prescribing is to be found in a Royal College of Psychiatrists' report on the use of licensed medicines for unlicensed applications in psychiatric practice (Royal College of Psychiatrists, 2007).

The use of a drug off-label represents an area of potentially increased risk since the MHRA has not examined the risks and benefits of using the medicine in these circumstances. Should the patient suffer an adverse event from the drug, liability would rest with the prescriber and/or their employers unless they can demonstrate that they have acted responsibly in accordance with a respectable, responsible body of professional opinion and in the best interests of the patient. In some instances use of a drug off-label is commonplace and is listed in national prescribing guidelines.

An example of this would be the use of sodium valproate as a treatment for acute mania and in the prophylaxis of bipolar disorder. Use in these circumstances is known as 'near label'. At the other end of the spectrum lies 'far label' prescribing where use of the drug is not supported by an evidence base and does not form a part of recognised psychiatric prescribing practice. 'Far label' prescribing is, of course, potentially more risky than 'near label' prescribing.

The off-label use of psychotropic medicines by psychiatrists is very common. In one survey, 65% of senior psychiatrists reported prescribing medication off-label within the previous month, most commonly for an unlicensed indication (Lowe-Ponsford & Baldwin, 2000). In a survey of psychotropic prescribing for psychiatric in-patients in England, the most frequent unlicensed indications were olanzapine for a psychotic illness other than schizophrenia and sodium valproate prescribed for an affective disorder (Douglas-Hall *et al*, 2001). Since this survey was conducted the licensed indications for olanzapine have been extended to include the treatment and prophylaxis of bipolar disorder.

In psychiatric secure settings, off-label prescribing is likely to be even more common than in general psychiatry because of the highly specialist and complex nature of the patients and the difficult-to-treat nature of some disorders. In a survey of prescribing for young people detained in conditions of medium security, 68% of psychotropic prescribing was off-label, most commonly because the indication was off-label (Haw & Stubbs, 2010). Antipsychotics and antiepileptics prescribed as mood stabilisers were the two most commonly used off-label classes of drugs, with aggression and post-traumatic stress symptoms being the most frequent target symptoms. Other examples of off-label prescribing in secure settings include the use of high-dose antipsychotics for treatment-resistant schizophrenia, antipsychotics for the treatment of behavioural and psychiatric symptoms of dementia (BPSD) and drugs prescribed as part of the acute management of acutely disturbed and violent behaviour, so-called rapid tranquillisation. The following sections examine the off-label use of medication in a number of special patient groups. The list is not intended to be comprehensive. The main class of drugs involved are antipsychotics.

Use of antipsychotics in the treatment of behavioural and psychiatric symptoms of dementia

Behavioural and psychiatric symptoms of dementia are common, affecting 50–80% of patients (Lyketsos *et al*, 2002) and usually manifesting as such behaviours as aggression, agitation, disinhibition and wandering. While non-pharmacological treatments, such as behavioural management programmes and complementary therapies, undoubtedly have an important role to play, where symptoms are severe and particularly troublesome drug treatment may be necessary to prevent harm to self or others. Available medications include cholinesterase inhibitors, memantine and most controversially antipsychotics. Only two antipsychotics, haloperidol and risperidone, are licensed for the management of BPSD but use of both first- and second-generation antipsychotics for BPSD is not recommended either by the MHRA (Duff, 2004) or by NICE (National Collaborating Centre for Mental Health, 2007). This is because of the associated increased morbidity and mortality from cerebrovascular disease and also from all-cause mortality (Kales *et al*, 2012). It has been estimated that antipsychotic drugs caused about 1800 deaths among people with dementia every year in the UK (Department of Health, 2009).

Antipsychotics have been very widely used in care and nursing homes to control BPSD, with a reported 25–40% of elderly residents in long-stay units having antipsychotics prescribed mainly for BPSD (Snowdon *et al*, 2005; Alanen *et al*, 2006). Their use has for some years been strongly discouraged because of the associated increased mortality and there is evidence that general practitioners' (GPs') prescribing of antipsychotics to patients with dementia has recently fallen (Zmietowicz, 2012). However, in specialist settings and where carefully conducted trials of other pharmacological and non-pharmacological measures have failed, low-dose atypical antipsychotics may have a role in the management of selected, particularly challenging patients. In a survey of prescribing for BPSD conducted in a tertiary referral centre in 2007, of the 50 patients with BPSD, 56% were receiving antipsychotics, most commonly olanzapine (Haw *et al*, 2008). Almost all patients had severe BPSD, were already receiving an antipsychotic at the time of admission to the tertiary referral centre, and the behaviours being targeted were mainly aggression and agitation. Audit of case note documentation showed generally satisfactory results, although with some room for improvement, for example in the documentation of off-label drug usage and screening for risk factors for cerebrovascular disease. Despite their widespread use in this selected patient group, it is of note that in the CATIE-AD study antipsychotic medication proved no more effective than placebo for the treatment of BPSD in Alzheimer's disease and discontinuation owing to adverse effects or intolerance favoured the placebo group (Schneider *et al*, 2006). However, the patients in this study were out-patients and therefore likely to experience much less behavioural disturbance than those in specialist in-patient care.

Use of clozapine in the treatment of borderline personality disorder

Borderline personality disorder (BPD) is characterised by instability in affective regulation, impulse control, interpersonal relationships and self-image. It is a commonly occurring and frequently severe disorder when found among patients in secure settings. The majority of patients are female and comorbid psychiatric diagnoses, such as schizophrenia and substance misuse, are very common (Haw & Stubbs, 2011). Treatment of BPD is largely psychosocial and good results have been reported with dialectical behaviour therapy (Linehan *et al*, 2006). The NICE guideline on the treatment and management of BPD (2011) states that medication should not be used specifically for BPD or its individual symptoms, although a Cochrane systematic review of pharmacotherapy for BPD reported some benefit for topiramate, lamotrigine and valproate as well as aripiprazole and olanzapine (Lieb *et al*, 2010). In a recent survey of male and female patients with BPD at a secure hospital, low-dose clozapine (median dose 275 mg daily) was the most frequently prescribed psychotropic drug for BPD (38% of patients were receiving it) (Haw & Stubbs, 2011). In only a minority of instances was the drug prescribed for psychotic symptoms. Instead, clozapine was being used to reduce arousal, aggression and self-harm.

Clozapine's licensed indications are, of course, restricted to treatment-resistant and treatment-intolerant schizophrenia. This is because treatment carries an approximately 1% risk of agranulocytosis (Kane *et al*, 1988). It has been promoted as a treatment for BPD for several decades (Chengappa *et al*, 1999), but the evidence base for its use is weak and is limited to case reports and case series and small open studies (Vohra, 2010; Frogley *et al*, 2013). In one small study use of clozapine in female medium secure BPD patients with comorbid mild intellectual disability was associated with a reduction in rates of self-injury and restraint (Fajumi *et al*, 2012). Prescribing clozapine for BPD is an area that merits further investigation in the form of randomised controlled trials (RCTs). In the meantime, clinicians should be mindful of the risk of agranulocytosis and also the serious metabolic side-effects of clozapine and only consider its use for patients with severe BPD unresponsive to other therapies. A thorough discussion of the risks and benefits of the drug with the patient is essential before commencing treatment.

Pharmacological management of aggression and agitation associated with acquired brain injury

Aggression and agitation are two neurobehavioural sequelae that can complicate rehabilitation following acquired brain injury. These symptoms are particularly troublesome, causing distress and disruption, and when severe frequently lead to institutional care. In a proportion of individuals, aggression continues for many years. Neurobehavioural therapy is key to the management of behavioural disturbance in acquired brain injury but drugs have also been used, albeit with limited evidence of benefit (Chew & Zafonte, 2009). No drugs are licensed for the treatment of aggression in acquired brain injury, although both chlorpromazine and haloperidol are licensed for the short-term management of psychomotor agitation. However, first-generation antipsychotics are not recommended in this patient population given their propensity to cause motor side-effects. A

Cochrane review of the pharmacological management of agitation and aggression in acquired brain injury identified only six RCTs in total and concluded that the best evidence of effectiveness was for beta-blockers (four RCTs), although the studies concerned were small, short-term and have not been replicated (Fleminger *et al*, 2006). Antipsychotics should be used with caution, since sedative medication can cause confusion and also because this patient population is thought to be at increased risk of developing neuroleptic malignant syndrome (Vincent *et al*, 1986). However, antipsychotics do have an established role in the management of comorbid disorders, such as organic delusional disorder and schizophrenia-like disorders. In clinical practice carbamazepine and valproate are commonly used to manage aggression, but again, hard evidence of benefit to this patient group is lacking and well-designed RCTs are needed. Evidence-based guidelines for the pharmacological treatment of neurobehavioural sequelae of traumatic brain injury have been published by the Neurobehavioral Guidelines Working Group *et al* (2006).

Rapid tranquillisation

Rapid tranquillisation is the use of sedative medication to calm the patient sufficiently to minimise the risk they pose to themselves or to others. According to NICE (2005), rapid tranquillisation includes the administration of oral as well as parenteral sedation and the use of as required (p.r.n.) medication as well as medication specifically written up for the occasion. Together with physical measures such as seclusion and physical restraint, rapid tranquillisation is a treatment of last resort, only employed when de-escalation measures have failed to resolve acutely disturbed behaviour.

The evidence base for the use of particular drugs in rapid tranquillisation is relatively weak. Research in this area is bedevilled by the acutely ill nature of the patient group such that they are generally too unwell to give informed consent to take part in RCTs and so trials tend to be conducted on patients with only a modest level of behavioural disturbance. NICE (2005) have issued guidance as to preferred drugs to be used. Oral medication should be offered first, before moving to intramuscular if the patient is refusing medication. The intramuscular route is to be preferred to intravenous on the grounds of safety. If psychosis is absent, NICE advises lorazepam, while in the presence of psychotic symptoms an antipsychotic together with a benzodiazepine is recommended, intramuscular olanzapine being an alternative (it cannot be given concurrently with benzodiazepines). In practice, where the administration of a single dose of sedative p.r.n. medication to a mildly agitated patient ends and rapid tranquillisation begins is not clear and this leads nursing staff to be unclear as to when and how frequently the patient should have their vital signs monitored.

Rapid tranquillisation requires that the patient undergoes careful physical monitoring of temperature, pulse, blood pressure and respiratory rate until they are ambulatory. Monitoring may be difficult and can potentially place nursing staff at risk of assault, for example if the patient has been aggressive and is unpredictable and therefore being nursed in seclusion. Pulse oximetry should be applied if the patient is asleep or unconscious since rapid tranquillisation drugs can cause respiratory depression. In the case of benzodiazepines this can be reversed by intravenous flumazenil, though repeated injections may be necessary since many benzodiazepines have longer half-lives than flumazenil. Further details of recommended medication for rapid tranquillisation can be found in the *Maudsley Prescribing Guidelines in Psychiatry* (Taylor *et al*, 2012) and in the NICE clinical guideline on the short-term management of disturbed/ violent behaviour (NICE, 2005). Most of the drugs commonly used for rapid tranquillisation are being used off-label but their use in this context is supported by national guidelines and widespread clinical practice.

Use of antipsychotics for challenging behaviour in people with intellectual disabilities

Challenging behaviour in the absence of mental illness is the presenting problem of some patients with intellectual disability in secure services (many patients have comorbid mental disorders, although these may be difficult to diagnose in the presence of intellectual disabilities). The term 'challenging behaviour' encompasses a range of harmful behaviours including aggression, self-injury, destructiveness and stereotyped repetitive behaviours. Psychological interventions in the form of behavioural modification programmes have traditionally been applied to manage such behaviours, but antipsychotics are also commonly prescribed, despite there being little evidence from drug trials that the benefits outweigh the risks. The use of antipsychotics in this patient group is particularly controversial because of the vulnerable nature of individuals with intellectual disability. In a Cochrane review on the subject, only nine RCTs were identified and the authors concluded that these provided no evidence of whether antipsychotics help or harm adults with intellectual disability and challenging behaviour (Brylewski & Duggan, 2004). In one RCT comparing risperidone, haloperidol and placebo no significant differences were found between the three groups (Tyrer *et al*, 2008). The authors concluded that antipsychotics should no longer be regarded as an acceptable routine treatment for aggressive challenging behaviour in people with intellectual disability. Again, in this patient group there are problems with generating new evidence because of the significant challenges associated with recruiting people who lack the mental capacity to give informed consent to participate in research studies.

A number of studies have carried out programmed withdrawal of antipsychotics from adults with intellectual disabilities with varying degrees of success (see, for example, Ahmed *et al*, 2000; Stevenson *et al*, 2004). It would appear that a variable proportion of patients can have their antipsychotic withdrawn without deterioration in their behaviour, although some do relapse. The risks of using antipsychotics in this particular patient group include an increased susceptibility to developing movement disorders and also seizures and detrimental effects on learning and cognitive function (Brylewski & Duggan, 2004). Starting dose should be low with slow titration to the target dose, which should in general be lower than that for adults with psychosis and without intellectual disability. Some clinicians favour low-dose risperidone, which now has a licence for the short-term treatment of persistent aggression in children and adolescents with intellectual disabilities. If the antipsychotic proves ineffective or if the side-effects outweigh the benefits, it should be slowly withdrawn.

Prescribing for children and young people

It has for some years been recognised that children and young people are not just small adults but have specific prescribing needs. The publication of a *British National Formulary for Children* since 2005 has been a welcome addition for those prescribing for young people. Unfortunately, for ethical and other reasons, few drug trials are conducted on children and hence evidence of safety and efficacy in this patient population has often had to be extrapolated from adults. In some cases, this has had unfortunate consequences. For example, it is now known that antidepressants prescribed for the treatment of depression are less effective and more likely to initially increase suicidal behaviour in young people than in adults and this has led to warnings and restrictions on their use in those aged less than 18 years of age (MHRA, 2004).

Young people in secure settings have a wide variety of diagnoses including complex post-traumatic stress disorder (PTSD), intellectual disabilities, autism spectrum disorders (ASD), conduct disorder and early-onset schizophrenia. They frequently have comorbidity of psychiatric disorders. Prescribing is mainly off-label and the main classes of drugs prescribed are antipsychotics and anti-epileptics as mood stabilisers (Haw & Stubbs, 2010). The commonest off-label indications are aggression and complex PTSD. Several first-generation (chlorpromazine, haloperidol and trifluoperazine) and some second-generation antipsychotics (risperidone and aripiprazole) are licensed for use in adolescents, although in practice second-generation drugs are used (Haw & Stubbs, 2010).

For children and young people with ASD and maladaptive behaviours, low-dose risperidone has a good evidence base in terms of efficacy, although children and young people seem particularly sensitive to weight gain and other metabolic side-effects (Sharma & Shaw, 2012). There is some, though lesser, support for the use of aripiprazole, this drug having a lesser propensity to cause metabolic side-effects (Ching & Pringsheim, 2012). Propranolol may be useful in reducing arousal and aggression in young people with ASD and there is emerging evidence that it can improve performance on some tasks of cognition (Narayanan *et al*, 2010).

Treatment-resistant schizophrenia

Defining treatment resistance

Although there is no universally accepted definition of treatment resistance in schizophrenia, many clinicians use those developed by Juarez-Reyes *et al* (1995) – failure to respond to at least two antipsychotic drugs equivalent to 600 mg of chlorpromazine per day for more than 4 weeks – and Kane *et al* (1988) – no demonstrable improvement after three periods of treatment with antipsychotics (from two or more different chemical classes) in the previous 5 years equivalent to 1000 mg per day of chlorpromazine for 6 weeks and patients had had no episodes of good functioning in the previous 5 years. Using these criteria, Kane *et al* (1988) reported the incidence of treatment-resistant schizophrenia to be 20%. Brenner and Merlo (1995) propose that treatment resistance be considered one end of a spectrum of antipsychotic drug response rather than being a separate entity from treatment-responsive schizophrenia, full remission in this disorder being uncommon.

Prognostic factors predicting poor treatment response

The following factors have been identified as being associated with a poor treatment response in schizophrenia: severe symptoms at the time of initial diagnosis, longer duration of untreated psychosis and insidious onset of illness, slow and insidious progression, poor adherence to treatment with medication, prominent negative symptoms, cognitive deficits, chronic substance misuse and comorbid mental illness (Ballon & Lieberman, 2010).

Pharmacological management

Is the patient truly resistant to treatment?

Several issues need to be addressed before assuming non-response to antipsychotic medication. Is the diagnosis of schizophrenia correct or does the patient have another diagnosis that requires different treatment? Has the patient been prescribed adequate doses of antipsychotics for sufficient duration of time? Does the patient fully adhere to their medication? It may be helpful to switch to a liquid preparation to improve adherence and plasma level monitoring may also be of assistance. An alternative strategy would be to switch to a depot antipsychotic. A further factor that can lead to apparent treatment resistance is ongoing illicit drug misuse. This can be detected by urinary drug screen, hair or nail clipping analysis. Finally, it needs to be considered whether the patient is experiencing side-effects which are masking a clinical response. For example, use of a high-potency first-generation antipsychotic can cause severe extrapyramidal side-effects or akathisia, which may present as negative symptoms or agitation respectively.

Clozapine

Clozapine is the antipsychotic of choice for treatment-resistant schizophrenia. Its benefits in this context were demonstrated by the seminal paper of Kane *et al* (1988). Clozapine has additional benefits to patients in secure settings given its anti-suicidal (Meltzer *et al*, 2003) and anti-aggressive effects (Glazer & Dickson, 1998). Some authors argue that clozapine should be used earlier in the course of the illness, after failure to respond to a single second-generation antipsychotic (Agid *et al*, 2007), but clozapine has a range of potentially serious side-effects, including agranulocytosis (highest incidence in the first 18 weeks of treatment), seizures, myocarditis, hypotension, bowel perforation, pulmonary embolus and metabolic side-effects. In addition, patients commonly complain of troublesome hypersalivation and sedation, which though not medically serious can result in patients stopping the drug.

Clozapine therapy requires close haematological monitoring and slow dosage titration. A low pre-treatment neutrophil count in a patient of African or African–Caribbean descent may indicate a diagnosis of benign ethnic neutropenia. In this condition the proportion of marginated neutrophils – those deposited next to blood vessel walls – is higher than in people of Caucasian origin. A haematologist should be consulted to confirm this diagnosis since patients with benign ethnic neutropenia have a different (lower) reference range for white cell count and so treatment with clozapine is generally possible. Lithium can be used to increase the white cell count, although it does not protect against neutropenia. An alternative to lithium is granulocyte colony-stimulating factor (G-CSF), which stimulates the neutrophil count and can be used to help maintain the neutrophil count within the reference range as well as being used in the treatment of agranulocytosis (Spencer *et al*, 2012).

If clozapine has to be discontinued because of neutropenia, advice should be sought from a haematologist with a special interest in clozapine therapy as to whether re-challenge with clozapine is advisable. A third of patients who have to stop clozapine because of neutropenia or agranulocytosis will again develop a blood dyscrasia if clozapine is re-introduced and on this occasion the dyscrasia generally occurs more rapidly and is more severe than on the first occasion (Dunk *et al*, 2008).

Not all patients respond to clozapine monotherapy. The management of clozapine-resistant schizophrenia is well reviewed by Kerwin & Bolonna (2005). Before considering clozapine augmentation strategies it is first necessary to consider whether any of the following factors are operating: poor adherence to therapy, ongoing substance misuse and, more fundamentally, whether clozapine has been prescribed in an adequate dosage and for sufficient duration. Although there is thought to be no direct relationship between clozapine plasma level and clinical response, it is generally held that a plasma level of 350–450 ng/mL should be achieved before deeming the patient to be a clozapine non-responder (Perry *et al*,

1991; Potkin *et al*, 1994). In some patients the response to clozapine is delayed by several months and on this basis it is generally accepted that clozapine monotherapy should be tried for 6 months.

Clozapine augmentation strategies

Clozapine augmentation with a second antipsychotic is a commonly tried strategy when clozapine monotherapy has failed. The improvement found is generally quite small and this clinical impression has been confirmed by a meta-analysis (Taylor & Smith, 2009). As Kerwin & Osborne (2000) have pointed out, clozapine lacks high-potency dopamine receptor blockage and so a logical next step would be to augment its effect with a highly selective dopamine receptor blocker such as sulpiride or amisulpride. Positive results have been reported from small RCTs for both sulpiride and amisulpride augmentation (Shiloh *et al*, 1997; Assion *et al*, 2008). Augmentation with a second antipsychotic can also help lower the dose of clozapine and hence reduce the side-effect burden. Most reports have involved aripiprazole and in one small study it was possible to reduce clozapine dosage (Karunakaran *et al*, 2007). In addition, 18 out of 24 patients lost weight (on average 5 kg).

Where clozapine augmentation with a second antipsychotic is not successful, augmentation of clozapine with other agents should be considered. The strongest evidence of benefit exists for lamotrigine, which reduces glutamate release and increases γ-aminobutyric acid (GABA) (there is thought to be hyperfunction of glutamate in schizophrenia). Although there have been a number of negative small studies, their meta-analysis suggests a moderate effect size (Tiihonen *et al*, 2009). The evidence of benefit for other augmentation strategies, such as valproate and topiramate, is less convincing. Alternative suggested options for augmenting clozapine can be found in the Maudsley guidelines (Taylor *et al*, 2012). The authors comment that the outcome of such strategies is usually disappointing.

High-dose antipsychotic prescribing and antipsychotic polypharmacy

When treating resistant schizophrenia that has failed to respond to clozapine and clozapine augmentation strategies or where treatment with clozapine has been refused or is not possible, clinicians sometimes resort to high-dose antipsychotic prescribing in an attempt to improve a patient's mental state and behaviour. One strategy is to increase the dosage of a single antipsychotic beyond the maximum recommended by the BNF in the hope of achieving a remission. The more common high-dose prescribing practice is to add in a second antipsychotic, the combined percentage dose of both antipsychotics exceeding 100% (see the widely adopted method of calculating total percentage dose described by Yorston & Pinney, 1997). This practice is known as combined antipsychotics or antipsychotic polypharmacy.

High-dose prescribing is more prevalent in secure settings than on open acute wards and its use is associated with aggression (Lelliott *et al*, 2002).

The combination of a depot antipsychotic with an oral atypical is commonly used in low and medium security (Bains & Nielssen, 2003; Haw & Stubbs, 2003). The presence of a depot ensures adherence to at least part of the treatment regime. Although there are a number of case reports describing improvements on high-dose therapy, the evidence base for this strategy is weak and there is a lack of well-conducted RCTs. Neither does high-dose prescribing have a pharmacological rationale, since dopamine receptors are usually fully saturated at conventional dosages. High-dose prescribing and concurrent use of more than one antipsychotic (other than when changing medication or when augmenting clozapine with a second antipsychotic) is not recommended by the Royal College of Psychiatrists (2014) or the NICE guideline on schizophrenia (NICE, 2009). However, many clinicians report improvement in symptoms and behaviour when using high dosages and combination therapy with individual patients and so these strategies would seem reasonable to try, providing more evidence-based options have been tried and failed (Haw & Stubbs, 2003). High-dose and combination treatment leads to a greater side-effect burden than conventional dose monotherapy and there have been concerns about QTc prolongation and sudden death as well as metabolic side-effects and neuroleptic malignant syndrome (Royal College of Psychiatrists, 2014). Patients thus require careful physical health monitoring of ECG, temperature, pulse, blood pressure, BMI, lipids and glucose. Target symptoms should be assessed, preferably using standardised rating scales, and the response to treatment (or lack of it) should be documented in the case notes.

The antipsychotic most commonly used in above-BNF dosages is olanzapine but there is little evidence of its efficacy over conventional doses of antipsychotics. In an RCT involving young adults with early-onset schizophrenia, olanzapine in a dose of up to 30 mg daily was compared with clozapine (Kumra et al, 2008a,b). Clozapine proved more efficacious than olanzapine, although both groups of patients suffered prominent metabolic side-effects. In a small RCT of patients with treatment-resistant schizophrenia or schizoaffective disorder, high-dose olanzapine (25–45 mg/day) was found to be as efficacious as clozapine on most outcome measures, though weight gain was greater than with clozapine (Meltzer et al, 2008). Thus, high-dose olanzapine may be worth a therapeutic trial where treatment with clozapine is not possible. It is recommended that high-dose strategies be tried for a period of 3 months and if there are no definite signs of improvement after this time the dose should be reduced back to within-the-BNF-recommended range (Royal College of Psychiatrists, 2014).

Conclusions

The pharmacological management of specialist patient groups in secure care settings commonly involves off-label prescribing. When using a drug off-label the prescriber should familiarise themselves with the evidence base for such use and be confident that the risk–benefit ratio is favourable. Both antipsychotic polypharmacy and high-dose antipsychotic prescribing for treatment-resistant schizophrenia are common in secure settings, despite there being a paucity of evidence for their efficacy and concerns about side-effects and safety. It is essential that prescribers keep up to date with the pharmacological management of specialist patient groups, including relevant national guidance. Where decisions about drug treatment are not clear cut, a second opinion may be indicated. Patients should be as fully involved in treatment decisions as is possible, including discussion on the likely benefits, side-effects and risks of each proposed drug.

References

Agid, O., Remington, G., Kapur, S., et al (2007) Early use of clozapine for poorly responding first-episode psychosis. *Journal of Clinical Psychopharmacology*, **27**, 369–373.

Ahmed, Z., Fraser, W., Kerr, M.P., et al (2000) Reducing antipsychotic medication in people with learning disability. *British Journal of Psychiatry*, **176**, 42–46.

Alanen, H.M., Finne-Soveri, H., Noro, A., et al (2006) Use of antipsychotic medications among elderly residents in long-term institutional care: a three-year follow-up. *International Journal of Geriatric Psychiatry*, **21**, 288–295.

Assion, H.J., Reinbold, H., Lemanski, S., et al (2008) Amisulpride augmentation in patients with schizophrenia partially responsive or unresponsive to clozapine: a randomized, double-blind, placebo-controlled trial. *Pharmacopsychiatry*, **41**, 24–28.

Bains, J.J.S. & Nielssen, O.B. (2003) Combining depot antipsychotic medications with novel antipsychotics in forensic patients: a practice in search of a principle. *Psychiatric Bulletin*, **27**, 14–16.

Ballon, J.S. & Lieberman, J.A. (2010) Advances in the management of treatment-resistant schizophrenia. *Focus*, **8**, 475–487.

Brenner, H.D. & Merlo, M.C. (1995) Definition of therapy-resistant schizophrenia and its assessment. *European Psychiatry*, **10** (suppl. 1), s11–17.

Brylewski, J. & Duggan, L. (2004) Antipsychotic medication for challenging behaviour in people with learning disability. *Cochrane Database of Systematic Reviews*, **3**, CD000377.

Chengappa, K.N., Ebeling, T., Kang, J.S., et al (1999) Clozapine reduces severe self-mutilation and aggression in psychotic patients with borderline personality disorder. *Journal of Clinical Psychiatry*, **60**, 477–484.

Chew, E. & Zafonte, R.D. (2009) Pharmacological management of neurobehavioral disorders following traumatic brain injury – a state-of-the-art review. *Journal of Rehabilitation Research and Development*, **46**, 851–879.

Ching, H. & Pringsheim, T. (2012) Aripiprazole for autism spectrum disorders (ASD). *Cochrane Database of Systematic Reviews*, **5**, CD009043.

Day, J.C., Wood, G., Dewey, M., et al (1995) A self-rating scale for measuring neuroleptic side-effects: validation in a group of schizophrenic patients. *British Journal of Psychiatry*, **166**, 650–653.

Department of Health (2009) *The Use of Antipsychotic Medication for People with Dementia: Time for Action*. Department of Health.

Douglas-Hall, P., Fuller, A. & Gill-Banham, S. (2001) An analysis of off-licence prescribing in psychiatric medicine. *Pharmaceutical Journal*, **267**, 890–891.

Duff, G. (2004) *Atypical Antipsychotic Drugs and Stroke*. Medicines and Healthcare Products Regulatory Agency.

Dunk, L.R., Annan, L.J. & Andrews, C.D. (2008) Rechallenge with clozapine following leucopenia or neutropenia during previous therapy. *British Journal of Psychiatry*, **188**, 255–263.

Fajumi, T., Manzoor, M. & Carpenter, K. (2012) Clozapine for use in women with borderline personality disorder and co-morbid learning disability. *Journal of Learning Disabilities and Offending Behaviour*, **3**, 6–11.

Fleminger, S., Greenwood, R.R.J. & Oliver, D.L. (2006) Pharmacological management for agitation and aggression in people with acquired brain injury. *Cochrane Database of Systematic Reviews*, **4**, CD003299.

Frogley, C., Anagnostakis, K., Mitchell, S., *et al* (2013) A case series of clozapine for borderline personality disorder. *Annals of Clinical Psychiatry*, **25**, 125–134.

General Medical Council (2013a) *Good Medical Practice*. GMC.

General Medical Council (2013b) *Good Practice in Prescribing and Managing Medicines and Devices*. GMC.

Glazer, W.M. & Dickson, R.A. (1998) Clozapine reduces violence and persistent aggression in schizophrenia. *Journal of Clinical Psychiatry*, **59** (suppl. 3), s8–14.

Haupt, D.W. & Newcomer, J.W. (2001) Hyperglycemia and antipsychotic medication. *Journal of Clinical Psychiatry*, **62** (suppl. 27), s15–26.

Haw, C. & Stubbs, J. (2003) Combined antipsychotics for 'difficult-to-manage' and forensic patients with schizophrenia: reasons for prescribing and perceived benefits. *Psychiatric Bulletin*, **27**, 449–452.

Haw, C. & Stubbs, J. (2010) Off-label psychotropic prescribing for young persons in medium security. *Journal of Psychopharmacology*, **24**, 1491–1498.

Haw, C. & Stubbs, J. (2011) Medication for borderline personality disorder: a survey at a secure hospital. *International Journal of Psychiatry in Clinical Practice*, **15**, 280–285.

Haw, C., Stubbs, J. & Yorston, G. (2008) Antipsychotics for BPSD: an audit of prescribing practice in a specialist psychiatric inpatient unit. *International Psychogeriatrics*, **20**, 790–799.

Healy, D. & Nutt, D. (1998) Prescriptions, licence and evidence. *Psychiatric Bulletin*, **22**, 680–684.

Juarez-Reyes, M.G., Shumway, M., Battle, C., *et al* (1995) Effects of stringent criteria on eligibility for clozapine among public mental health clients. *Psychiatric Services*, **46**, 801–806.

Kales, H.C., Kim, H.M., Zivin, K., *et al* (2012) Risk of mortality among individual antipsychotics in patients with dementia. *American Journal of Psychiatry*, **169**, 71–79.

Kane, J., Honigfeld, G, Singer, J., *et al* (1988) Clozapine for the treatment-resistant schizophrenic: a double-blind comparison with chlorpromazine. *Archives of General Psychiatry*, **45**, 789–796.

Karunakaran, K., Tungaraza, T.E. & Harborne, G.C. (2007) Is clozapine–aripiprazole combination a useful regime in the management of treatment-resistant schizophrenia? *Journal of Psychopharmacology*, **21**, 453–456.

Kerwin, R.W. & Bolonna, A. (2005) Management of clozapine-resistant schizophrenia. *Advances in Psychiatric Treatment*, **11**, 101–108.

Kerwin, R.W. & Osborne, S. (2000) Antipsychotic drugs. *Medicine*, **28**, 23–25.

Kumra, S., Kranzler, H., Gerbino-Rosen, G., *et al* (2008a) Clozapine and 'high-dose' olanzapine in refractory early-onset schizophrenia: a 12-week randomized and double-blind comparison. *Biological Psychiatry*, **63**, 524–529.

Kumra, S., Kranzler, H., Gerbino-Rosen, G., *et al* (2008b) Clozapine versus 'high-dose' olanzapine in refractory early-onset schizophrenia: an open-label extension study. *Journal of Child and Adolescent Psychopharmacology*, **18**, 307–316.

Lelliott, P., Paton, C., Harrington, M., *et al* (2002) The influence of patient variables on polypharmacy and combined high dose of antipsychotic drugs prescribed for inpatients. *Psychiatric Bulletin*, **26**, 411–414.

Lieb, K., Völlm, B., Rücher, G., *et al* (2010) Pharmacotherapy for borderline personality disorder: Cochrane systematic review of randomised trials. *British Journal of Psychiatry*, **196**, 4–12.

Linehan, M.M., Comtois, K.A., Murray, A.M., *et al* (2006) Two-year randomized controlled trial and follow up of dialectical behaviour therapy vs therapy by experts for suicidal behaviors and borderline personality disorder. *Archives of General Psychiatry*, **63**, 757–766.

Lowe-Ponsford, F. & Baldwin, D.S. (2000) Off-label prescribing by psychiatrists. *Psychiatric Bulletin*, **24**, 415–417.

Lyketsos, C.G., Lopez, O., Jones, B., *et al* (2002) Prevalence of neuropsychiatric symptoms in dementia and mild cognitive impairment: results from the cardiovascular health study. *JAMA*, **288**, 1475–1483.

Medicines and Healthcare Products Regulatory Authority (2004) *Selective Serotonin Reuptake Inhibitors (SSRIs): Overview of Regulatory Status and CSM Advice Relating to Major Depressive Disorder (MDD) in Children and Adolescents Including a Summary of Available Safety and Efficacy Data*. MHRA.

Meltzer, H.Y., Alphs, L., Green, A.I., *et al* (2003) Clozapine treatment for suicidality in schizophrenia: International Suicide Prevention Trial (InterSePT). *Archives of General Psychiatry*, **60**, 82–91.

Meltzer, H.Y., Bobo, W.V., Roy, A., *et al* (2008) A randomised, double-blind comparison of clozapine and high-dose olanzapine in treatment-resistant patients with schizophrenia. *Journal of Clinical Psychiatry*, **69**, 274–285.

Narayanan, A., White, C.A., Saklayen, S., *et al* (2010) Effect of propranolol on functional connectivity in autism spectrum disorder – a pilot study. *Brain Imaging Behavior*, **4**, 189–197.

National Collaborating Centre for Mental Health (2007) *Dementia: a NICE-SCIE Guideline on Supporting People with Dementia and Their Carers in Health and Social Care (CG42)*. NICE.

National Institute for Clinical Excellence (2005) *Violence: The Short-Term Management of Disturbed/Violent Behaviour in In-Patient Psychiatric Settings and Emergency Departments*. NICE.

National Institute for Health and Clinical Excellence (2009) *Schizophrenia: Core Interventions in the Treatment and Management of Schizophrenia in Adults in Primary and Secondary Care*. NICE.

National Institute for Health and Clinical Excellence (2011) *Borderline Personality Disorder: Treatment and Management*. NICE.

Neurobehavioral Guidelines Working Group, Warden, D.L., Gordon, B., *et al* (2006) Guidelines for the pharmacologic treatment of neurobehavioral sequelae of traumatic brain injury. *Journal of Neurotrauma*, **23**, 1468–1501.

Perry, P.J., Miller, D., Arndt, S.V., *et al* (1991) Clozapine concentrations and norclozapine plasma concentrations and clinical response of treatment-refractory schizophrenic patients. *American Journal of Psychiatry*, **148**, 231–235.

Potkin, S.G., Bera, R., Gutaskeram, B., *et al* (1994) Plasma clozapine concentrations predict clinical response in treatment-resistant schizophrenia. *Journal of Clinical Psychiatry*, **55** (suppl. B), s133–136.

Royal College of Psychiatrists (2007) *Use of Licensed Medicines for Unlicensed Applications in Psychiatric Practice (CR142)*. RCPsych

Royal College of Psychiatrists (2009) *Good Psychiatric Practice, 3rd edn (CR154)*. RCPsych.

Royal College of Psychiatrists (2014) *Consensus Statement on High-Dose Antipsychotic Medication (CR190)*. Royal College of Psychiatrists.

Schneider, L.S., Tariot, P.N., Dagerman, K.S., *et al* (2006) Effectiveness of atypical antipsychotic drugs in patients with Alzheimer's disease. *New England Journal of Medicine*, **355**, 1525–1538.

Sharma, A. & Shaw, S.R. (2012) Efficacy of risperidone in managing maladaptive behaviors for children with autistic spectrum disorder: a meta-analysis. *Journal of Pediatric Health Care*, **26**, 291–299.

Shiloh, R., Zemishiany, Z., Aizenberg, D., *et al* (1997) Sulpiride augmentation in people with schizophrenia partially responsive to clozapine: a double-blind placebo-controlled study. *British Journal of Psychiatry*, **171**, 569–573.

Snowdon, J., Day, S. & Baker, W. (2005) Why and how antipsychotic drugs are used in 40 Sydney nursing homes. *International Journal of Geriatric Psychiatry*, **20**, 1146–1152.

Spencer, B.W., Williams, H.R., Gee, S.H., *et al* (2012) Granulocyte Colony Stimulating Factor (G-CSF) can allow treatment with clozapine in a patient with severe benign ethnic neuropaenia (BEN): a case report. *Journal of Psychopharmacology*, **26**, 1280–1282.

Stevenson, C., Rajan, L, Reid, G., *et al* (2004) Withdrawal of antipsychotic drugs from adults with intellectual disabilities. *Irish Journal of Psychological Medicine*, **21**, 85–90.

Taylor, D. & Smith, L. (2009) Augmentation of clozapine with a second antipsychotic – a meta-analysis of randomized, placebo-controlled studies. *Acta Psychiatrica Scandinavica*, **119**, 419–425.

Taylor, D., Paton, C. & Kapur, S. (2012) *The Maudsley Prescribing Guidelines in Psychiatry*. Wiley-Blackwell.

Tiihonen, J., Wahlbeck, K. & Kiviniemi, V. (2009) The efficacy of lamotrigine in clozapine-resistant schizophrenia: a systematic review and meta-analysis. *Schizophrenia Research*, **109**, 10–14.

Tyrer, P., Oliver-Africano, P., Ahmed, Z., *et al* (2008) Risperidone, haloperidol, and placebo in the treatment of aggressive challenging behaviour in patients with intellectual disability: a randomised controlled trial. *Lancet*, **371**, 57–63.

Vincent, F.M., Zimmerman, J.E. & Van Haren, J. (1986) Neuroleptic malignant syndrome complicating closed head injury. *Neurosurgery*, **18**, 190–193.

Vohra, A.K. (2010) Treatment of severe borderline personality disorder with clozapine. *Indian Journal of Psychiatry*, **52**, 267–269.

Yorston, G. & Pinney, A. (1997) Use of high dose antipsychotic medication. *Psychiatric Bulletin*, **21**, 566–569.

Zmietowicz, Z. (2012) Number of dementia patients rises while GPs' prescribing of antipsychotics falls. *BMJ*, **345**, e4861.

CHAPTER 17

Human rights in secure psychiatric care

Catherine Penny and Tim Exworthy

Introduction

In recent years human rights have become increasingly relevant to all areas of public life. People with mental illness who pose a risk to others are among the most vulnerable members of our society, and special attention must be paid to protecting their rights. At the same time their rights often require careful balancing with the rights of others who may be adversely affected by their behaviour. This chapter introduces the European Convention on Human Rights and the associated Human Rights Act 1998, which enacts the Convention in UK law. It then focuses on the articles of the Convention most relevant to mental health practice, particularly in secure psychiatric care, and identifies the implications for clinicians.

The European Convention on Human Rights

The United Nations (UN) was formed in October 1945 and in 1948 its Universal Declaration of Human Rights was adopted by member states, partly as an attempt to protect against a repetition of the atrocities of World War II. The Council of Europe, founded in 1949, was also formed with this aim in mind, and its European Convention on Human Rights and Fundamental Freedoms came into force the following year. The other major contemporary influence on the Convention was the considerable anxiety of Western European leaders about the spread of communism across Eastern Europe. Articles 1 to 14 of the Convention are presented in Box 17.1, with those most relevant to mental health practice in bold.

Initially, two separate entities ensured that the Convention was followed, the European Commission of Human Rights and the European Court of Human Rights, but since 1999 the Court alone has ruled on Convention violations. Currently, 47 states are contracting parties to the Convention, including many of the post-communist Eastern European countries.

> **Box 17.1** Articles 1–14 of the European Convention on Human Rights, with those most relevant to mental health practice highlighted
>
> 1 The High Contracting Parties are obliged to secure to everyone within their jurisdiction the following rights:
> 2 **the right to life;**
> 3 **freedom from torture;**
> 4 freedom from slavery;
> 5 **the right to liberty;**
> 6 the right to a fair trial;
> 7 freedom from retrospective criminal law;
> 8 **the right to respect for private and family life;**
> 9 freedom of thought, conscience and religion;
> 10 freedom of expression;
> 11 freedom of assembly and association;
> 12 the right to marry and found a family; and
> 13 the right to an effective remedy if their rights are violated.
> 14 **The enjoyment of the rights and freedoms set forth in this Convention must be secured without discrimination on any ground.**

The European Court of Human Rights

There are 47 judges, one per contracting party. They can sit in various combinations; the largest chamber, the Grand Chamber of 17 judges, hears the most important cases. The Court rules first on the admissibility of claims of human rights violations. An application is only admissible where:

- The applicant is a victim – either direct or indirect – of an alleged violation. Where an individual has died, close family members are considered indirect victims and an Article 2 application is made (*McCann v UK (App no 18984/91)* (1995) 21 EHRR 97). Family members of those who have been detained, or relatives of physically or mentally incapable victims such as young children or people with a mental disorder may also be seen as indirect victims (*Paton v UK* (1981)). An application cannot usually be brought by a third party. However, if an individual lacks legal capacity to instruct a lawyer, for example through the operation of guardianship law, and lacks mental capacity to instruct a lawyer, the Court may allow applications to be brought by family members or carers (for example, *HL v UK (App no 45508/99)* (2005) 40 EHRR 32).
- The applicant has suffered a significant disadvantage because of the alleged violation.
- The applicant is not anonymous. The applicant can request that their identity be anonymised in any judgments, but their identity will not be concealed from the respondent state.

- The application is not incompatible with the Convention, manifestly ill founded, or an abuse of the right of application.
- The applicant has exhausted the available domestic remedies.
- Not more than 6 months has passed since the date of the final decision of a domestic court or since the day after the applicant becomes aware of the act or decision about which they are complaining.

If an application is held admissible, the Court examines the merits of the case. It can investigate by visiting the site of an alleged violation and can hear oral evidence, but most cases are decided on documentary evidence alone. The Court's judgments include its rulings on the alleged violations of the Convention, and the defendant state is expected to put an end to any breach and restore as far as possible the situation before the breach. The Court may also make 'just satisfaction' awards for damages, costs or expenses to injured parties; or may order specific measures, such as release from detention, or more general measures, for the defendant state to implement.

The Court has a serious problem with delays, and currently has a huge backlog of cases. In total, 99 900 applications were pending following allocation to a judicial formation on 31 December 2013 (Council of Europe, 2014); the largest number originated from Russia, followed by Italy, Ukraine and Serbia. In 2011–2012, the UK chaired the Council of Europe and argued for greater procedural efficiency and for an increased focus on the most serious violations. In January 2012, UK Prime Minister David Cameron suggested that some Court findings against the UK, including in the areas of terrorism (for example, *Othman (Abu Qatada) v UK (App no 8139/09)* (2012) 55 EHRR 1) and prisoner voting (*Hirst v UK (No 2) (App no 74025/01)* (2006) 42 EHRR 41), reflected 'not enough account... being taken of democratic decisions by national parliaments' and led to 'anxiety that the concept of human rights [was] being distorted' (Cameron, 2012).

Enforcement of the Convention

Contracting parties generally wish to adhere to the Convention and to be seen to do so; as a result, they usually act proactively to avoid violations. An adjudication by the Court that the Convention has been breached puts moral and reputational pressure on the defendant state to follow the judgments made and to avoid future similar breaches. If the state ignores a Court judgment, then, at least in theory, the Council of Europe, the overarching administrative body for the Convention, could expel it from membership. In practice, the Council's Committee of Ministers, comprising the foreign secretaries of the contracting parties, primarily uses peer pressure to enforce the Convention. The execution of Court judgments is kept under review by the Committee.

The Council of Europe's Commissioner for Human Rights is mandated to promote awareness of and respect for human rights in the member states.

The Commissioner visits states and publishes performance reports in areas of concern, and provides advice on how to better adhere to the Convention. Despite difficulties with enforcement, the Convention is widely regarded as the most effective international human rights agreement in the world.

Proportionality

The idea of proportionality is a dominant theme in the Convention. The Court has noted that 'inherent in the whole of the Convention is a search for a fair balance between the demands of the general interest of the community and the requirements of the protection of the individual's fundamental rights' (*Soering v UK (App no 14038/88)* (1989) 11 EHRR 439 [89]). Such a fair balance is struck by the application of the principle of proportionality.

The margin of appreciation

The doctrine of the 'margin of appreciation' means that states are allowed some freedom in how they interpret the requirements of the Convention. For example, what is an accepted clinical practice in mental healthcare in one state may not be so in another.

The Human Rights Act

The Human Rights Act 1998 ('the Act'), which came into force in 2000, incorporates the Convention into UK domestic law. According to section 2 of the Act, the decisions of the Court and the European Commission of Human Rights must be taken into account by UK courts when making decisions about Convention rights. According to section 3, UK courts must interpret domestic legislation 'so far as it is possible to do so' in a manner compatible with the Convention. If they cannot, then they may make a declaration of incompatibility (section 4). Some commentators believe that judges have changed UK law to fit the Convention more closely than Parliament intended.[a] Section 6 states that: 'It is unlawful for a public authority to act in a way which is incompatible with a Convention right'. The mental health tribunal, National Health Service (NHS) trusts and employees, and non-NHS organisations and employees when they are caring for NHS patients are considered 'public authorities'. Section 8 gives the power to UK courts to award remedies for breaches of Convention rights: UK citizens can now bring a legal action in respect of an alleged breach in the UK courts rather than going directly to the European

---

a. See, for example, HC 873-ii *Uncorrected Transcript of Oral Evidence of Lord Judge and Lord Phillips of Worth Matravers to Joint Committee on Human Rights*, 15 November 2011 (http://www.parliament.uk/documents/joint-committees/human-rights/JCHR%2015%20November%20transcript.pdf).

Court. According to section 19 of the Act, when introducing a new bill to Parliament, the government must make a statement about its compatibility with the Convention.

Convention rights

In this section we discuss the five articles of the Convention most relevant to mental healthcare in secure environments and the right to free elections covered by Protocol 1, Article 3 of the Convention, and their implications for clinicians.

Article 2: The right to life

Suicide

Contracting parties to the Convention have both a negative duty not to kill and a positive duty to take active steps to safeguard life. This positive duty involves a general obligation to enact legislative and implement administrative frameworks to protect life in all settings, including in hospitals. It also involves an operational obligation to take special precautions when a person is detained, whether that is in police custody, prison, an immigration centre or hospital. The state must do all that it reasonably can to safeguard the lives of those within its care where they know, or ought to know, of the existence of a real and immediate risk to life. The UK Supreme Court has ruled that mentally unwell voluntary in-patients, as well as patients detained under the Mental Health Act 1983, are entitled to these special precautions because of their vulnerability and due to the fact that they may be detained should they try to leave hospital (*Rabone v Pennine Care NHS Foundation Trust* [2012] UKSC 2). In the *Rabone* case, it was held that because Melanie Rabone's psychiatrist's decision to allow her leave from hospital was 'one that no reasonable psychiatric practitioner would have made, the trust failed to do all that could reasonably have been expected to prevent the real and immediate risk of Melanie's suicide'. As a result it was concluded that her right to life had been violated. This case highlights the importance of competent documented risk assessment and care planning.

One of the implications of the *Rabone* judgment is that inquests involving the suicide of a mental health in-patient – whether detained or voluntary – will now be conducted as an 'Article 2 inquest'. Such inquests are more likely than others to involve a jury, a narrative verdict, expert witness evidence and legally represented family members. Clinicians required to give evidence can expect to be questioned in relation to possible gross failures and lack of basic medical attention, as would occur in other inquests, but also about whether there was a real ('substantial or significant') and immediate ('present and continuing') risk to life and whether appropriate precautions were taken. Future cases may extend the requirement to protect patients further, for example to: those subject to a community treatment order, conditional discharge or deprivation of liberty safeguards authorisation; those on section 17 leave from hospital; those who have an intellectual disability and require physical healthcare; or those who have delirium caused by a physical illness for which they are being treated.

Homicide

The positive obligation to safeguard life extends to protecting citizens from being killed by another individual (*Osman v UK (App no 23452/94)* (2000) 29 EHRR 245). The European Court held that, for there to be a violation of the right to life in these circumstances, it must be established, first that the authorities knew or ought to have known at the time of the event of a real and immediate risk to the life of an identified individual or individuals from the criminal acts of a third party; and second, that they failed to take measures within the scope of their powers which, judged reasonably, might have been expected to avoid that risk. In this case, a teacher, Paul Paget-Lewis, had become obsessed with his pupil, Ahmet Osman. He followed Ahmet home, was suspected of having committed various acts of vandalism against the Osmans' property (although there was insufficient evidence to charge him), wrote graffiti on the school premises seeking to undermine Ahmet's friendship with another pupil, and crashed his car into a vehicle that the other pupil was travelling in. Eventually he stole a shotgun, sawed off both barrels, went to the Osmans' home, shot Ahmet and fatally shot his father before going on to shoot a deputy headmaster and fatally shoot the deputy headmaster's son. When he was arrested by the police, he was reported to have said 'Why didn't you stop me before I did it, I gave you all the warning signs?' The Court held that there was no Article 2 violation because it was not the case that the police knew or ought to have known that there was a real and immediate threat to Ahmet and his father's lives from the teacher.

Though there was held to be no Article 2 violation in this case, it raises challenging questions for healthcare professionals about a possible duty to a third party whose life may be at risk from a patient (Gavaghan, 2007). Professionals may have a duty to detain a patient, to breach confidentiality in order to warn a potential victim, or to take other 'measures within the scope of their powers' where the *Osman* criteria are met. Prior to *Osman*, it was clear that healthcare professionals could depart from their duty of confidentiality if a patient posed a serious threat to a third party (see *W v Egdell* [1990] 1 All ER 835 (CA)). Following *Osman*, it appears that they might sometimes have a duty to breach confidentiality to avoid violating Article 2. This possible new duty to share information to protect others brings the situation in Europe closer to that in much of the USA and in other common law jurisdictions. In a famous US case, Prosenjit Poddar murdered Tatiana Tarasoff after telling his psychologist about his violent and obsessive thoughts about her. The psychologist had informed the police that he was concerned that Prosenjit might hurt Tatiana: the Supreme Court of California held that he had had a duty to warn Tatiana himself (*Tarasoff v The Regents of the University of California* (1976) 17 Cal 3d 430). Following a submission from the American Psychiatric Association the court revised their initial decision in a second judgment from a 'duty to warn' the endangered party to a 'duty to protect'.

It appears that UK healthcare professionals would be under a duty to breach confidentiality to protect others only in certain, highly specific circumstances. It is rarely possible to predict who will be seriously violent and when, so it would be rare that a professional would or should know that a patient poses a real and immediate risk to someone else's life. Also, the duty applies to 'an identified individual or individuals' (*Osman v UK* (2000)) rather than to potential victims in general, or even a group of potential victims such as children. Mental health professionals are generally concerned about whether a patient will be violent to someone rather than whether they will be violent to a named individual. Finally, the duty only applies where breaching confidentiality might reasonably be expected to protect life: often it is unclear how a disclosure would reduce the risk the patient poses to the potential victim. If a professional is considering breaching confidentiality because of their concern about harm to a third party, they should also weigh their duty to share this information with their duty to protect their patient's life, since warning a potential victim or their family could result in pre-emptive action that puts the patient's own life at risk.

Assisted dying

The right to life does not entail a right to assisted death (*Pretty v UK (App no 2346/02)* (2002) 35 EHRR 1). Assisting another to die by suicide remains a crime in the UK under the Suicide Act 1961.

Article 3: Freedom from torture

According to Article 3 of the Convention, 'No one shall be subjected to torture or to inhuman or degrading treatment or punishment'. The Court has said that treatment can be construed as inhuman if it causes 'intense physical or mental suffering' in its victims; and degrading if it is 'such as to arouse [...] feelings of fear, anguish and inferiority capable of humiliating and debasing them and possibly breaking their physical or moral resistance' (*Ireland v UK (App no 5310/71)* (1978) 2 EHRR 25). Torture occurs where 'suffering of the particular intensity and cruelty implied by the word ['torture']' is inflicted (*Ireland v UK* (1978)). As with the right to life, there can be no derogation from this right. Member states have a positive duty to take active measures to protect people from torture and a negative duty not to engage in torture.

Insufficient medical treatment

In *Keenan v UK (App no 27229/95)* (2001) 33 EHRR 38, the applicant's son, Mark Keenan, who had been diagnosed with paranoid schizophrenia and a personality disorder, had died by suicide while serving a prison sentence. Susan Keenan's Article 2 complaint was rejected on the basis that the authorities had responded in a reasonable way to his conduct by placing him on watch in the healthcare area of the prison when he expressed suicidal thoughts. However, her Article 3 complaint was accepted, because overall Mark had not been effectively monitored – in the 10 days prior to his death there had been no entries in his medical notes – and because he had not had sufficient psychiatric input into his assessment and treatment and had been punished for an assault on prison staff with 7 days' segregation when mentally unwell. These failings were held to amount to inhuman and degrading treatment and punishment.

In *MS v UK (App no 24527/08)* (2012) 55 EHRR 23, a man with an intellectual disability had been arrested and detained in a police station under section 136 of the Mental Health Act 1983. He was clapping loudly, shouting, banging on the door, banging his head against the wall of his cell and licking the wall; he had lowered his trousers and waved his testicles about. He was assessed as displaying clear signs of mental illness and as requiring a transfer to a psychiatric intensive care unit or medium secure hospital. However, a suitable bed could not be found and he remained in the police station without treatment for more than the permitted 72 hours. The Court held that his situation had been degrading and had therefore resulted in a breach of Article 3. This finding may have implications for the care of those prisoners who have untreated psychosis and whose transfer to hospital is delayed because of problems arranging assessment by local mental health professionals or because of failure to agree on or find a suitable bed (Forrester *et al*, 2009). In in-patient mental healthcare, Article 3 may be violated by serious neglect in any aspect of care.

Medical treatment without consent

From 1972 to 1984, Istvan Herczegfalvy was compulsorily detained in prison and hospital in Austria. He went on hunger strike and was force-fed. He did not consent to any treatment but was given antipsychotic medication against his will. Because of his aggression, mechanical restraints were used to administer the treatment: on one occasion he was tied to a bed and kept in handcuffs for more than 2 weeks. The Court held that there had not been a violation of Article 3 and that 'the established principles of medicine are admittedly in principle decisive in such cases; as a general rule, a measure which is a therapeutic necessity cannot be regarded as inhuman or degrading'. However, it added that 'the Court must nevertheless satisfy itself that the medical necessity has been convincingly shown to exist' and noted that 'the position of inferiority and powerlessness which is typical of patients confined in psychiatric hospitals calls for increased vigilance in reviewing whether the Convention has been complied with' (*Herczegfalvy v Austria* (1993) 15 EHRR 437). This case provides a vivid example of European human rights jurisprudence setting a minimum standard of care; though some Court judgments set demanding standards, others like this one indicate minimum standards which are surpassed by the domestic law of most of the contracting parties to the Convention.

In *R (Wilkinson) v The Responsible Medical Officer Broadmoor Hospital* [2001] EWCA Civ 1545, a man with a personality disorder whose responsible medical officer (now responsible clinician) thought he had symptoms that would be helped by antipsychotic treatment argued that Articles 2, 3 and 8 would be violated if he were forced to have the treatment. The second opinion appointed doctor (SOAD) agreed that the treatment could be given, but an independent doctor instructed by the patient's solicitor thought that it should not. The Court of Appeal of England and Wales held that treatment of a protesting patient under the Mental Health Act is a potential infringement of their rights under Articles 3 and 8. Furthermore, it held that in some cases involving a controversial treatment the court should hear oral evidence from the doctors involved in order to come to its own view, even where treatment has been authorised in line with the procedural safeguards of the Mental Health Act. In *R (B) v Dr SS* [2006] EWCA Civ 28, a patient who had capacity had been treated without consent for bipolar affective disorder under the Mental Health Act: the Court of Appeal held that his Article 3, 8 and 14 rights had not been breached. To date there are no UK cases where treatment with medication for mental disorder without consent has been held to breach the Convention.

Seclusion

Colonel Munjaz, a patient detained in Ashworth high secure hospital, was kept in seclusion for several extended periods, the longest lasting 18 days. Ashworth had its own seclusion policy with less frequent patient reviews than the Mental Health Act Code of Practice advised. The Court of Appeal held that the Code of Practice exists to protect patients, including their Article 3 right not to be subjected to inhuman or degrading treatment, commenting that 'There is no doubt that seclusion is capable of amounting to the 'inhuman or degrading treatment or punishment' which is prohibited by Article 3' (*R (Munjaz) v Mersey Care NHS Trust* [2003] EWCA Civ 1036). While Ashworth's departure from the Code of Practice was deemed unlawful by the Court of Appeal, the House of Lords later reversed their judgment, holding that Ashworth was entitled to have its own policy (*R (Munjaz) v Mersey Care NHS Trust* [2005] UKHL 58).

Deportation

In *D v UK (App no 30240/96)* (1997) 24 EHRR 423, D, a resident of Saint Kitts and Nevis, had been found to be carrying £120000 worth of cocaine on arrival at a London airport. While in prison serving his sentence he developed AIDS. He was later released on licence and the government planned to deport him back to Saint Kitts. By then, his AIDS was at a very advanced stage and the European Court held that returning him to his homeland, where there was no or limited healthcare, would amount to inhuman treatment and therefore a violation of Article 3.

There have not, at the time of writing, been any successful cases arguing against deportation on the grounds that inadequate mental healthcare in the receiving country would lead to a breach of Article 3. In *Bensaid v UK (App no 44599/98)* (2001) 33 EHRR 10, the deportation from the UK to Algeria of a patient with schizophrenia was held not to breach Articles 3 or 8. The Grand Chamber of the Court held that it is only in 'very exceptional' cases that withdrawal of treatment as a result of deportation would constitute a violation of Article 3 (*N v UK (App no 26565/05)* (2008) 47 EHRR 39).

Protecting others

It may be that healthcare professionals' duty to protect third parties, as set out in *Osman*, would extend to preventing torture. For example, if a professional knew that a patient with a sexual interest in children was planning to assault a known child, then he might have a legal duty to take reasonable steps to protect the child.

Article 5: The right to liberty

Article 5 is a limited right: for certain classes of people the right to liberty is restricted in some circumstances. Article 5(1) states that 'Everyone has the right to liberty and security of person. No one shall be deprived of his liberty save in the following cases and in accordance with a procedure prescribed by law'. Of direct relevance to secure psychiatric care is the case of 'the lawful detention... of persons of unsound mind', which is expressly permitted by Article 5(1)(e). Thus the detention of persons of unsound mind requires a procedure prescribed by law (meaning that it is accessible and the consequences for a given action are foreseeable), and that detention is lawful (conforming to both domestic law and the Convention). Article 5 is 'designed to ensure that no-one should be arbitrarily dispossessed of his liberty' (*Schiesser v Switzerland (App No 7710/76)* (1979) 2 EHRR 417).

The Convention draws a distinction between restriction and deprivation of liberty (*Guzzardi v Italy (App No 7367/76)* (1981) 3 EHRR 333) – the requirements of Article 5 apply only to the latter. Moreover, most patients admitted to psychiatric hospitals enter voluntarily without formal procedures and have the right to leave if they so choose. However, almost without exception, patients in secure hospitals will be subject to detention pursuant to mental health legislation, most frequently the Mental Health Act. European case law has not defined 'unsoundness of mind' but the Court has been prepared to accept a broad interpretation. This 'margin of appreciation' allows individual countries considerable freedom as to how they frame the criteria for detention within their jurisdiction. The leading case in this regard is *Winterwerp v the Netherlands (App No 6301/73)* [1979] 2 EHRR 387, which required three criteria to be met.

1   The person must be reliably shown to be of unsound mind on the basis of objective medical judgement. The word 'reliably' requires a degree of predictability that different doctors will arrive at the same or a similar diagnosis; but the Convention does not require adherence to a particular classification system. The judgement can be exercised by those with a general medical qualification and is not limited to specialists in psychiatry. Following the 2007 amendments to the Mental Health Act 1983, while a medical judgement is required to authorise the initial detention, other mental health professionals, trained to be approved clinicians, can apply for its renewal.

2   The mental disorder must be of a kind or degree to warrant compulsory confinement. This sets a threshold of severity to justify depriving a person of their liberty and is replicated by the phrase 'nature or degree' in the Mental Health Act 1983. Confinement may be necessary either for treatment of the mental disorder or, alternatively, to prevent them causing harm to others (*Hutchinson Reid v UK (App No. 50272/99)* (2003) 37 EHRR 9).

3   The validity of continued confinement depends on the persistence of the mental disorder. This criterion recognises that mental disorders can wax and wane in their manifestations over time and that the severity required to justify compulsory confinement might not persist following a period of hospitalisation and treatment.

While these criteria clarify who might be deprived of their liberty, the question of what exactly constitutes a deprivation of liberty is more problematic. The Court has addressed this issue on a number of occasions. Being detained does not necessarily mean being restricted to the physical confines of the hospital or clinic, and indeed it does not apply only to those subject to domestic mental health legislation. Deprivation of liberty pursuant to Article 5 is 'an autonomous concept under the Convention, that is, whether a measure is defined as detention under national law is not the decisive factor in deciding on whether a person's Convention rights have been violated' (Bartlett *et al*, 2007).

Principles to determine deprivation of liberty

In examining whether a person has been deprived of their liberty the Court has consistently followed a set of principles set out in many judgments, including the domestic case of *Ashingdane v UK (App No 8225/78)* (1985) 7 EHRR 528: 'the starting point must be the specific situation of the individual concerned and account must be taken of a whole range of factors such as the type, duration, effects and manner of implementation of the measure in question'. This is often referred to as the objective element in the determination as to whether a state of deprivation of liberty exists.

To it can be added a subjective element, namely that the person has not consented to his confinement, assuming they have the capacity to do so. The third element is that the state, either directly or indirectly, is involved and responsible for the deprivation of liberty (*Storck v Germany (App No 61603/00)* (2005) 43 EHRR 96). While it is seldom the case that a single factor would be sufficient to define an individual as being deprived of their liberty, a key issue is whether others exercise 'complete and effective control' over the individual. In the Bournewood case (*HL v UK* (2005)), the carers of HL, a young man with autism admitted informally to psychiatric hospital, were not permitted to visit him at all in case he would want to leave with them at the end of the visit. The Court held there had been a violation of Article 5 in this case, and the UK Parliament responded by introducing the Deprivation of Liberty Safeguards in England and Wales, which came into force in 2009.

It used to be thought that a fourth element, concerning the use of an appropriate comparator (the 'relevant comparator'), was needed to determine whether a deprivation of liberty had occurred. In the domestic Cheshire West case the Court of Appeal had held that the question of whether there had been a deprivation of liberty required comparison not to an adult without a disability, but to 'an adult of similar age with the same capabilities as X, affected by the same condition or suffering the same inherent mental and physical disabilities and limitations as X' (*Cheshire West and Cheshire Council v P* [2011] EWCA Civ 1257). The Supreme Court rejected this approach. It held that determination as to whether a deprivation of liberty existed or not is blind to a person's disability. Instead the 'acid test' is whether the person is 'under continuous supervision and control and [is] not free to leave'.

The purpose of detention pursuant to Article 5(1)(e) is not punitive and, consequently, an individual must be detained in an appropriate therapeutic environment (*Aerts v Belgium* (2000) 29 EHRR 50). However, European jurisprudence has been blind to the level of security in which the person is detained. In an early case before the Court, Leonard Ashingdane argued that his continued detention in a high security hospital, a result of a failure to transfer him due to a long-running industrial dispute at the receiving hospital where he would have resided on an open ward, amounted to a violation of his rights under Article 5. The Court disagreed (*Ashingdane v UK* (1985)): Article 5 permitted challenges to detention but not to the type of regime in which the person was detained (Bartlett *et al*, 2007: p. 35). It has been a long-standing feature of domestic law that, for lawfully detained persons, additional degrees of confinement, such as solitary confinement, speak to the conditions of detention and do not constitute a deprivation of the 'residual liberty' of the person. In the judgment in the case of Colonel Munjaz, the European Court made the general observation that 'a substantial period of unnecessary seclusion of a mentally disordered patient, involving total deprivation of any residual liberty that the patient may have within the hospital, is capable of amounting to an unjustified deprivation of liberty'; however, this had not occurred in this case (*Munjaz v UK (App No 2913/06)* [2012] ECHR 1704). Regular reviews are necessary to ensure that seclusion is terminated as soon as it is no longer appropriate.

Article 5(4) contains a procedural safeguard against continued, inappropriate detention: 'Everyone who is deprived of his liberty by arrest or detention shall be entitled to take proceedings by which the lawfulness of his detention shall be decided speedily by a court and his release ordered if the detention is not lawful'. Thus a detained patient has a right to periodically challenge his detention before a court, in England and Wales the first-tier tribunal (mental health). To function as a court the relevant body has to be independent of the parties involved and has to have court-like attributes, including a procedure that allows the patient to present their own case and to challenge the case against them. The Convention does not require a public hearing but such a hearing can be permitted (*AH v West London Mental Health NHS Trust and another* [2010] UKUT 264 (AAC) and [2011] UKUT 74 (AAC)). A second attribute in order to be considered a court is the ability to order the person's discharge if the conditions for detention are not met. Initially, mental health tribunals had no power to independently order the discharge from detention of a patient detained pursuant to a restricted hospital order (sections 37 and 41, Mental Health Act 1983), that power being reserved solely to the Secretary of State, the relevant government minister. An early case before the European Court, *X v UK (App No 7215/75)* (1981) 4 EHRR 188 confirmed the need for a tribunal to have the ability to exercise a similar power and the law was thus amended. More recently, the first Remedial Order under the Human Rights Act 1998 reversed the burden of proof in tribunal hearings so that it falls to the detaining authority to demonstrate that the required conditions for detention exist (following the domestic case of *R v MHRT, ex parte KB and seven others* [2002] EWHC Admin 639).

The procedural safeguard of Article 5(4) calls for the decision on the continuation of detention to be made 'speedily'. There have been a series of cases that collectively set down the time parameters within which the decision must be made (*R v MHRT, ex parte KB and seven others* [2002]), allowing for more leeway in second or subsequent applications to the tribunal.

Another aspect of the safeguard Article 5(4) affords against inappropriate detention was explored in the IH case (*R v Secretary of State for the Home Department and another, ex parte IH* [2003] UKHL 59).This involved a restricted patient, detained in a high secure hospital, who was given a deferred conditional discharge at his tribunal hearing. Not all of the conditions could be met because it was not possible to find a forensic psychiatrist willing to supervise him in the community as part of the conditions of the discharge. However, under the existing law, the tribunal was unable to revisit its decision. The House of Lords (as it was then) held that a deferred conditional discharge was a provisional decision, and the tribunal should monitor implementation of the conditions and if necessary reconvene to consider how any difficulties could be overcome and the case satisfactorily concluded.

Article 8: The right to a private life

According to Article 8, 'Everyone has the right to respect for his private and family life, his home and his correspondence'. As a qualified right interference is permitted if it is 'in accordance with the law and is necessary in a democratic society in the interests of national security, public safety or the economic wellbeing of the country, for the prevention of disorder or crime, for the protection of health or morals, or for the protection of the rights and freedoms of others' (Article 8(1)). The phrase 'necessary in a democratic society' subsumes the principle of proportionality and aims to protect individuals from arbitrary decision-making. The burden lies on the state to justify an interference as being proportionate.

Confidentiality

The disclosure of confidential information about a patient without their capacitous consent to anyone outside of the care team may violate Article 8 unless it is a necessary and proportionate response to a particular situation. However, there would be no violation where the patient does not have capacity to consent and the disclosure is judged to be in their best interests (Mental Capacity Act 2005 sections 2–4). Neither would a violation occur where there is a specific legal obligation to disclose reports to the mental health tribunal when a patient's case is to be considered (to the Care Quality Commission in relation to patients who have been treated on the basis of a certificate issued by a SOAD) or to the Secretary of State for Justice on restricted patients (Department of Health, 2015). Further, it would be appropriate to disclose information necessary for action allowed by the Mental Health Act to safely and securely convey a patient to hospital under its authority; or to find and return a patient who is absent without leave; or to transfer responsibility for a patient who is subject to the Mental Health Act from one team to another (Department of Health, 2015). Also, it would be appropriate to disclose some information to a patient's nearest relative when the patient is detained under the Mental Health Act or made subject to supervised community treatment, or discharged from either circumstance (Department of Health, 2015). The Mental Health Act regulations also require nearest relatives to be informed of the renewal of a person's detention, extension of supervised community treatment and transfer from one hospital to another. However, these duties to inform nearest relatives are not absolute and, in almost all cases, information is not to be shared if the patient objects or if sharing the information is not practicable, including on the grounds that it would have a detrimental impact on the patient that is disproportionate to any advantage to be gained (if this were to happen, this would amount to a violation of the patient's Article 8 right to privacy). It may not be a violation to disclose limited information about the discharge of certain mentally disordered offenders detained in hospital to their victims. These victims also have the right to make representations about the discharge of the patient who victimised them (Domestic Violence, Crime and Victims Act 2004).

If there is an overriding public interest in line with one of the permissions for interference mentioned in Article 8, disclosure is allowed. This would include situations where a patient poses a serious risk to another person, as discussed for Article 2, or where disclosure would prevent a serious crime. The public interest in such disclosure must be balanced against both the rights of the patient and the public interest in maintaining trust in a confidential healthcare service. Even in cases where there is no overriding public interest in disclosing detailed clinical information about a patient's state of health, there may nevertheless be an overriding public interest in sharing more limited information about the patient's current and past mental health problems if doing so will help ensure properly informed risk management (Department of Health, 2015). Carers and other individuals who give personal information to professionals also have a right to expect that it will be treated confidentially and not passed on to anyone unless either there is an overriding reason that makes it necessary to do so and there is legal authority to do so, or the individual was made aware that someone (often the patient if the information is about them) would be informed and did not object.

Other interferences with the right to a private life

An individual's private and family life can encompass all aspects of their living circumstances. Some of the interventions used in the management of patients in secure psychiatric care may interfere with that right, including, *inter alia*, monitoring telephone calls and mail; restricting access to telephones, IT equipment and the internet; using handcuffs when escorting a patient out of the secure environment (e.g. to court); seclusion, restraint and compulsory administration of treatment; searching of patients, their belongings and their visitors; and dietary limitations and restrictions on smoking. As case law has evolved, a four-pronged 'Huang test' of proportionality has emerged, which can be considered by any individual or organisation deciding whether to use these, or any other, interventions that interfere with a person's private life (*Huang v Secretary of State for the Home Department* [2007] UKHL 11):

1   Does the policy or measure in question pursue a sufficiently important objective?
2   Is the rule or decision under review rationally connected with that objective?
3   Are the means adopted no more than necessary to achieve that objective?

4   Does the measure achieve a fair balance between the interests of the individual(s) affected and the wider community (i.e. a question of whether a measure constitutes a proportionate means of achieving a legitimate aim)?

Using this test may mean settling for the least restrictive of a series of restrictive therapeutic interventions. The 'least restrictive principle' is seen throughout the Mental Health Act 1983 and the Mental Capacity Act 2005.

Article 14: Freedom from discrimination

Article 14 provides that 'the rights and freedoms set forth in this Convention shall be secured without discrimination on any ground'. This includes discrimination on the ground of mental disorder. Article 14 applies to both the rights listed in Box 17.1 (see p. 270) and other rights agreed to by the state concerned. In the UK, this includes the rights in the 'First Protocol' to the Convention – the right to protection of property, the right to education and the right to free elections.

Protocol 1, Article 3: The right to free elections

Article 3 of the First Protocol asserts that states 'undertake to hold free elections at reasonable intervals by secret ballot, under conditions which will ensure the free expression of the people in the choice of the legislature'. Since the Representation of the People Act 2000 was enacted, patients detained under the civil provisions of the Mental Health Act and remanded prisoners transferred to hospital under the Act have, in addition to voluntary patients, been entitled to vote. Patients can register to vote from hospital. Further, the Electoral Administration Act 2006 means that patients can now vote in person from hospital. Sentenced prisoners who have been transferred to hospital cannot vote: the government has said that prisoners will not be given the vote, despite the European Court's decision in *Hirst v UK* (No 2) (2006) that a blanket ban on prisoners voting breached Article 3 of the First Protocol. A study by McIntyre *et al* (2012) suggests that these legislative changes have led to an increase in in-patients registering to vote. However, the researchers found that, in Westminster, psychiatric adult in-patients who were eligible to vote were only half as likely to register as the general population and half as likely to vote if registered. Informational and physical barriers are problematic. The researchers found that nine out of ten patients who were not registered to vote either did not know that they could do so or did not know how to register. Staffing and transportation issues on the day of an election may prevent patients attending a polling station. There are other barriers too: symptoms of illness such as delusions, anxiety or reduced motivation; a lack of confidence in making a voting decision; or a belief that the political system does not value them. Participation in elections may lessen the social exclusion and inequality that many psychiatric patients face. Hospitals should provide written guidance to both staff and patients on eligibility criteria, voting rights and the process of registration well before elections, and should support and encourage patients to register and vote.

Conclusions

Human rights law has many implications for the care and treatment of patients in secure psychiatric settings. The current chapter is not exhaustive but provides an overview of the key issues and challenges that face practitioners. We should understand the Convention and the Human Rights Act, and their associated case law, so that we can fulfil our duty to ensure that patients, including when at their most vulnerable, can fully enjoy their human rights.

References

Bartlett, P., Lewis, O. & Thorold, O. (2007) *Mental Disability and the European Convention on Human Rights (International Studies in Human Rights, volume 90)*. Martinus Nijhoff Publishers.

Cameron, D. (2012) *Speech by UK Prime Minister David Cameron to the Council of Europe Parliamentary Assembly (January 25, 2012)*. TSO (The Stationery Office). Available at: http://www.number10.gov.uk/news/european-court-of-human-rights/ (accessed January 2015).

Council of Europe (2014) *European Court of Human Rights Annual Report 2013*. Registry of the European Court of Human Rights.

Department of Health (2015) *Mental Health Act 1983: Code of Practice*. TSO (The Stationery Office).

Forrester, A., Henderson, C., Wilson, S., *et al* (2009) A suitable waiting room? Hospital transfer outcomes and delays from two London prisons. *Psychiatric Bulletin*, **33**, 409–412.

Gavaghan, C.A. (2007) Tarasoff for Europe? A European Human Rights perspective on the duty to protect. *International Journal of Law and Psychiatry*, **30**, 255–267.

McIntyre, J., Yelamanchili, V., Naz, S., *et al* (2012) Uptake and knowledge of voting rights by adult in-patients during the 2010 UK general election. *Psychiatrist*, **36**, 126–130.

Cases

Aerts v Belgium (2000) 29 EHRR 50.

AH v West London Mental Health NHS Trust and another [2010] UKUT 264 (AAC) and [2011] UKUT 74 (AAC).

Ashingdane v UK (App No 8225/78) (1985) 7 EHRR 528.

Bensaid v UK (App no 44599/98) (2001) 33 EHRR 10.

Cheshire West and Cheshire Council v P [2011] EWCA Civ 1257.

D v UK (App no 30240/96) (1997) 24 EHRR 423.

Guzzardi v Italy (App No 7367/76) (1981) 3 EHRR 333.

Herczegfalvy v Austria (1993) 15 EHRR 437.

Hirst v UK (No 2) (App no 74025/01) (2006) 42 EHRR 41.

HL v UK (App no 45508/99) (2005) 40 EHRR 32.

Huang v Secretary of State for the Home Department [2007] UKHL 11.

Hutchinson Reid v UK (App No. 50272/99) (2003) 37 EHRR 9.

Ireland v UK (App no 5310/71) (1978) 2 EHRR 25.

Keenan v UK (App no 27229/95) (2001) 33 EHRR 38.

McCann v UK (App no 18984/91) (1995) 21 EHRR 97.

MS v UK (App no 24527/08) (2012) 55 EHRR 23.

Munjaz v UK (App No 2913/06) [2012] ECHR 1704.

N v UK (App no 26565/05) (2008) 47 EHRR 39.

Osman v UK (App no 23452/94) (2000) 29 EHRR 245.

Othman (Abu Qatada) v UK (App no 8139/09) (2012) 55 EHRR 1.

Paton v UK (App no 8416/78) (1981) 3 EHRR 408.

Pretty v UK (App no 2346/02) (2002) 35 EHRR 1.

Rabone v Pennine Care NHS Foundation Trust [2012] UKSC 2.

R (B) v Dr SS [2006] EWCA Civ 28.

R v MHRT, ex parte KB and seven others [2002] EWHC Admin 639.

R v Secretary of State for the Home Department and another, ex parte IH [2003] UKHL 59.

R (Munjaz) v Mersey Care NHS Trust [2003] EWCA Civ 1036.

R (Munjaz) v Mersey Care NHS Trust [2005] UKHL 58.

R (Wilkinson) v The Responsible Medical Officer Broadmoor Hospital [2001] EWCA Civ 1545.

Schiesser v Switzerland (App No 7710/76) (1979) 2 EHRR 417.

Soering v UK (App no 14038/88) (1989) 11 EHRR 439 [89].

Storck v Germany (App No 61603/00) (2005) 43 EHRR 96.

Tarasoff v The Regents of the University of California (1976) 17 Cal 3d 430.

W v Egdell [1990] 1 All ER 835 (CA).

Wilkinson v UK (App no 14659/02) [2006] ECHR 1171.

Winterwerp v the Netherlands (App No 6301/73) [1979] 2 EHRR 387.

X v UK (App No 7215/75) (1981) 4 EHRR 188.

CHAPTER 18

Quality assurance and clinical audit in secure psychiatric care

Fiona Mason, David Thomas and Lesley Wilson

Introduction

In this chapter we will briefly describe clinical audit as an essential quality assurance tool within healthcare generally, with a focus on its potential application within secure psychiatric environments. Some practical tools and suggestions are provided.

Ensuring quality of service delivery is fundamental to the protection and effective treatment of patients. Despite this, academics and clinicians have struggled to agree how to define quality care. This may in part relate to the diversity of stakeholders; service users, commissioners, regulatory bodies and healthcare professionals all have a vested interest in the quality of services and yet can have very differing views on what is important and how this should be measured. Within secure services there are additional stakeholders to consider such as the Ministry of Justice, previous victims and the general public. Professor Lord Darzi defined high-quality care as care that is as 'safe and effective as possible' and 'care [that] is personal to each individual' (Department of Health, 2008); this definition was expanded by the National Quality Board (Department of Health, 2011a) to define three areas of quality as clinical effectiveness, safety and patient experience, emphasising that all three were equally important. Since the time of Florence Nightingale and the Crimean War, clinical audit has had a part in a modern health service, yet it was not until the 1989 White Paper, *Working for Patients* (Department of Health, 1989), that it rose to prominence. With the more recent development of the National Health Service (NHS) standard contract (Department of Health, 2011b) and the requirement for healthcare providers to substantiate the effectiveness of the care and treatment they provide, the focus for clinical audit has shifted to support the quality governance agenda. It is now essential that all healthcare organisations develop processes and systems to enable responsible managers and authorities to be assured that quality care is delivered; such systems encompass clinical or healthcare governance, one component of which is clinical audit.

What is continuous quality improvement in healthcare?

It is possible to make some assumptions. First, all healthcare providers wish to be known as good-quality providers; second, quality is a relative term and what is considered good quality today is likely to be outdated and of lesser quality in years to come. Based on these assumptions it is reasonable to assume that all healthcare providers strive towards some level of continuous quality improvement (CQI), if only to maintain a stable reputation for good quality. But what is quality in healthcare – is it safety, clinical effectiveness and the patient experience? Is there a single definition or will it remain mercurial, changing shape with time and the assessor's perspective? The Health Foundation, an independent UK charity that works to continuously improve the quality of healthcare, in its booklet *Quality Improvement Made Simple*, suggests:

> 'Improving quality is about making healthcare more safe, effective, patient centred, timely, efficient and equitable' (Health Foundation, 2010).

It expands on the definition, stating that:

- safe is the avoidance of harm from care intended to help
- effective means based on scientific knowledge (evidence), which produces clear benefit
- person-centred means respectful and responsive to an individual's needs and values
- timely means reducing potentially harmful delays
- efficient means avoiding waste
- equitable is consistent quality irrelevant of an individual's characteristics.

But what of organisational quality improvement? McLaughlin & Kaluzny (1999) suggest that:

> 'Continuous quality improvement (CQI) is a structured organisational process for involving personnel in planning and executing a continuous flow of improvement to provide quality healthcare that meets or exceeds expectations' (p. 3).

They propose seven common characteristics that an organisation which prioritises CQI should possess:

1. linkage between quality and the strategic plan
2. a quality board
3. training programmes
4. processes to identify and implement improvements
5. quality improvement teams
6. support for process design and analysis
7. policies that motivate and involve staff in quality improvement.

Perhaps more simply, Shortell *et al* (1995: p. 377) say: 'What really matters is whether or not a hospital has a culture that supports quality improvement work and an approach that encourages flexible implementation.' Specifically for this chapter, we shall focus on the use of clinical audit as a key tool for the identification of potential weakness within secure psychiatric services.

What is quality in a secure psychiatric care environment?

Patients in secure services are generally subject to detention under the Mental Health Act 1983 (amended 2007). The revised Mental Health Act Code of Practice (Department of Health, 2015) outlines five overarching principles: (1) least restrictive option and maximising independence, (2) empowerment and involvement, (3) respect and dignity, (4) purpose and effectiveness, and (5) efficiency and equity. In its annual report the Care Quality Commission (2010*a*), the independent regulator of health and adult social care services in England, noted a number of general recommendations relevant to secure psychiatric settings; they highlighted the need to:

- implement the Royal College of Psychiatrists' (2011) standards on the use of emergency detention by the police (Section 136)
- address over-occupancy, ensure appropriate staffing levels and skill mix on mental health wards
- ensure standards on low secure units are applied
- ensure policies on patient involvement are implemented
- ensure universal access to independent mental health advocacy
- review the priority given to social circumstances and quality of reports served to mental health (review) tribunals
- review practices and documentation regarding the use of control and restraint and seclusion
- improve practice in relation to assessment and recording of capacity and consent.

More specific to secure psychiatric services, the Department of Health published *Best Practice Guidance: Specification for Adult Medium-Secure Services* (Department of Health, 2007), which led to the development of the Quality Network for Forensic Mental Health (QNFMH). The focus on safety, effectiveness and patient experience was broadened within the specification to include standards relating to security, accessible and responsive care, the care environment and public health, as outlined in Table 18.1.

The document also described how additional stakeholders for secure services, namely the public and the criminal justice system, view the concepts of care provision. The QNFMH developed standards for medium secure services, which were reviewed and updated in 2014 (Royal College of Psychiatrists' Centre for Quality Improvement, 2014), where the groupings used complement the Department of Health (2007) best practice guidance (Table 18.2). Some but not all the standards have specific subsections.

Table 18.1 Standards headings

Section	Focus
A. Safety	Patient safety is enhanced by the use of healthcare processes, working practices and systemic activities that prevent or reduce the risk of harm to patients. Patients are detained in safe and secure environments, which also protects those they may harm
B. Clinical and cost effectiveness	Patients achieve healthcare benefits that meet their individual needs through healthcare decisions and services based on what assessed research evidence has shown provides effective clinical outcomes
C. Governance	Managerial and clinical leadership and accountability, as well as an organisation's culture, systems and working practices, ensure that probity, quality assurance, quality improvement and patient safety are central components of all the activities of a healthcare organisation
D. Patient focus	Healthcare is provided in partnership with patients, their carers and relatives, respecting their diverse needs, preferences and choices, and in partnership with other organisations (especially social care organisations) whose services have an impact on patient well-being
E. Accessible and responsive care	Patients receive services as promptly as possible, have choice in access to services and treatments, and do not experience unnecessary delay at any stage of service delivery or of the care pathway
F. Care environment and amenities	Care is provided in environments that promote patient and staff well-being and respect for patients' needs and preferences, in that they are designed for the effective and safe delivery of treatment, care or a specific function, provide as much privacy as possible, are well maintained and are cleaned to optimise health outcomes for patients
G. Public health	Programmes and services are designed and delivered in collaboration with all relevant organisations and communities to promote, protect and improve the health of the population served and reduce health inequalities between different population groups and areas

Source: Department of Health (2007).

In 2012, the Department of Health completed a consultation as part of a review of the existing 2002 national minimum standards for general adult services in psychiatric intensive care units and low secure environments (Department of Health, 2002). This review led to the publication of *Low Secure Services* (Department of Health, 2012) and the formulation of an accreditation process for psychiatric intensive care services. The

Table 18.2 Quality Network for Forensic Mental Health standards

Standards	Subsection
Patient safety	• Physical security • Procedural security • Relational security • Safeguarding children and vulnerable adults
Patient experience	• Patient focus • Family and friends • Environment and facilities
Clinical effectiveness	• Patient pathways and outcomes • Physical healthcare • Workforce
Governance	• Governance

Source: Royal College of Psychiatrists' Centre for Quality Improvement (2014).

Department of Health (2011c) has also published specific guidance on high-security psychiatric services. In addition to these standards, all healthcare providers within England are subject to registration through the Care Quality Commission (CQC). Any Department of Health secure service standards must therefore be interpreted alongside the CQC *Specialist Mental Health Services: Provider Handbook* (Care Quality Commission, 2014). The key lines of enquiry are outlined in Table 18.3 (see p. 292).

Clinical quality assurance should be underpinned by the use of clinical indicators and outcome measures, both generic and disease specific (Mainz, 2003). However, mental health services have struggled to identify robust valid and reliable indicators. It may be that some generic service indicators also apply to secure services. For example, Wettstein (2005) listed a range of quality indicators, measures and outcomes specific to psychiatry, including:

- time until treatment
- adequacy (effectiveness) of treatment
- frequency and duration of seclusion or restraint
- symptomatic improvement or remission
- functional status, return to employment
- complications (e.g. criminal justice involvement or suicidal behaviour).

In the UK one widely used mental health outcome measure is the Health of the Nation Outcome Scales (HoNOS; James, 2002), with an adapted version, HoNOS-secure developed and validated for secure services (Dickens *et al*, 2007; Sugarman *et al*, 2009). The indicators in the HoNOS-secure focus more on the patient's risk assessment across multiple domains, such as risk to self and others, risk from others, need

Table 18.3 CQC key lines of enquiry

Safe People are protected from abuse and avoidable harm	• What is the track record on safety? • Are lessons learned and improvements made when things go wrong? • Are there reliable systems, processes and practices in place to keep people safe and safeguard from abuse? • How are risks to people who use services assessed, and their safety monitored and maintained? • How well are potential risks to the service anticipated and planned for in advance?
Effective People's care, treatment and support achieves good outcomes, promotes a good quality of life and is based on the best available evidence	• Are people's needs assessed and care and treatment delivered in line with legislation, standards and evidence-based guidance? • How are people's care and treatment outcomes monitored and how do they compare with other services? • Do staff have the skills, knowledge and experience to deliver effective care and treatment? • How well do staff, teams and services work together to deliver effective care and treatment? • Do staff have all the information they need to deliver effective care and treatment to people who use services? • Is people's consent to care and treatment always sought in line with legislation and guidance? • Are people subject to the Mental Health Act 1983 (MHA) assessed, cared for and treated in line with the MHA and Code of Practice?
Caring Staff involve and treat people with compassion, kindness, dignity and respect	• Are people treated with kindness, dignity, respect and compassion while they receive care and treatment? • Are people who use services and those close to them involved as partners in their care? • Do people who use services and those close to them receive the support they need to cope emotionally with their care, treatment or condition?
Responsive Services are organised so that they meet people's needs	• Are services planned and delivered to meet the needs of people? • Do services take account of the needs of different people, including those in vulnerable circumstances? • Can people access care and treatment in a timely way? • How are people's concerns and complaints listened and responded to and used to improve the quality of care?
Well-led The leadership, management and governance of the organisation assures the delivery of high-quality person-centred care, supports learning and innovation, and promotes an open and fair culture	• Is there a clear vision and a credible strategy to deliver good quality? • Does the governance framework ensure that responsibilities are clear and that quality, performance and risks are understood and managed? • How does the leadership and culture reflect the vision and values, encourage openness and transparency and promote good quality care? • How are people who use the service, the public and staff engaged and involved? • How are services continuously improved and sustainability ensured?

Source: CQC (2014) Appendix B: Key lines of enquiry. In *Specialist Mental Health Services: Provider Handbook*. © Care Quality Commission 2013. Reproduced with permission.

for physical security and safely staffed living environment, and leave arrangements. By modifying the original twelve HoNOS scales and developing a separate 'security scale' of seven additional ratings, it has been possible to measure and monitor change in outcomes and change in the need for physical, relational and procedural security measures. The HoNOS-secure can be used within prisons, secure in-patient and community forensic services (Sugarman *et al*, 2009). Sugarman & Kakabadse (2008) also proposed a model of healthcare governance for secure services built on the concepts of rights, risks and recovery, with an integrative strategic approach covering policy, training and audit. Drawing together the themes from the available literature, we propose qualitative and quantitative measures that may help define quality within a secure psychiatric setting (Table 18.4).

Table 18.4 Proposed qualitative and quantitative measures of quality within secure psychiatric care

Theme	Aspect
Patient safety	• Risk assessments (self-harm, harm to others, leave, etc.) • Seclusion, control and restraint practices and documentation • Physical healthcare (including side-effects) • Investigation and learning from serious incidents • Mental health and mental capacity assessments • Consent • Rights-based risk reduction training
Patient experience	• Involvement in service development and evaluation • Involvement in care planning • Recovery-centred care • Information in multiple and suitable formats • Supporting independence • Respecting privacy and dignity • Respecting individual diversity and culture • Access to advocacy
Clinical effectiveness	• Clear policies and procedures based on robust evidence • Monitoring implementation of and adherence to clinical guidelines • Care programme approach implemented with clear documentation of care planning and progress • Competent motivated staff • Clinical supervision for all staff
Security	• Physical, relational and procedural security of premises • Clear procedures for ensuring restricted or contraband items are not brought in • Functioning alarm systems for both patients and staff

Clinical audit and quality assurance

Clinical audit is a:

> 'quality improvement cycle that involves measurement of the effectiveness of healthcare against agreed and proven standards for high quality, and taking action to bring practice in line with these standards so as to improve the quality of care and health outcomes' (Brain *et al*, 2011: p. 1).

Often described as a cycle, clinical audit has very specific stages. The Healthcare Quality Improvement Partnership (2009) has redefined the traditional audit cycle and proposed four clear stages to clinical audit (Fig. 18.1).

Stage 1. Preparation and planning

Key questions the clinical auditor needs to ask themselves when preparing and planning an audit are:

- What do I audit?
- How do I successfully involve my colleagues?
- How will I collect the data?
- How will I analyse the data?
- Who do I need to feedback to (internally and externally)?
- How will I feedback?
- Who do I need 'buy in' from to implement any changes?

A comprehensive audit proposal form should allow the auditor to explore these questions and find solutions before the audit commences.

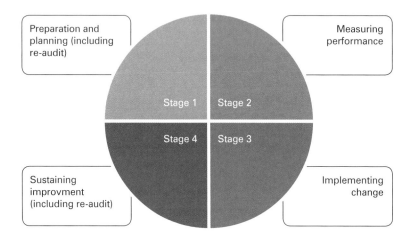

Fig. 18.1 HQIP four stages of clinical audit (2009)
Reproduced with kind permission of Healthcare Quality Improvement Partnership.

Topic selection

The background and role of the auditor is likely to heavily influence the subject area. Other factors that might influence topic selection include anecdotal evidence, concerns about a current practice or new guidance, and professional requirements. Resource allocation to support audits will need to be considered against competing priorities. Table 18.5 suggests a number of audit subjects relevant to secure psychiatric services. These have been mapped to relevant guidance and standards for the audit, and potential questions suggested for the audit tool. All audits can be used as evidence for CQC's outcome 16 (Care Quality Commission, 2010*b*) and standard 169 for medium secure units (Royal College of Psychiatrists' Centre for Quality Improvement, 2014) as these relate to assessing and monitoring the quality of service provision.

Involving others in planning

Planning with others can markedly improve the success of the audit; if clinicians and other stakeholders (as outlined in Fig. 18.2) are involved early, they are more likely to take an active interest and feel ownership of an audit, and they are then more likely to act on the results. When reviewing the results it may be useful to consider the potential impact of this involvement through the Hawthorne effect, whereby individuals consciously improve their practice as they are being monitored.

All potential stakeholders should be considered when planning the membership of an audit design team and Fig. 18.2 illustrates the wide variety of other groups that the clinical auditor may wish to consider, depending on the circumstances.

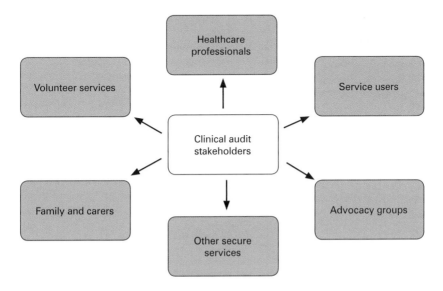

Fig. 18.2 Potential stakeholders in clinical audit.

Table 18.5 Suggested audits and audit questions within secure psychiatric care

Suggested audit	National standards and regulations	Potential audit questions
Leave for detained patients	MHA section 17 CQC outcome 4 MSU 49	• Has a risk assessment been completed? • Has the patient's registered clinician agreed to the leave? • Was a copy of the authorisation given to the patient? • Was a copy given to any relevant carers or family? • Is there consistency in the use of the documentation? • Were the terms of the leave adhered to?
Risk assessment of harm to self or others	MSU 77, 107, 122, 123, 145, 164 CQC outcome 4 NHSLA 6.3	• Has a risk assessment been completed within 24 hours of admission? • Has the risk assessment been reviewed? • Is the outcome of the risk assessment reflected in the individual's care plan? • If at risk of harm, is the patient on enhanced observations? • Does the observation level reflect the risk level? • Has the patient's medication been reviewed to reflect the risk assessment? • Have therapeutic interventions been implemented to reflect risk assessment?
Potential ligature points	NHSLA 4.1 CQC outcome 10	• Are there any potential ligature points in the areas patients can access? • Are these areas supervised or non-supervised? • Are the patients on the unit being assessed for the risk of self-harm?
Mental capacity assessment	MCA 2005 CQC outcome 7	• Has a formal mental capacity assessment been undertaken? • Is the assessment fully documented? • Are assessments reviewed as appropriate? • Do the care plans reflect the results of the capacity assessment?
Consent to treatment	CQC outcome 2 MHA part 4 MSU 65 MHAC	• Has a mental capacity assessment been completed? • Has the mental capacity assessment been reviewed? • Is there evidence that the patient has consented to treatment if they have capacity? • Have the risks and benefits of the treatment been fully explained to the patient? • Have the risks and benefits discussions been documented? • Are the risks and benefits identified accurate? • Has the patient been given the opportunity to ask questions about their treatment? • Has the patient had the time to digest the information before consenting? • Has written information on treatment been given?

Table 18.5 *contd*

Suggested audit	National standards and regulations	Potential audit questions
		• Is the appropriate person taking consent? • Is the information available in various formats to support language, cognitive impairments etc.?
SOADs	MHA part 4 CQC outcome 2 MHAC	• Has a SOAD been requested? • Is the assessment of the SOAD documented? • Has the patient's condition been reviewed since the last assessment by the SOAD?
Privacy and dignity while under observation	CQC outcome 1 NHSLA 6.5 MHAC MSU 114 NICE quality standard	• Is the observation level for the patient appropriate? • Does the patient feel their privacy or dignity has been maintained? • Has the observation level been explained to the patient so they understand why their privacy may not be maintained?
Access to meaningful activity while on an MSU	MSU 105, 106, 127 CQC outcome 1 NICE quality standard	• How many hours of meaningful activity does each patient receive? • Is the patient involved in deciding what meaningful activity they undertake? • What activities does the service offer patients? • Does the patient have a weekly timetable of activities? • Does the ward display information on activities available? • Is there any evidence of any activities being cancelled in the past month? • Are patients attending their planned activities and if not, what is preventing this from happening? • Are activities discussed in the community meeting? • Are activities risk assessed to be used in a secure psychiatric care setting? • Are patients involved with the future planning and commissioning of activities? • Do the activities reflect the recovery ethos?
CPA review	CQC outcome 1, 4 MSU 133, 134, 135 NICE quality standard	• Was the patient involved in the planning of their review? • Was the patient able to bring an advocate? • Were all relevant people invited? • Did the relevant people attend? • Were all the necessary reports/information available at the review? • Were the reports fully completed and consistent? • Are the reports up to date? • Were all people involved able to participate and voice their opinions? • Were decisions made fully agreed?

Table 18.5 *contd*

Suggested audit	National standards and regulations	Potential audit questions
Individual care planning following assessment	CQC outcome 1 MSU 124, 126, NICE quality standard	• Was an assessment completed on admission? • Was an initial care plan devised within 24 hours of admission? • Is there a multidisciplinary care plan in the patient notes? • Does the care plan reflect all the issues raised in the assessment? • Is there evidence that the patient has been involved in the development of their care plan? • Has the patient signed the care plan? • Does the patient have a copy of the care plan? • Has the care plan been updated in the past month? • Can all staff, including temporary staff, access the care plan? • Is the care plan recovery focused? • Does the care plan reflect the physical/relational security requirements of the service user?
Access to independent mental health advocates	MHAC MSU 89 CQC outcome 1	• Is there any evidence that the patient has been in contact with an independent mental health advocate? • Are the contact details of the local advocacy service readily available/displayed on the unit? • Does the advocacy service understand the care, treatment and support options available to the patient?
Management of aggression and violence	MSU 42 NICE CG25 NHSLA 2.8 CQC outcome 4	• Is there a risk assessment related to the patient's potential violent behaviour? • Has the risk assessment been reviewed? • Has the patient been advised of actions to be taken should they become violent? • Has the patient been involved in developing an advance directive detailing their preferred strategies should they become violent? • Does the record detail justification for the use of any rapid tranquillisation or seclusion?
Use of restraint and seclusion	MHAC MSU 43, 117 CQC outcome 7	• Is there documentation of multidisciplinary reviews during a seclusion event? • Was de-escalation appropriately used prior to seclusion? • Is the seclusion room a safe environment? • Was the restraint or seclusion event reported via an incident reporting system?
Rapid tranquillisation	NHSLA 6.7 NICE quality standard CQC outcome 7	• Are there clear prescribing guidelines for rapid tranquillisation? • Have the guidelines been adhered to?

Table 18.5 *contd*

Suggested audit	National standards and regulations	Potential audit questions
		• Have the staff been trained on rapid tranquillisation?
		• Was rapid tranquillisation necessary?
		• Had all other option been explored?
		• Has post-tranquillisation observations been documented?
		• Have any abnormal observations been escalated?

CQC, Care Quality Commission (2014) (see also Table 18.3); MCA, Mental Capacity Act; MHA, Mental Health Act 1983; MHAC, *Monitoring the Use of the Mental Health Act in 2009/10* (Care Quality Commission, 2010a); MSU, *Standards for Medium Secure Services* (Royal College of Psychiatrists' Centre for Quality Improvement, 2014); NHSLA, *NHSLA Risk Management Standards 2012-13* (NHS Litigation Authority, 2012); NICE, National Institute for Health and Care Excellence guidance reference or quality standard; SOAD, second opinion appointed doctor.

The audit team should, where possible, involve relevant stakeholders to agree the topic, developing its focus, suggesting aspects of the topic to be audited, highlighting areas of concern from their experience, agreeing on the standards to be used, supporting audit design, participating in data collection and publicising the audit among their peers. When involving other stakeholders in the audit process, the lead needs to ensure that they understand the process and their role within it. Involvement can take many forms and does not have to be time consuming or resource intensive. Targeted focus groups can allow the auditor to gather a large amount of information in a relatively short period, while using virtual groups via e-mail can give stakeholders time to consider the audit and comment.

Setting standards

The aspect which sets audit apart from other quality assurance processes is the measurement against standards. As discussed, there are a number of nationally recognised standards within secure psychiatric care that can be used for audit purposes. Alongside these, clinical guidelines published by the UK National Institute for Health and Care Excellence (NICE) often have an audit criteria appendix, with an associated audit tool. Where standards are not already developed, auditors will need to develop their own, bearing in mind that they are:

- clear, unambiguous statements
- defined with specific inclusion and exclusion criteria
- referenced to the research evidence or to national or local policy
- SMART: Specific, Measurable, Achievable, Realistic and Timely
- developed through a consultative process with the relevant stakeholders.

Stage 2. Measuring performance

Once standards have been agreed, the auditor is ready to plan data collection and analysis. Typically a number of questions arise that the auditor needs to consider when planning this stage of the audit, for instance:

- Do I collect prospective or retrospective data?
- Can I collect the data from the patient's records?
- Do I need to include others – family, staff?
- How do I score and record the data?
- Do I need others to help collect the data?
- Does data collection require clinical knowledge?
- How will I analyse the data?

For many audits it will not be possible to collect data from the entire potential cohort and clinical audit teams frequently ask 'How many individuals do I need to include to make my results valid?' This is not an easy question to answer. It will be guided by the nature of the topic of the audit, the size and nature of the potential patient pool and of course resources. Searching the internet for 'optimum sample size determination' will identify a number of tools freely available online and advice can be sought from the organisation's clinical audit or research teams. Besides the size of the sample, the nature of sampling can vary and can include simple random sampling, systematic random sampling, stratified random sampling and cluster sampling. *An Introduction to Statistics for Clinical Audit* (Moore *et al*, 2011) gives a detailed description and guide on how to use these various types of sampling systems. The aim for the auditor when considering these questions is to ensure that the sample represents the population to which the results will be generalised.

Collating data

Following a review of patient identifiable information by the Caldicott Committee in 1997, the Department of Health published six Caldicott Principles to enable control and safeguard of such information (Department of Health, 1997). These principles were revised in 2013 with a seventh principle being added (Table 18.6; Department of Health, 2013). Although the principles primarily relate to patient-identifiable information, it is best practice that the auditor should ensure they are followed.

Traditionally, clinical audit has focused on quantitative data, but used closed questions with little room for comments; this trend has slowly begun to change with auditors being encouraged to seek more open qualitative responses and surveying patients' views as part of the audit. Analysis of qualitative data can be more challenging but this should not prevent an auditor from undertaking such analysis when appropriate. The challenge is greatest when data collection is shared between a number of people; all data collectors must have the same understanding of the tool and terminology to ensure consistency and inter-rater reliability. However the data are collated,

Table 18.6 Caldicott principles: considerations within clinical audit

Caldicott principles	Application in clinical audit
1. Justify the purpose	• Is the audit necessary? • Will the audit benefit patient care?
2. Don't use personal confidential data unless it is absolutely necessary	• Person-identifiable information, relating to both patient and staff, should not be collated in an audit
3. Use the minimum necessary personal confidential data	• Only collect the information you need • When collecting demographics consider the potential to identify an individual by their characteristics
4. Access to personal confidential data should be on a strict need-to-know basis	• Does the person collating the data usually have access to records? • Are they bound by a code of confidentiality? • Are they able to interpret the data in the records accurately? • Is the audit collating only what it needs?
5. Everyone with access to personal confidential data should be aware of their responsibilities	• Are all auditors collating the same information? • Do auditors know what to do if they discover evidence of poor practice? • Do auditors understand what person-identifiable data are? • Do auditors know how to store or where to send the data once collated? • How long will the raw data be kept once the report has been agreed?
6. Comply with the law	• Data Protection Act 1998 • Health and Social Care Act 2012 • Code of conduct and regulations from professional bodies
7. The duty to share information can be as important as the duty to protect patient confidentiality	• Do auditors know what to do if they discover evidence of poor practice? • The success of an audit relies on the auditor sharing the findings to ensure practice is improved

Source: Department of Health (2013).

the audit plan and final report need to clearly describe the process and define ambiguous terminology; this ensures that any re-audit undertaken will follow the same methodology.

Data analysis

Data analysis in audit does not need to be complicated; most deal with summary variables, percentages, means, modes or medians and the ranges or standard deviations. A variety of statistical tests, depending on the nature of the data, can be used to check for evidence of statistically significant differences or change; however, these can add confusion for some readers, whereas statistical significance can and often is different to clinical significance. Auditors need to be careful when comparing results with previous audits, focusing especially on the methodology and samples to ensure comparability for interpretation and decision-making.

Stage 3. Implementing change

Once the results are known and gaps in compliance indentified, auditors need to ensure that the results are effectively communicated back to all the relevant stakeholders in a timely and engaging fashion; the style used often needs to be tailored to the audience to ensure maximum impact, discussion and effective action-planning.

Audit report

Each organisation should have an approved audit report template, though these vary greatly. As a minimum, the auditor needs to ensure that the whole audit process is clearly described, to allow all the stakeholders to fully understand the process and results so that re-audits can be undertaken in a similar manner. We recommend that an effective audit report should have distinct sections to guide the reader through the document. Suggested sections and content are outlined below.

Title page

This should include:

- audit title (make this clear and concise)
- service/division
  - if the report relates to one service only, then this should be clearly documented
  - if the audit is organisation wide, it is useful to state this
- audit date
  - date of the report
  - period of data collection
- audit author (name and designation of the person writing the audit)
- lead auditor (if different to the audit author, name and designation)
- professions involved (if this has been a multidisciplinary project, then state the other healthcare professions involved in the audit process)
- organisation's logo.

Executive summary

Not all audit reports will need an executive summary; some smaller, simpler audits are reasonably quick and easy to read. However, executive summaries are beneficial when communicating with senior management and decision makers, identifying the key findings and implications of the audit. The executive summary should include a condensed account of the reasoning behind the audit, the methodology and the key findings and recommendations. If the executive summary is particularly targeted at senior management, it is often useful to link the audit to the relevant contractual and regulatory requirements.

Introduction/background

This section should explain why the topic was chosen and what national and local drivers existed to support its selection. Within this section the auditor should refer to any national or local guidance that the audit relates to.

For example: 'The organisation recently reviewed and updated its clinical guidance on rapid tranquillisation following the published NICE guidance'.

Aims and objectives

The report needs to document a clear audit aim. The objectives detail how the audit will be conducted to achieve the stated aim.

For example: 'The aim of the audit is to provide assurance that the recently published clinical guideline on rapid tranquillisation has been fully implemented. The objectives are to:

1   ensure that rapid tranquillisation is prescribed as per the guideline
2   ensure post-tranquillisation observations are undertaken and recorded in the service user's notes
3   ensure that relevant staff have received training in the use and monitoring of rapid tranquillisation'.

Standards

Within this section the author should refer to the standards against which the audit is conducted. Rather than stating all the standards individually, the reader needs to know where the standards came from – were they from national guidance, pre-existing audits, local policy or developed locally. If the last, the author should detail the development, consultation and ratification of the standards.

For example: 'The standards were based on NICE Clinical Guideline 136 and the Mental Health Act 1983'.

Methodology

This section should detail how the audit was conducted, including sampling, services included, audit tool used, data sources, nature of the data, data collection period, who collected the data, where and how data were collated, who analysed the data, how they were analysed, who compiled the report and how this was shared with stakeholders (Box 18.1).

If any data were excluded during the audit, then the reasoning behind this needs to be clearly documented. When this section is complete it is useful to ask a colleague who has not been involved in the audit to read it through and comment whether they could repeat the audit based purely on the information given. If they cannot, then something has been missed.

Box 18.1 Example of audit report methodology section

'All records from service users who had received rapid tranquillisation in the past 2 months, April and May 2012, were audited using the audit tool in appendix 1. The audit was undertaken by the link pharmacist and the ward manager for the unit involved in the tranquillisation. The audit took place on the ward using the electronic notes and prescription charts.

Training data were obtained from the organisation's training and development team who record attendance on a local database.

The audit team provided data inputting and analysis using the organisation's electronic software.

The report was compiled jointly between the head of pharmacy and the head of clinical services and was ratified by the operational committee. The report has been published on the organisation's internal internet site and presented at the local shared learning from audit event.

All units were given copies of their individual reports to allow for localised action-planning, which contributed to the organisation-wide action plan.

Table 18.7 Example: Standard – The rapid tranquillisation prescription adheres to the local policy

Criteria	Adherence, n (%)
Dosing	12 (75)
Route of administration	16 (100)
Appropriate clinician prescribed	12 (75)

Table 18.8 Example: Audit of rapid tranquillisation action plan

Date of action plan: July 2012		Monitored by: risk management committee		
Recommendation	**Action required**	**Required by date**	**Responsible person**	**Status/update**
1. Awareness of correct dosages needs to be increased in all prescribers of rapid tranquillisation	I. Develop and offer awareness sessions for prescribers II. Record attendance at awareness sessions III. Include information of dosages in pharmacy newsletter	Nov 2012	Head of Pharmacy	

Results

The first line in this section should advise the reader of the number of cases audited; if a sampling method was used, then the total population figure from which it was drawn should be stated. If possible, contrast the audited population against the wider one on key demographic variables to show that it is representative (Table 18.7).

Results should be presented clearly and, where possible, compared with previous audit data to show changes in compliance. The use of simple charts and graphics usually facilitates reader understanding.

Individual professionals or units within a service should not be identified; audit is about improvement, not performance management. If a breakdown by ward or clinician is required, as is now increasingly the case, then they should be allocated an anonymised code and individually advised of their code.

Findings

The findings section is the author's opportunity to discuss the results and identify the key themes and observations. The report should highlight areas of good practice as well as areas that need improvement.

For example: '100% of prescriptions audited showed that the appropriate route of administration was used, however, 25% used incorrect dosages.'

Recommendations

The recommendations should be based on the findings of the audit. They should be shared and agreed with all the stakeholders, as this enables the development of a robust action plan.

For example, recommendations could be phrased: 'Awareness of correct dosages needs to be increased in all prescribers involved in rapid tranquillisation'.

Action plan

All audit reports should contain an action plan, which should be based on the SMART approach. Although not traditionally included in action plans, it may be beneficial to review the financial impact of the actions required.

A clearly defined process for monitoring and reporting on the action plan should be agreed at the development stage to ensure actions and learning from the audit are not lost (Table 18.8).

Stage 4. Sustaining improvement

The aim of clinical audit is to improve care and health outcomes for patients, thus driving up quality; this improvement needs to be sustained.

Once the actions have been completed and after an opportunity for practice to change, a re-audit should be planned to complete the audit cycle. There is no clear guide as to how frequently to re-audit as this can depend on the nature of the potential failure, the intensity of actions required and practicality (how long it will take to embed any new systems or paperwork).

Feedback to services should continue throughout the re-audits to ensure staff are aware of changes and improvements and where developments are still required. Once compliance has been consistently achieved, it may be considered that there is no added benefit to continue auditing that specific area. Auditors should be encouraged to share their learning with other services, both internally and externally. Sharing the audit reports can allow for benchmarking with similar services.

Conclusions

By undertaking regular and appropriate clinical audits healthcare organisations can have a clear view of gaps in service provision. Undertaking the audit is not enough; the ultimate aim of audit is to develop practices and improve care. To provide assurance to the organisation's board there is a requirement to ensure that the process of clinical audit is robust and follows best practice.

Clinical audit is a critical quality assurance tool within secure psychiatric care environments, as it is in any other clinical setting: helping the quality of care provision to develop, for care to become safer, more effective, more patient centred, timely, efficient and equitable. To do so fully, audit should be undertaken within a quality improvement infrastructure consisting of:

- linkage to a strategic plan
- a quality board
- training programmes
- processes to identify and implement improvements
- formation of quality improvement teams
- support for process analysis and design
- policies that enable and motivate staff involvement in quality improvement.

Clinical audit must be structured to ensure reproducibility and cyclical to support continuous improvement. It must support individual professional development and organisational governance. To support clinicians, teams and healthcare organisations, clinical audit must have an accessible specialist resource to coordinate the work and to support its integration into everyday clinical activity.

References

Brain, J., Schofield, J., Gerrish, K., *et al* (2011) *A Guide for Clinical Audit, Research and Service Review*. Healthcare Quality Improvement Partnership.

Care Quality Commission (2010*a*) *Monitoring the Use of the Mental Health Act in 2009/10*. CQC.

Care Quality Commission (2010*b*) *Essential Standards of Quality and Safety*. CQC.

Care Quality Commission (2014) *Specialist Mental Health Services: Provider Handbook*. CQC.

Department of Health (1989) *Working for Patients*. Department of Health.

Department of Health (1997) *Report on the Review of Patient-Identifiable Information (The Caldicott Report)*. Department of Health.

Department of Health (2002) *National Minimum Standards for General Adult Services in Psychiatric Intensive Care Units and Low Secure Environments*. Department of Health.

Department of Health (2007) *Best Practice Guidance: Specification for adult medium-secure services*. Department of Health.

Department of Health (2008) *High Quality Care For All: NHS Next Stage Review Final Report*. TSO (The Stationery Office).

Department of Health (2011a) *NHS Standard Contract 2012/13*. Department of Health.

Department of Health (2011b) *Quality Governance in the NHS, National Quality Board Advice and Recommendations*. Department of Health.

Department of Health (2011c) *Guidance on the High Security Psychiatric Services (Arrangements for Safety and Security at Ashworth, Broadmoor and Rampton Hospitals)*. Department of Health.

Department of Health (2012) *Low Secure Services: Good Practice Commissioning Guide, Consultation Draft*. Department of Health.

Department of Health (2013) *Information: To Share or Not To Share, Government Response to the Caldicott Review*. Department of Health.

Department of Health (2015) *Mental Health Act 1983: Code of Practice*. TSO (The Stationery Office).

Dickens G., Sugarman, P. & Walker, L. (2007) HoNOS-secure: a reliable outcome measure for users of secure and forensic mental health services. *Journal of Forensic Psychiatry & Psychology*, **18**, 507–514.

Health Foundation (2010) *Quality Improvement Made Simple*. Health Foundation.

Healthcare Quality Improvement Partnership (2009) *The Criteria and Indicators of Best Practice in Clinical Audit*. HQIP.

James, M. (2002) The use of Health of the Nation Outcome Scales (HoNOS) in routine clinical practice by NHS mental health service providers in England: a summary of findings. *Approach*, **23**, 13–16.

Mainz, J. (2003) Methodology matters: defining and classifying clinical indicators for quality improvement. *International Journal for Quality in Health Care*, **15**, 523–530.

McLaughlin, C.P. & Kaluzny, A.D. (1999) Defining quality improvement: past, present and future. In *Continuous Quality Improvement in Health Care: Theory, Implementation and Applications*, 2nd edn, pp. 3–33. Jones & Bartlett.

Moore J., Smith M. & Barwick, M. (2011) *An Introduction to Statistics for Clinical Audit*. Healthcare Quality Improvement Partnership.

NHS Litigation Authority (2012) *NHSLA Risk Management Standards 2012-13 for NHS Trusts providing Acute, Community, or Mental Health & Learning Disability Services and Non-NHS Providers of NHS Care*. NHSLA.

Royal College of Psychiatrists (2011) *Standards on the Use of Section 136 of the Mental Health Act 1983 (England And Wales)* (CR159). Royal Collete of Psychiatrists.

Royal College of Psychiatrists' Centre for Quality Improvement (2014) *Quality Network for Forensic Mental Health Services: Standards for Medium Secure Services*. RCPsych CCQI.

Shortell, S.M., O'Brien, J.L., Carman, J.M., *et al* (1995) Assessing the impact of continuous quality improvement/total quality management: concept versus implementation. *Health Services Research*, **30**, 377–401.

Sugarman, P. & Kakabadse, N.K. (2008) A model of mental health governance. *International Journal of Clinical Leadership*, **16**, 17–26.

Sugarman, P., Walker, L. & Dickens, G. (2009) Managing outcome performance in mental health using HoNOS: experience at St Andrew's Healthcare. *Psychiatrist*, **33**, 285–288.

Wettstein, R. (2005) Quality and quality improvements in forensic mental health evaluations. *Journal of the American Academy of Psychiatry and the Law*, **33**, 158–175.

CHAPTER 19

Psychological support following violent assault and trauma: what works for staff in secure settings?

Annette Greenwood and Carol Rooney

Introduction

At the heart of quality healthcare for patients is the principle that an employing organisation should ensure appropriate support and care for its staff. This can pose significant challenges for services, including those providing secure care for people with mental disorder where there is increased risk of harm occurring to staff during their daily practice. In the UK, secure mental health services provide care for patients who have enduring serious mental health problems and a history of convictions and/or challenging behaviour. The Nursing in Secure Environments scoping study (United Kingdom Central Council for Nursing, Midwifery and Health Visiting, 1999) highlighted that patients' mental disorder and offending patterns pose intense demands on nurses because they are required to maintain empathic relationships while also focusing on risk management, including the prevention and management of violence and aggression. Further, patients may expose staff to other behaviours that are potentially distressing, for example severe self-harm and accounts of traumatic abuse.

Research suggests that educational interventions can be effective in reducing some of the effects that working with potentially violent patients has on the therapeutic relationship. Dickinson & Hurley (2012) reviewed the literature and reported that staff working in secure environments often experience strong negative emotional reactions towards patients, which can lead to antipathy and alienation. They have suggested that educational programmes should be provided to promote the building of therapeutic alliances and to increase understanding. According to Howard *et al* (2009), training and support for staff may increase self-efficacy and thus reduce burnout. They have called for longitudinal research to increase understanding of the relationship between violence and burnout. A number of studies have recommended that staff in secure services should be provided with effective support structures (Kirby & Pollock, 1995; Coffey & Coleman, 2001; Mason, 2002).

Despite the acknowledgment of a need for support, there has been little clear guidance about implementing any specific support model. This chapter describes the development and content of a new support model (ASSIST) for staff working in secure mental health services and the support services based on that model. We describe the contextual factors underlying the need for the ASSIST model, including the nature and prevalence of aggression and violence against healthcare staff in mental health settings and specifically in secure care. We outline the potential physical and psychological consequences of exposure to aggression and violence and identify why this is a priority for action at local service and national policy levels. We describe the emergence and development of policy in the UK that is directed at providing support for staff and minimising adverse effects of violence once it has occurred. We then look at the development and implementation of the ASSIST psychological first aid model (Greenwood *et al*, 2012) at a large provider of secure mental health services. In addition, we discuss how an in-house trauma response service delivers support for staff who have been seriously assaulted, threatened or traumatised at work. We conclude by presenting data about use of the service and explain how we have embedded the concept of psychological first aid into organisational thinking.

Violence and aggression in healthcare

Incidence of aggression and violence

The NHS Security Management Service (2010) reported that one in three National Health Service (NHS) staff (32%) have been verbally abused or threatened by a patient in the past 12 months. One in 20 (5%) have been physically assaulted by a patient and 1% have been assaulted by a member of the public. Almost 165 000 NHS employees working in the 388 UK trusts participated in the Care Quality Commission's 8th annual staff survey during the final quarter of 2011 (Care Quality Commission, 2011). The survey covered all occupational groups, including medical and nursing staff, other clinical professionals, and clerical and hotel services staff. Eight per cent of staff reported experiencing physical violence perpetrated by patients, relatives or members of the public in the previous year. Fifteen per cent had been subjected to bullying, harassment and abuse. The figures for violence were highest for front-line clinical staff (12%), particularly workers in ambulance trusts (18%) and mental health trusts (15%). More than half (53%) of staff who had experienced physical abuse said they had been physically assaulted by a patient or a member of the public on one occasion in the past 12 months, whereas one in three (34%) reported that this had occurred on two to five occasions. Around one in four staff working in acute environments reported experiencing emotional and/or psychological distress as a result of verbal abuse. This was roughly the same proportion of staff who reported emotional and/or psychological distress following an incident of physical assault, suggesting that the effects of verbal abuse may be underestimated.

Potential effects of violence and aggression

The Care Quality Commission (2011) review found that following the experience of physical or verbal abuse staff reported that they experienced one or more of the following:

- felt less safe in the workplace
- experienced less job satisfaction
- suffered a short-term physical injury
- had taken time off work.

Erdos & Hughes (2001) found that those staff working in mental health environments who spent the most time with patients were at greatest risk of experiencing an assault, and those at the highest risk were the nursing personnel. They examined the repercussions of violent episodes and found that minor injuries resulted in reduced duties or time off work. However, a small number of staff sustained life-threatening injuries, including fractures, lacerations or loss of consciousness. Forty-five percent of staff in their study took time off work following an assault and 65% of this group described themselves as taking up to a year to fully recover. Some victims reported symptoms suggestive of post-traumatic stress disorder (PTSD), including increased startle response, changes in sleep patterns, increased body tension and generalised body soreness.

Bowers' (2002) study of nurses working with patients diagnosed with personality disorder in secure environments identified that nurses had a heightened concern for their own physical safety, with one describing how he had fists clenched with keys in between his fingers when walking up an alleyway near to his home, in case anyone jumped out at him. Others described how they had increased their home security, becoming more careful about locks and fitting security devices. Other nurses reported coming home feeling stressed, being uncommunicative when they first arrived home, and found it difficult to relax or switch off. This type of stress seemed to be associated with violent incidents on the ward, verbal abuse, confrontations, self-mutilation by patients, complaints and investigations. Nurses reported occasions when they had increased their alcohol and tobacco consumption, experienced insomnia, nightmares and occasionally dreaded coming in to work. Experiencing violence in the workplace is a major cause of direct trauma for mental health staff working in secure units, leading to a range of effects: bio-physiological, cognitive, emotional and social effects (Greenwood et al, 2012).

Bio-physiological effects

Anxiety or fear is the most frequently reported bio-physiological effect of workplace violence. Fear may relate to the workplace or to patients, fear of permanent effects of the assault or of becoming dependent on others (Lanza, 1983; Hauck, 1993).

Cognitive effects

These include threats to personal pride, but reports of feeling humiliated, intimidated or harassed have also been noted (Lanza *et al*, 1991; Hauck, 1993). Others report experiencing denial or rationalisation and disbelief at the incident (Chambers, 1998). Guilt, self-blame or shame are commonly cited reactions to aggression reported in a majority of studies. Hauck (1993) found that some nurses feel guilty where they perceive that they could have handled the situation in a more appropriate way.

Emotional effects

A frequently reported emotional response is anger. This may be self-directed or anger towards superiors or the employing organisation (Hauck, 1993). Various threats to personal integrity or pride are reported, with some victims perceiving themselves as disrespected, unappreciated, violated, robbed of their rights (Gates *et al*, 1999), humiliated (Lanza *et al*, 1991) or intimidated, harassed and threatened (Fry *et al*, 2002).

Social effects

Assaults can affect or undermine the nurse–patient relationship and lead to avoidance of patients, self-doubt about the quality of their work and feelings of insecurity at work (Flannery *et al*, 1994; Chambers, 1998).

Stress and burnout in secure mental healthcare

Burnout is the outcome of a prolonged response to chronic interpersonal and job stressors (Sullivan, 1993; Maslach, 2003). The syndrome comprises elements of reduced personal accomplishment, depersonalisation and emotional exhaustion (Maslach *et al*, 1996). Depersonalisation is associated with negative, cynical attitudes and feelings towards patients (Maslach *et al*, 1996). Emotional exhaustion involves staff feeling they can no longer give of themselves psychologically because of depleted resources (Leiter & Maslach, 2006).

Work that involves close involvement and intensive interactions with others can sometimes lead to burnout (Rohland, 2000; Kilfedder *et al*, 2001) and burnout is an acknowledged syndrome of the helping professions (Tillett, 2003). Numerous factors have been associated with high levels of staff stress and burnout in care environments, including team climate (Rose & Schelewa-Davies, 1996), staff support (Ito *et al*, 1999), coping strategies (Mitchell & Hastings, 2001), service user characteristics (Hatton *et al*, 1995) and staff personality (Rose *et al*, 2003). The forensic setting is frequently singled out as a particularly stressful area of care (Kirby & Pollock, 1995). A number of interrelated factors are key to the development of emotional exhaustion in staff and will be discussed now.

Patient diagnosis and presentation

A significant proportion of patients in forensic services will have the diagnosis of borderline personality disorder and this patient group is likely to be highly interpersonally demanding. A diagnosis of borderline personality disorder is associated with less sympathetic and more pessimistic responses to challenging behaviour among staff (Bowers, 2003). Gallop *et al* (1989) showed that mental health professionals feel particularly alienated from patients with this diagnosis. There is also evidence that the function of aggression differs between patients. Schizophrenia is associated with aggression whose antecedent is institutional demands (e.g. to attend sessions), whereas personality disorder is associated with attainment of tangible benefits, that is instrumental aggression (Daffern & Howells, 2007). If disturbed behaviour is linked to personality disorder, in contrast to serious mental illness, nursing staff are more likely to believe that the patient acted out of free choice and are more likely to advocate moral censure (Crichton, 1997). The clinical presentation of patients in secure environments can be particularly complex and challenging, and these patients themselves can be the source of significant stress and psychological challenges to staff. Smith & Hart (1994) showed that intense encounters with angry patients could lead to nurses disconnecting and withdrawing from patients. Within a forensic setting, where there is increased confinement, the interpersonal context is likely to be a critical determinant of the therapeutic capability of the in-patient environment (Brunt & Rask, 2005). According to Nathan *et al* (2007), if discord in relationships is not addressed, cognitive biases may be reinforced, resulting in the development of therapeutically damaging styles of interaction. For example, clinical staff may respond to some manifestations of psychopathology, such as self-harm, differently on the grounds that it is 'behavioural' or driven by 'attention-seeking'.

Patient gender

Self-harm is notably more common in women in-patients in secure forensic units (Coid *et al*, 2001). Responses to self-harm are more likely to involve increased supervision or observations, which can increase anxiety. High levels of stress among observing staff are frequently reported in the literature (Barre & Evans, 2002; Westhead *et al*, 2003). A study of the differences in levels of burnout between staff working in male and female medium secure units (Nathan *et al*, 2007) showed that burnout increased significantly in staff in female wards over time, particularly in relation to emotional exhaustion and depersonalisation.

Type of aggression displayed

There is evidence that men display more physical aggression than women, while women are more likely to employ relational aggression (Leschied *et al*, 2001; Archer & Coyne, 2005; Conway, 2005). The latter is more subtle and covert and can invade the interpersonal space of staff more continuously;

consequently, staff are drawn into more emotionally charged relationships (Nathan *et al*, 2007).

Staff personality

Chung & Harding (2009) found that the personality traits of staff working in a secure intellectual disability service could predict both risk of burnout and psychological well-being even after controlling for their perception of patients' challenging behaviour. Using the five global personality traits identified by Costa & McCrae (1992) (neuroticism, extraversion, openness to experience, agreeableness, conscientiousness) they found that particular personality traits predict burnout components differently. Specifically, depending on their level of agreeableness, neuroticism and extraversion, staff perceive their patients' challenging behaviour as more or less stressful and translate it into a threat or less than a threat, and will subsequently respond to it with emotional reactions (burnout). This suggests that testing for personality types could be helpful in staff selection processes in secure care and that education should involve the interaction between personal characteristics and aggression.

Staff self-efficacy

Self-efficacy, or the self-perception of one's own ability to manage tasks, has been suggested as having a moderating role in stress responses in the workplace (Jimmieson, 2000). Hastings & Brown (2002) found that low levels of self-efficacy in relation to managing patients' violent behaviour were associated with negative emotional reactions to challenging behaviour in secure intellectual disability services. Howard & Hegarty (2003) suggest that staff support can serve as a moderator of staff responses to violence. This finding is consistent with research suggesting that staff support may reduce stress levels (Crawford, 1990; Burke & Greenglass, 1993). This reinforces the benefits of providing training packages that improve staff confidence in ability to manage aggressive behaviour.

The interplay of these factors suggests that staff who are most at risk of developing emotional exhaustion are those working with patients diagnosed with personality disorder, staff working with women and with those who express therapeutic nihilism.

The psychological well-being of healthcare staff

In the UK, interest in the psychological well-being of healthcare staff has developed considerably over the past 20 years. This interest stemmed from studies of stress and burnout in nurses, doctors and psychologists (Cushway, 1992; Greenwood, 1997) that informed a Department of Health strategy for all NHS staff. The resulting paper, *Working Together – Securing a Quality Workforce for the NHS* (Department of Health, 1998) was an important step forward which stated that all NHS staff in England should have access to counselling services by April 2000. It is now a requirement for all NHS trusts who wish to gain Foundation status to offer such a service. In the early 2000s, the Royal College of Nursing commissioned a guidance document, *Counselling for Staff in Health Service Settings: A Guide for Employers and Managers* (Greenwood, 2002), which went some way towards ensuring that counselling services met a minimum quality standard.

Greenwood's work in the early 1990s, while employed at a number of large acute NHS trusts, was to develop and provide psychological support for staff who had been affected by a major incident that caused or threatened serious harm to human welfare. Examples of major incidents within the NHS at that time included criminal acts by healthcare staff that resulted in patient harm or death, including the case of the nurse Beverly Allitt (Clothier *et al*, 1994). Psychological support services for staff at this time were predominantly based on the technique of psychological debriefing as developed by Mitchell (1983). Mitchell was a US masters student and part-time paramedic whose systematic debriefing technique aimed to reduce the incidence, duration and severity, or impairment, caused by traumatic stress (Everly & Mitchell, 1999). By the late 1990s the debriefing model had been adapted for use in a range of organisations including, in the UK, the NHS and police service, and in response to major civil disasters (Rick & Briner, 2012). Psychological debriefing has, over the years, attracted much criticism within the academic literature and indeed the National Institute for Health and Care Excellence (NICE) (NICE, 2005) does not recommend psychological debriefing as a treatment for traumatised people, rather suggesting 'watchful waiting'. Research on managing workplace trauma conducted for the UK Health and Safety Executive (Rick *et al*, 1998*a,b*) further challenged the role of psychological debriefing and its usefulness in post-incident support. Rick *et al*'s (1998*b*) research in particular focused on how in some occupations exposure to traumatic events may be inevitable. Indeed, for nursing and clinical staff working in a secure mental health hospital this is the case. Rick and colleagues suggest that while the literature area follows major disasters, less is researched about the less 'headline friendly' trauma resulting from the daily work of individuals working within organisations, including banks and hospitals.

According to Tehrani (2004), 'the law attempts to protect employees by placing a duty of care on the employer' (p. 62). Indeed, the Health and Safety at Work etc Act 1974 specifies that an employing organisation has the responsibility to proactively prevent psychological harm occurring to their employees through the work they carry out. To meet this duty the employer has to put in place a number of policies and procedures, including ensuring that there are adequate risk assessments, safe practices and post-trauma support for employees who become involved in traumatic events. The Management of Health and Safety at Work Regulations 1999 specifically require organisations to carry out risk assessments to ensure psychological risks are minimised (Kinder & Rick, 2012: p. 336).

More generally, there has been a significant development in the concept of well-being. Indeed, the concept of psychological well-being has been acknowledged as important by the UK government's recent Office for National Statistics incorporation of well-being metrics (Office for National Statistics, 2012). The notion of health rather than sickness has been further developed by Dame Carol Black, the then National Director for Health and Work. Her report, *Working for a Healthier Tomorrow* (Department for Work and Pensions, 2008a), focused on the health and well-being of the working-age population. Black's main thesis is that work is intrinsically good for mental health and well-being. The key areas that have thus been identified for intervention from this report are:

- the need for clear guidance on how to improve health in the workplace
- the unsatisfactory nature of the sick note (the sick note with its connotations of illness and disability has now been replaced by a fitness for work note)
- the importance of extending occupational health service provision to all employees and the need to tackle misconceptions about mental ill health in the workplace.

Dame Black's publication highlights the importance of creating a healthy workforce as well as the potential benefits for staff, patients and the NHS in particular, by endorsing the link between good work and good health. The NHS *Health and Well-being (Final Report)* ('the Boorman review') states: 'it is essential that staff health and well-being is properly embedded as a priority in the NHS Operating Framework and is included in the Care Quality Commission and Monitor assessment and reporting frameworks' (Department of Health, 2009: p. 22). This was an important review which highlighted the need for healthcare organisations within the UK to provide robust and professional support services for staff. Secure mental healthcare services need to be able to deal with the traumatic nature of the work of nurses and other clinical staff who often care for aggressive and violent patients.

All these developments have shifted the responsibility for supporting healthcare staff to the employer, which is a positive move for all healthcare staff. In the next section we will describe how we have taken this idea and transformed the concept to reflect the needs of staff working on secure mental health wards.

The 'ASSIST' psychological first aid model

Development phase

In the context of the policy changes outlined so far, in this section we describe the development of a psychological support model for staff at a large UK provider of secure care. St Andrew's Healthcare is a charity and one of the largest providers of secure mental health in the UK, with

1000 beds across four locations and over 4000 staff. In 2007 the charity identified that staff who work with aggressive and violent patients may at times need professional support. The support should be provided by a professional with experience of working with traumatised staff and who should be able to develop a service reflecting both the needs of the staff and of the organisation. St Andrew's Healthcare has a national reputation for caring for high-risk, aggressive and violent patients. A starting point for the service was the appointment in March 2009 of a trauma service manager, an experienced counselling psychologist, with 17 years of psychological trauma support within the NHS in the UK (A.G.), to lead and develop on the project. This commitment by the organisation to acknowledge the need for staff support and to provide resources for the development of the service were key factors in its success.

A scoping exercise involving more than 400 staff was an important part of identifying the design and implementation of the new 'trauma response' service. Historically, the response to potential trauma was reported to have been *ad hoc*, with no systematic follow-up or rigorous service evaluation. During this consultation phase staff reported that '[violence] happens anyway', but did recognise the need to do something. One senior nurse who had been subject to an assault stated:

> 'I remember feeling "why me" and then feeling, why am I tearful and unable to cope? I always thought that I was a strong person and could cope with anything so why was I in such a state? I also began to question my belief in my job role, what I had said or done wrong for this to happen to me; was I in the right job? Could I go back to the unit where this patient remained? I seemed to have lost me, and was afraid I would not return.'

Staff reported that they wanted a service that valued them, that was confidential and provided a place that they could access easily. An important factor for staff involved in the scoping study was that anyone providing psychological support needed to understand the precise organisational culture and context of working on a locked ward in secure mental healthcare and not simply apply general knowledge about stress and burnout.

Understanding the organisational context

The consultation therefore highlighted important factors about violence and aggression in secure mental healthcare that should be considered when planning support services. Some assaults occur during restraint when staff use physical techniques to de-escalate a situation and relocate the patient to an environment where they are less likely to harm themselves, other patients or the staff. Staff report being most traumatised when they believe there is no way out of a situation or when they perceive that they are going to die. Each member of staff on the ward has a personal alarm system which they can activate when they feel threatened by a patient. Pulling the alarm alerts other staff to respond and help deal with the incident, but a few minutes or seconds can seem a long time when a patient has a member of staff in a head lock. All staff joining the organisation attend a week's induction where every aspect of working in secure environment wards is covered. New starters are also given a local induction by the ward staff to orientate them to the clinical area and receive a full 'handover' of information about the patients in their care. All the staff attend ongoing training in the first 6 months of employment and each year attend training in physical restraint and breakaway techniques.

The ASSIST model

As a result of the consultation, a psychological framework was employed that considered recent government reports (Department for Work and Pensions, 2008a,b; NHS Health and Wellbeing Review Team, 2009) and that drew on the NICE guidelines for supporting people who have experienced a traumatic event. The framework is underpinned by an organisation-wide policy that informs managers and staff about how the service operates. The model builds on the latest directives and research, which suggest that work is beneficial to mental health and that an early return to work helps to build resilience and personal growth (Department for Work and Pensions, 2008a,b).

Psychological first aid

The ASSIST model is not a treatment for PTSD, but a psychological first aid intervention that provides quick, accessible and structured support and promotes psychological well-being. It builds on an individual's natural ability to recover from a traumatic incident and employs 'watchful waiting', as suggested by NICE (2005) for staff who have signs and symptoms of post-traumatic stress. Staff presenting with symptoms of PTSD are referred onward for specialist psychological assessment and treatment. The ASSIST psychological first aid model is underpinned by six principles (Greenwood *et al*, 2012):

1   Assessment of the individual or groups needs context and background. A function checklist is employed to assess psychological awareness and response to possible psychological triggers.

2   Structured sessions provide the individual with an understanding of the impact of psychological trauma and information of normal signs and symptoms and possible reactions.

3   Strategies to help cope with the psychological impact of the signs and symptoms of trauma are discussed.

4   Information regarding ongoing support is available via a 24/7 helpline provided by an external employee assistance programme.

5   Signposting and referrals to specialist help and treatment for staff who have continued frequency of signs and symptoms or who report life difficulties related to trauma reactions.

6   The model takes account of the individual's natural resilience and ability for psychological growth and recovery.

Access to psychological first aid

All serious assaults within the organisation resulting in injury are recorded on a Reporting of Injuries, Diseases and Dangerous Occurrences Regulations (RIDDOR; Health and Safety Executive, 2012) form and are reported to the health and safety team. Serious incidents are defined as those leading to 3 or more days' sickness absence as a result of assault. Where possible, the RIDDOR form is completed by the injured member of staff, who rates the severity of their injury on a scale from 1 to 5. This score is guided by the hospital's classification of events chart which includes a severity table that takes account of the impact from level 1 'no harm' to level 5 'highly serious'. The severity levels were developed from guidance in the National Patient Safety Agency (2008) classification systems. Staff who self-report a level 3 or above event are offered a non-compulsory appointment with the trauma advisor and, additionally, staff may self-refer.

Staff are offered an appointment within 3–5 working days of an incident where possible, but in the event of a more serious event may be seen with 24 hours. The ASSIST psychological first aid response model provides within the first session an assessment of psychological well-being and function. A focus on normalisation of the assault or trauma forms a key part of the session rather than a counselling approach because talking therapies can embed the trauma further and potentially traumatise the counsellor vicariously (Guy & Guy, 2009). A leaflet outlining signs and symptoms of post-traumatic stress and normal reactions to trauma is provided. Staff attendees frequently report that being given an understanding and information on typical reactions to trauma helps them to recover and take back some control in the recovery process. Further information is given on what support is available to them out of hours, with the contact details of an employee assistance programme with 24/7 helpline and the option to self-refer for one-to-one counselling if needed. This programme is delivered by qualified counsellors with training in dealing with traumatic events.

Follow-up and return to work

Follow-up sessions to monitor and support an early return to work when fit are provided where needed. In most cases staff do return to work within 2 weeks of their physical injuries healing. Returning to work should be a managed process with the first assessment for fitness to work being completed by the staff member's general practitioner. They are then seen by the hospital's occupational health nurse and their ward/line manager. The occupational health nurse will provide a phased return to work plan, detailing the number of hours per day to be worked and the level of clinical engagement with patients. This will be reviewed by the manager to assess when the person can return to full duties.

One of the main challenges for staff who have experienced a traumatic event in their workplace is that they will have to return to the site of the event. This is a similar challenge to the one faced by first responders such as firefighters and paramedics. However, the main difference for staff who work on the locked secure mental health wards is that the patient who assaulted them will, in most cases, still be present. This adds a different dimension for the returning member of staff to deal with. It is quite normal for people who have been traumatised to develop phobic reactions and fears associated with the event site and this may be exacerbated in these circumstances.

The ASSIST model supports the practice of ongoing contact between the injured staff member and his or her line manager at an early stage and throughout any period of sickness absence following an assault. This contact helps maintain the link with work and can reassure the injured party, many of whom report feeling guilty about not being at work and letting their colleagues down. Rick *et al* (2006), in their longitudinal study of traumatised post office staff, found that an empathic approach from the line manager was the single factor most associated with perceived level of support on the day of the incident. Part of the trauma response felt by staff who have been assaulted can include feelings of fear and guilt; giving staff permission to be off on sick leave and recover pays dividends because those staff are more likely to return to work, maintain their role within the team and provide patients with continuity of care in the future.

Supporting infrastructure

Alongside the ASSIST model is an organisational policy that outlines how staff and managers can access the support needed. Ease of access to the service has been improved by installation on all personal computers within the organisation of a desktop icon that can be used to obtain contact details for the trauma response service. In times of emotional distress, contact information should be readily accessible in a quick and confidential manner. In addition, the ASSIST model is supported by organisational infrastructure through the provision of trauma awareness training for new staff. This prepares them for patient contact and helps their understanding of the environment of a secure locked ward. The sessions include an outline definition of post-traumatic stress, a brief overview of the development of the field of psychological trauma, how it affects individuals and what the signs and symptoms are. The focus is on information and normalisation of traumatic reactions to serious assaults and threats in a secure mental health in-patient environment. The staff attending the sessions also discuss examples of traumatic incidents that have happened at work. These sessions have been well attended and the evaluation feedback has been very positive. Managing risk is high on the agenda for all clinical staff. Serious injury can mean that staff may not be able to return to their job role, which does cause a lot of anxiousness and uncertainty and can result in staff returning to work too soon.

Conclusions

We have described a model of organisational support structures that has been developed for staff working within the context of a secure mental health environment. In the 3 years since April 2009, a total of 480 staff members have accessed the trauma response service following a serious violent incident. A key element of the success of the ASSIST model has been the recognition that any staff support systems need to be integrated into organisational management structures. The positioning of the trauma service centrally with direct communication links to health and safety, clinical risk, human resources and occupational health services has enabled the development of an accessible model of support that is fully embedded in the systems and structures of the organisation. The trauma service manager is a member of the health and safety and serious untoward incidents review groups, and is able to bring elements of lessons learned directly from staff reports and incorporate organisational learning into practice, with the ability to respond quickly to serious incidents, being part of the emergency response plan structures. We have identified two areas of future research, which should add to the development and refinement of both staff support structures and management practices in secure environments. These are the process of psychological recovery of staff after serious violent assault by patients and elements which support the development of psychological resilience. Further understanding of these crucial areas would assist in the development of support structures designed to meet the particular needs of staff working in secure environments.

References

Archer, J. & Coyne, S.M. (2005) An integrated review of indirect, relational and social aggression. *Personality and Social Psychology Review*, **9**, 212–230.

Barre, T. & Evans, R. (2002) Nursing observations in the acute in-patient setting, a contribution to the debate. *Mental Health Practice*, **5**, 10–14.

Bowers, L. (2002) *Dangerous and Severe Personality Disorder: Response and Role of the Psychiatric Team*. Routledge.

Bowers, L. (2003) Manipulation: search for an understanding. *Journal of Psychiatric and Mental Health Nursing*, **10**, 329–334.

Brunt, D. & Rask, M. (2005) Patient and staff perceptions of the ward atmosphere in a Swedish maximum security forensic psychiatric hospital. *Journal of Forensic Psychiatry and Psychology*, **16**, 263–276.

Burke, R.J. & Greenglass, E. (1993) Work stress, role conflict social support and psychological burnout among teachers. *Psychological Reports*, **73**, 371–380.

Care Quality Commission (2011) *NHS staff have their say as the results of national survey are published*. CQC, 16 March.

Chambers, N. (1998) 'We have to put up with it – don't we?' The experience of being the registered nurse on duty, managing a violent incident involving an elderly patient. *Journal of Advanced Nursing*, **27**, 429–436.

Chung, M.C. & Harding, C. (2009) Investigating burnout and psychological well-being of staff working with people with intellectual disabilities and challenging behaviour: the role of personality. *Journal of Applied Research in Intellectual Disabilities*, **22**, 549–560.

Clothier, C., MacDonald, C.A. & Shaw, D.A. (1994) *The Allitt Inquiry: Independent Inquiry Relating to Deaths and Injuries on the Children's Ward at Grantham and Kesteven General Hospital During the Period February to April 1991*. HMSO.

Coffey, M. & Coleman, M. (2001) The relationship between support and stress in forensic community mental health nursing: an investigation of its causes and effects. *Journal of Advanced Nursing*, **34**, 397–407.

Coid, J., Kahtan, N. & Gault, S. (2001) Medium secure forensic psychiatry services: comparison of seven English health regions. *British Journal of Psychiatry*, **178**, 55–61.

Conway, A.M. (2005) Girls, aggression and emotional regulation. *American Journal of Orthopsychiatry*, **75**, 334–339.

Costa, P.T. & McCrae, R.R. (1992) *Revised NEO Personality Inventory (NEO-PI) and NEO Five Factor Inventory (NEO-FFI) Professional Manuals*. Psychological Assessment Resources.

Crawford, J.V. (1990) Maintain staff morale: the value of a staff training and support network. *Mental Handicap*, **18**, 48–51.

Crichton, J. (1997) The response of nursing staff to psychiatric in-patient misdemeanour. *Journal of Forensic Psychiatry*, **8**, 36–61.

Cushway, D. (1992) Stress in clinical psychology trainees. *British Journal of Clinical Psychology*, **31**,169–179.

Daffern, M. & Howells, K. (2007) Antecedents for aggression and the function analytic approach to the assessment of aggression and violence in personality disordered patients within secure settings. *Personality and Mental Health*, **1**, 126–137.

Department for Work and Pensions (2008a) *Working for a Healthier Tomorrow: Dame Carol Black's Review of the Health of Britain's Working Age Population*. TSO (The Stationery Office).

Department for Work and Pensions (2008b) *Improving Health and Work: Changing Lives. The Government's Response to Dame Carol Black's Review of the Health of Britain's Working Age Population*. TSO (The Stationery Office).

Department of Health (1998) *Working Together – Securing a Quality Workforce for the NHS*. Department of Health.

Department of Health (2009) *NHS Health and Well-being (Final Report)*. Department of Health.

Dickinson, T. & Hurley, M. (2012) Exploring the antipathy of nursing staff who work within secure healthcare facilities across the United Kingdom to young people who self-harm. *Journal of Advanced Nursing*, **68**, 147–158.

Erdos, B. & Hughes, D. (2001) Emergency psychiatry: a review of assaults by patients against staff at psychiatric emergency centres. *Psychiatric Services*, **52**, 1175–1177.

Everly Jr, G.S. & Mitchell, J.T. (1999) *Critial Incident Stress Management (CISM): A New Era and Standard of Care in Crisis Intervention*. Chevron.

Flannery, R.B., Hanson, M.A. & Penk, W.E. (1994) Risk factors for psychiatric in-patient assaults on staff. *Journal of Mental Health Administration*, **21**, 24–31.

Fry, A.J., O'Riordan, D., Turner, M., *et al* (2002) Survey of aggressive incidents experienced by community mental health staff. *International Journal of Mental Health Nursing*, **11**, 112–120.

Gates, D.M., Fitzwater, E. & Meyer, U. (1999) Violence against caregivers in nursing homes: expected, tolerated, and accepted. *Journal of Gerontological Nursing*, **4**, 12–22.

Gallop, R., Lancee, W. & Garfinkel, P. (1989) How nursing staff respond to the label 'borderline personality disorder'. *Hospital and Community Psychiatry*, **40**, 815–819.

Greenwood, A. (1997) Stress and EAP counsellor. In *Handbook of Counselling in Organizations* (eds M. Carroll & M. Walton): pp. 260–272. Sage.

Greenwood, A. (2002) *Counselling for Staff in Health Service Settings: A Guide for Employers and Managers*. Royal College of Nursing.

Greenwood, A., Rooney, C. & Ardino, V. (2012) ASSIST: a model for supporting staff in secure healthcare. In *International Handbook of Workplace Trauma Support* (eds R. Hughes, A. Kinder & C.L. Cooper): pp. 87–104. Wiley-Blackwell.

Guy, K. & Guy, G. (2009) Psychological trauma: the Rewind trauma intervention model: counselling at work. *British Association for Counselling and Psychotherapy*, **Spring**, 19–22.

Hauck, M. (1993) *Die Wut bleibt – Gewalt von Patienten gegenüber Pflegenden [The Anger Remains – Patient Violence Towards Nurses]*. Kaderschule für die Krankenpflege, Aarau.

Hastings, R.P. & Brown, T. (2002) Behavioural knowledge, causal beliefs and self-efficacy as predictors of special educators' emotional reactions to challenging behaviours. *Journal of Intellectual Disability Research*, **46**, 144–150.

Hatton, C., Brown, R., Caine, A., *et al* (1995) Stressors, coping strategies and stress related outcomes among direct care staff in staffed houses for people with learning disabilities. *Mental Handicap Research*, **8**, 252–270.

Health and Safety Executive (2012) *A Guide to the Reporting of Injuries, Diseases and Dangerous Occurrences Regulations 1995*. UK Health and Safety Executive.

Howard, R. & Hegarty, J.R. (2003) Violent incidents and staff stress. *British Journal of Developmental Disabilities*, **99**, 3–21.

Howard, R., Rose, J. & Levenson, V. (2009) The psychological impact of violence on staff working with adults with intellectual disabilities. *Journal of Applied Research in Intellectual Disabilities*, **22**, 538–548.

Ito, H., Kurita, H. & Shiiya, J. (1999) Burnout among direct care staff members of facilities for persons with mental retardation in Japan. *Mental Retardation*, **37**, 477–481.

Jimmieson, N.L. (2000) Employee reactions to behavioural control under conditions of stress: the moderating role of self-efficacy. *Work and Stress*, **14**, 262–280.

Kilfedder, C.J., Power, K.G. & Wells, T.J. (2001) Burnout in psychiatric nursing. *Journal of Advanced Nursing*, **34**, 383–396.

Kinder, A. & Rick, J. (2012) Preparing for and managing trauma within organizations: how to rehabilitate employees back to work. In *International Handbook of Workplace Trauma Support* (eds R. Hughes, A. Kinder & C.L. Cooper): pp. 333–349. Wiley Blackwell.

Kirby, S. & Pollock, P.H. (1995) The relationship between a medium secure environment and occupational stress in forensic psychiatric nurses. *Journal of Advanced Nursing*, **22**, 862–867.

Lanza, M. (1983) The reactions of nursing staff to physical assault by a patient. *Hospital and Community Psychiatry*, **34**, 44–47.

Lanza, M., Kayne, H., Hicks, C., *et al* (1991) Nursing staff characteristics related to patient assault. *Issues in Mental Health Nursing*, **12**, 253–265.

Leiter, M.P. & Maslach, C. (2006) The impact of interpersonal environment on burnout and organizational commitment. *Journal of Organizational Behavior*, **9**, 297–308.

Leschied, A.W., Cummings, A.L., Van Brunschot, M., *et al* (2001) Aggression in adolescent girls: implications for policy, prevention and treatment. *Canadian Psychology*, **42**, 200–215.

Maslach, C. (2003) *The Cost of Caring*. ISHK Books.

Maslach, C., Jackson, S.E. & Leiter, M.P. (1996) *Maslach Burnout Inventory Manual*, 3rd edn. Consulting Psychologists Press.

Mason, T. (2002) Forensic psychiatric nursing: a literature review and thematic analysis of role tensions. *Journal of Psychiatric and Mental Health Nursing*, **9**, 511–524.

Mitchell, G. & Hastings. R.P. (2001) Coping, burnout and emotion in staff working in community settings for people with challenging behaviour. *American Journal of Mental Retardation*, **107**, 252–260.

Mitchell, J. (1983) When disaster strikes. *Journal of Emergency Medical Services*, **8**, 36–39.

Nathan, R., Brown, A., Redhead, K., *et al* (2007) Staff responses to the therapeutic environment: a prospective study comparing burnout among nurses working on male and female wards in a medium secure unit. *Journal of Forensic Psychiatry and Psychology*, **18**, 342–352.

National Institute for Health and Care Excellence (2005) *Post-Traumatic Stress Disorder (PTSD): The Management of PTSD in Adults and Children in Primary and Secondary Care (CG26)*. NICE.

National Patient Safety Agency (2008) *A Risk Matrix for Risk Managers*. NPSA.

NHS Health and Well-being Review Team (2009) *NHS Health and Well-Being, Final Report*. NHS.

NHS Security Management Service (2010) *Violence Against Frontline NHS Staff. Research Study Conducted for COI on Behalf of the NHS Security Management Service*. Ipsos Mori.

Office for National Statistics (2012) *Measuring National Well-Being: Life in the UK, 2012*. ONS (http://www.ons.gov.uk/ons/dcp171766_287415.pdf).

Rick, J. & Briner, R. (2012) Evidence-based trauma management for organizations: developments and prospects. In *International Handbook of Workplace Trauma Support* (eds R. Hughes, A. Kinder & C.L. Cooper): pp. 17–29. Wiley-Blackwell.

Rick, J., Perryman, S., Young, K., *et al* (1998a) *Workplace Trauma and Its Management: A Review of the Literature*. Health and Safety Executive Contract Report, 170/98.

Rick, J., Young, K. & Guppy, A. (1998b) *From Accidents to Assaults: How Organisational Responses to Traumatic Incidents Can Prevent Post-Traumatic Stress Disorder (PTSD) in the Workplace*. Health and Safety Executive Contract Report, 195/98.

Rick, J., O'Reagan, S. & Kinder, A. (2006) *Early Intervention Following Trauma: A Controlled Longitudinal Study at Royal Mail Group*. British Occupational Health Research Foundation Institute for Employment Studies.

Rohland, B.M. (2000) A survey of burnout among mental health center directors in a rural state. *Administration and Policy in Mental Health*, **27**, 221–237.

Rose, J. & Schelewa-Davies, D. (1996) The relationship between staff stress and team climate in residential services. *Journal of Learning Disabilities for Nursing, Health and Social Care*, **1**, 19–24.

Rose, J., David, G. & Jones, C., (2003) Staff who work with people who have intellectual disabilities: the importance of personality. *Journal of Applied Research in Intellectual Disabilities*, **16**, 267–278.

Smith, M.E. & Hart, G. (1994) Nurses' responses to patient anger: from disconnecting to connecting. *Journal of Advanced Nursing*, **20**, 643–651.

Sullivan, P.J. (1993) Occupational stress in psychiatric nursing. *Journal of Advanced Nursing*, **18**, 591–601.

Tehrani, N. (2004) *Workplace Trauma: Concepts, Assessment, and Intervention*. Brunner-Routledge.

Tillett, R. (2003) The patient within: psychopathology in the helping professions. *Advances in Psychiatric Treatment*, **9**, 272–279.

United Kingdom Central Council for Nursing, Midwifery and Health Visiting (1999) *Nursing in Secure Environments*. UKCC.

Westhead, J., Cobb, S., Boath, F., *et al* (2003) Feedback on constant observations. *Mental Health Nursing*, **12**, 14.

Index

Compiled by Linda English